Potentiality

Potentiality: Metaphysical and Bioethical Dimensions

EDITED BY JOHN P. LIZZA

Johns Hopkins University Press

Baltimore

© 2014 Johns Hopkins University Press
All rights reserved. Published 2014
Printed in the United States of America on acid-free paper

2   4   6   8   9   7   5   3

Johns Hopkins University Press
2715 North Charles Street
Baltimore, Maryland 21218-4363
www.press.jhu.edu

Library of Congress Cataloging-in-Publication Data

Potentiality : metaphysical and bioethical dimensions /
John P. Lizza, editor.
pages cm
Includes index.
ISBN-13: 978-1-4214-1174-3 (pbk. : alk. paper)
ISBN-10: 1-4214-1174-1 (pbk. : alk. paper)
ISBN-13: 978-1-4214-1178-1 (electronic)
ISBN-10: 1-4214-1178-4 (electronic)
1. Bioethics—Philosophy.   I. Lizza, John P., 1957–
editor of compilation.
QH332.P686 2014
176—dc23   2013016640

A catalog record for this book is available from the British Library.

Special discounts are available for bulk purchases of this book.
For more information, please contact Special Sales at 410-516-6936
or specialsales@press.jhu.edu.

Johns Hopkins University Press uses environmentally friendly
book materials, including recycled text paper that is composed
of at least 30 percent post-consumer waste, whenever possible.

CONTENTS

I would like to thank the staff of The Hastings Center, as inspiration for this work came while I was a visiting scholar at the Center in the summer of 2009. I have benefited greatly from my association with the Center for many years. I would also like to thank the Pennsylvania State System of Higher Education for a summer research grant that enabled me to work on this project. I am indebted to the conversations on potentiality that I have had with many of the contributors to this volume, my colleagues, and others, especially Allan Bäck, Daniel Callahan, Jason Eberl, David Hershenov, Joseph Jedwab, Bertha Alvarez Manninen, Mohan Matthen, Jennifer McKitrick, Alan Shewmon, and Tom Tomlinson. I thank them for their generous time, patience, and insights. I would also like to thank Laurel Delaney, secretary of the Philosophy Department at Kutztown University, for her help in assisting with obtaining materials and tireless proofreading, and two students, Crystal Williams and Jenn Dum, for their help with organizing materials and checking bibliographical references. Finally, I was fortunate to have a great editor in the person of Matt McAdam at Johns Hopkins University Press.

I gratefully acknowledge permission from the following authors and publishers to reprint material from previously published work:

Chapter 3. Joel Feinberg, "The Paradoxes of Potentiality," Appendix from Joel Feinberg, "The Rights of Animals and Unborn Generations," in William T. Blackstone, ed., *Philosophy & Environmental Crisis*, University of Georgia Press (1974): 67–68.

Chapter 4. Edward Covey, "Physical Possibility and Potentiality in Ethics," *American Philosophical Quarterly* 28:3 (1991): 237–44.

Chapter 5. Edward Langerak, "Listening to the Middle," *Hastings Center Report* 9:5 (1979): 24–28.

Chapter 7. Agata Sagan and Peter Singer, "The Moral Status of Stem Cells," *Metaphilosophy* 36:2–3 (2007): 265–84.

Chapter 8. Jeff McMahan, "Potential," in Jeff McMahan, *The Ethics of Killing,* Oxford University Press (2007): 302–29.

Chapter 9. Margaret Olivia Little, "Abortion and the Margins of Personhood," *Rutgers Law Journal* 39 (2008): 331–48.

Chapter 10. Bertha Alvarez Manninen, "Revisiting the Argument from Potential," *Philosophy, Ethics, and Humanities in Medicine* 2:7 (2007), www.peh-med.com /content/2/1/7.

Chapter 11. Don Marquis, "Are DCD Donors Dead?" *Hastings Center Report* 40:3 (2010): 24–31.

Chapter 13. John P. Lizza, "The Ethical Relevance of Active versus Passive Potentiality," *APA Newsletter on Philosophy and Medicine* 11:1 (2011): 22–28. www.apaonline .org/APAOnline/Publications/Newsletters/Past_Newsletters/Vol11/Vol_11.aspx.

Potentiality

Introduction

JOHN P. LIZZA

There has been a great deal of debate over the moral significance of the potentiality of human embryos and fetuses.[1] Indeed, the standard argument against abortion and the use of human embryonic stem cells for research appeals to the potentiality that the fetus has to develop characteristics, such as intellect and will, that we normally associate with personhood. It is argued that in virtue of this potentiality, the fetus has value and is deserving of some respect, if not all the rights and protections that are normally accorded to persons.

Potentiality has been less of an issue at the end of life, although it has figured in debate over the potential of individuals with total brain failure and those in permanent vegetative state. Because these individuals are thought to lack the potential for consciousness or any other mental function, proponents of a consciousness-related formulation of death argue that they are no longer living human beings or persons.[2] Potentiality has also been an issue in discussion of the meaning of *irreversibility* in the definition and determination of death, particularly in the case of non-heart-beating organ donation. In this context, "potentiality" and "irreversibility" may be complementary concepts in the sense that if some functions, such as circulation and respiration, can be said to be irreversibly lost, there is no potential for those functions to resume. Proponents of non-heart-beating organ donation and its critics disagree over whether the donors in these protocols are dead, that is, whether they have irreversibly lost circulatory and respiratory function. If they have not satisfied the criterion of death, critics argue that the removal of vital organs violates the "dead-donor rule" and is tantamount to vivisection.

This anthology aims to call attention to three main issues concerning consideration of potentiality in bioethical discussions in the hope that it will encourage further research. First, discussion of potentiality and its ethical significance is framed by assumptions about the nature of persons, for example, whether one adopts a substantive, qualitative, creative/transformative, or relational view of persons. Thus, the merits of arguments invoking potentiality in the bioethical context cannot be evaluated independent of consideration of alternative ontological views about persons. Second, recent philosophical work on the concept of dispositions needs to be taken into account in the analysis and evaluation of arguments invoking potentiality in the bioethical context. If potentialities are dispositions of a certain kind, then the work on dispositions needs to be integrated into the bioethical discussion. Indeed, the bioethical context may provide a way to test the plausibility of different accounts of dispositions or develop new theories of dispositions. Third, it is generally assumed that, if X has the potential to become Y, in some sense it must be possible for X to become Y. However, it is unclear what sense of "possibility" is being invoked in this assumption. Logical possibility seems inappropriate. However, if actual or realistic possibility is assumed, what kind of factors affect this possibility?

Persons and Potentiality: The Ontological Framing Problem

Contemporary arguments invoking potentiality in bioethics often rely on a concept of potentiality that has its roots in Aristotelian and Thomistic metaphysics. Grounding their view in an Aristotelian metaphysics in which things that exist by nature have innate principles to develop in certain ways, theorists such as Jason Eberl hold that the human fetus has the potential to develop characteristics, such as intellect and will, by virtue of the kind of thing it is. The potential to develop is thus construed as a power to effect change within a single substantial kind, where being a member of the kind with certain potentialities is what garners the being moral standing. This account of potentiality assumes that the zygote is the same individual substantive being or entity that later develops characteristics, such as intellect and will.[3]

In views such as Eberl's, *person* is treated as a substantial kind term and, when applied to human persons, is coextensive with the substantial kind term *human being*. Thus, by having the natural potential to develop personal characteristics, such as intellect and will, the fetus is an actual person at an early stage of development. In contrast to phase or qualitative sortal terms, like baker or mayor, which may apply at different times during the life history of a person, a person is a person throughout her life history. Accordingly, *fetus* is like *child, adolescent,* and *adult* in that all of these terms denote different phases in the life of a person. *Person,* however, denotes the substantial kind of which the others are phases or qualitative specifications. The mark of a substantial kind term is that it applies to the individual as long as it exists and categorizes the individual as the kind of thing it is in some fundamental sense. Thus, it is not that the fetus is worthy of moral consideration because its realization of such potential will make it an actual person in the future. Rather, the fetus is a person in virtue of its having such potential. The class of persons includes not only beings with the actual abilities of, say, intellect and will, but also beings with the natural potential for those abilities. Nonhuman animals, plants, and other beings are excluded from the class of persons, because they lack the potential for such abilities.[4,5]

Alternatively, *potential* and *potentiality* are frequently used in contexts far removed from a discussion of natural kinds. For example, someone might say, "Paavo has the potential to win several gold medals at the next Olympics," or "Helen has the potential to be a lead singer at the Metropolitan Opera." Appeal to such potentials may also be used to justify certain moral claims, such as "Paavo and Helen *should* continue to train." In these contexts, potentiality refers to some internal properties and to some degree of realistic possibility for some end to be realized. When "potentiality" is used in this way, the potential may be more dependent on *particular* internal characteristics and external factors than when it is used in the more Aristotelian sense of an innate property to develop in certain ways by virtue of being a member of a certain kind. In addition, the potentiality in question usually involves the realization of some accidental rather than essential property of whatever realizes the potential, for instance, Paavo becomes a gold medalist or Helen becomes an opera singer.

In this view, the potential to develop characteristics like intellect and will is interpreted as a human being (organism) becoming a person in the sense of acquiring the *quality* of being a person. *Person* is thus treated as a phase sortal or as a qualitative specification of some substance sortal, such as *human organism*. Moreover, to be a person at least requires consciousness and some type of mental life. Thus, to have any moral standing as a person, the being must minimally have the ability for consciousness. Since an early-term fetus has no mental life at all, no person would be denied rights or harmed by an abortion early in gestation. This psychological view of the person is most often associated with the philosopher John Locke ([1694] 1975) and has contemporary expression in the work of Derek Parfit (1986), Mary Anne Warren (1981), and Peter Singer (1993).

A third way to understand what is involved in the potential to develop intellect and will is to treat the development of whatever characteristics may be sufficient for personhood as involving the coming into existence of an entirely new substance. In this view, "person" is treated as a substance sortal, though it refers to a different substantive kind than the human being or human organism. Moreover, the person exists for some time contemporaneously with the human being or human organism. Jeff McMahan is a contemporary exponent of this view and sees the moral significance of a fetus's potential for developing into or creating a new person as bound up with the value of having new persons in the world.

Finally, there is a fourth option, which is to treat persons as essentially relational beings. In this view, persons are not defined exclusively by some natural, internal potential to develop in certain ways or by some actual abilities. Instead, persons are socially embedded and constructed; their identity is constituted in part by their relations to others.[6] The potential development or coming-to-be of a person cannot be understood independent of considerations of how the fetus is related to others, particularly the mother. The fetus's coming-to-be a person (or potentiality) is thus a relational phenomenon. Moreover, since relational factors affect an individual's potential to become a person, any moral standing associated with potentiality is thus affected by these same relational factors.

These observations on how alternative concepts of personhood are assumed in various arguments invoking "potentiality" pose a challenge to evaluating the bio-ethical arguments and counterarguments involving potentiality. In some cases, disagreement over the significance of potentiality stems from disagreement over the theory of "personhood" assumed in the discussion. Indeed, proponents of alternative views may be talking past each other because they assume different views of personhood. Thus, it may not be possible to evaluate the moral significance of claims about potentiality without evaluating alternative theories of personhood.

For example, two standard objections are often raised to the moral significance of a fetus's potential to develop characteristics that we associate with personhood. However, both of these objections assume that "person" is a phase or qualitative sortal term rather than a substantive one. Thus, if they are directed, as they usually are, against proponents of the potentiality argument who accept a species-defined or other substantive view about persons, these objections may miss their mark, since they may beg the question on the nature of persons.

The first objection holds that the fact that something may become a person is not a good reason for treating it now as a person. Peter Singer (1987) points out that, if it were, "Prince Charles, who is a potential King of England, would now have the rights of a King of England." Stanley Benn (1973, 102) uses a similar analogy: a president-elect may be a potential president but that is not a reason for treating a president-elect as an actual commander-in-chief. These analogies make sense because they employ phase sortal terms (*prince, king, president-elect, commander-in-chief*). In contrast, most proponents of the standard argument from potentiality hold that the fetus represents a phase in the development of a human being or person, just as childhood or adulthood are phases. Thus, that a fetus or child may become an adult does not entail that we should accord all of the same rights to the fetus and child that we do to adults. The fetus, child, and adult may have a right to life, but only the adult may have, for example, a right to vote. Proponents of the potentiality argument hold that *person* denotes the substance sortal of which *fetus* is a phase. Thus, a fetus does not become a person but is already a person in virtue of its inherent capacity to develop in certain ways.

By analogy, because "caterpillar" and "butterfly" denote phases of the kind Lepidoptera, it makes sense to say that a caterpillar is potentially a butterfly. Still, that alone is not a reason for attributing to caterpillars some properties of butterflies, for example, that they are winged. Yet it makes no sense to say that a caterpillar has the potential to be of the kind Lepidoptera. In virtue of its potential to develop into a butterfly, it already is. In the case of fetuses, proponents of the standard potentiality argument claim that certain rights and protections accord to persons at any stage in their development, and it is those rights and protections that apply to the fetus.

The second objection is a reductio ad absurdum argument about the significance of potentiality.[7] Critics of the argument from potentiality claim that to say that the fetus has the potential to become a person is to say that if certain things happen to it, it will eventually become a person. However, the same thing can be said about the unfertilized egg, sperm, and, perhaps with cloning technology, every human cell. If this is the case, then not only would abortion and contraception be wrong, but we might then be obliged to actualize all of the potential persons represented by those cells. Since the argument from potentiality seems to entail this absurd conclusion, it should be rejected.

This second objection also treats "person" as a phase sortal, rather than as a substance sortal, since personhood is understood as a property that something need not have throughout its life-history. However, proponents of the standard potentiality argument treat personhood as essential to things that are individuated and identified under the substance concept "person," and go on to argue that fetuses, but not unfertilized eggs and sperm, cannot be so individuated and identified. Unfertilized eggs and sperm are of a different kind. Again, parties in the debate are using "potentiality" in different ways due to a difference in how they understand the nature of persons. Thus, whether potentiality has moral significance may depend on prior ontological commitments about personhood. Its significance can therefore not be evaluated independent of the ontology of persons.

If one rejects the substantive account of person invoked in the standard potentiality argument that assumes that the fetus is the same individual as the later person, considerations of potentiality may nonetheless be morally relevant. Just as we might urge Paavo to continue to train since he has a realistic potential to compete in the Olympics or value the piece of marble because of its potential to become a sculpture by Michelangelo, we may value the potential of a fetus because it may take on the qualities of a person or become a person. However, as noted above, these considerations may be subject to the standard criticisms. Thus, if the fetus is not an actual person in virtue of its potential to develop in certain ways, Singer and Benn could argue that additional grounds must be given for why we think that they should be treated similarly. After all, potential presidents are not treated the same as actual presidents. Also, if the fetus has the potential to take on the qualities of a person or become a person, isn't the same true about the gametes and perhaps every somatic cell in the body, given the possibility of cloning? Since the gametes and somatic cells are not worthy of the respect accorded to persons and are not harmed if destroyed, there is no reason to think that the fetus is.

Structurally, moral arguments invoking potentiality that assume a qualitative or transformative/creative view of the development of a person are consequentialist. They appeal to the possibility of the actualization of a potential and argue that we are better off by doing what we can to promote the actualization of such a potential or at least not interfering with or deliberately preventing its actualization. Whether the fetus is the same individual as the later person and whether the fetus has an active or passive potentiality are irrelevant. What matters is the good produced by the promotion of future people. Thus, even if there is no unified organism in the case of an ovum about to be fertilized by a sperm and implanted into a womb and thus no individual with which to identify the future person, the potential for a future person to be produced in these circumstances may warrant protection of the process that will lead to its development or creation.

Such consequentialist justification for the protection of future persons may initially appear to be much weaker than the kind of justification available if the fetus can be identified with the later person. Indeed, the standard potentiality argument appeals to the harm done to a fetus prevented from enjoying the goods of life. Even if the potentiality argument is rejected because one rejects the substantive account of personhood that it assumes, once the personhood of a being is established, whenever that may be, a higher moral standing is generally accorded to that being. Thus, many who locate the onset of personhood during some point in the gestation of the fetus will oppose or restrict abortion after that point. Since the consequentialist argument assumes that what has merely the potentiality for intellect and will is not a person, the appeal to personhood status as a basis for protection cannot be invoked. Also, the development of the fetus may be in conflict with the exercise of rights of actual persons, such as the right of the mother to control her body. In cases in which the promotion of some good would involve a violation of the rights of an actual person, a strong case may be made on deontological and utilitarian grounds for protecting the rights of actual persons.

Yet even if one assumes that an individual right, such as the right to control one's body, need not be sacrificed for some utilitarian good, there still remains the ethical question of how one ought to exercise such a right. The long debate over abortion has focused on the question of rights: the right of the mother to control her body, the right of the fetus to live, and how to legally balance such rights. There has been a lot less discussion of how one ought to ethically exercise such rights. For example, while an adult has the legal right to gamble away the family's resources in Las Vegas, and many hold that it would be wrong for the government to interfere with the exercise of that right, it would be ethically wrong for an adult with family dependents to exercise the right to gamble in that way. Similarly, while a woman may have the right to abort a pregnancy, it does not necessarily follow that it would be right for her to do so, even if the fetus has no moral standing as a person, but (say) is a being with the potential to become one.

By analogy, consider the ethical considerations that could bear on a judgment to destroy a piece of marble that Michelangelo was about to work on. Suppose someone other than Michelangelo owned the marble and had the right to destroy it. Suppose this was the last piece of marble of a special type, size, and color that the owner had been supplying to Michelangelo and was needed to complete a composite sculpture that Michelangelo had worked on for years. Assume that if any other piece of marble were used, the entire composition would be ruined. Now, we can imagine various reasons for why the owner might refuse to provide Michelangelo with the marble. We might also accept some of these reasons on ethical grounds. For example, Michelangelo contracted to purchase the marble but then attempted to steal it. However, we might not accept others, for example, the owner destroyed the marble to spite Michelangelo and all the future generations who would have enjoyed the beauty of the completed sculpture. Even though the owner may have the right to destroy the marble, it would not be ethical to do so on such grounds.

It is in such a context that the ethical considerations of the potentiality of a fetus would need to be weighed, if the fetus's potentiality is understood in the sense of its becoming a person. In this context, the justification for abortion or the use of embryonic stem cells for research would lie in the details. We would need to consider the specific circumstances, motivations, and effects of the individual decisions to assess their ethical justification. Moreover, assuming one ought to consider the common good in one's ethical deliberations, consideration of whether abortion or the use of stem cells promoted the common good would be ethically relevant.

Potentiality and Dispositions

Although potentiality has figured prominently in the debate over issues in bioethics, it has not received the kind of focused logical, semantic, and metaphysical analysis that its centrality in the bioethical discussion warrants. Instead, the related concept of "disposition" has been an intense focus of recent philosophical discussion.

Disposition is perhaps most commonly used to refer to an individual's normal mood or temperament: "Our dog, Olga, had the sweetest disposition of anyone in the family." The term thus designates a character trait that will inevitably or habitually manifest itself in certain circumstances. Disposition may also refer to a physical property or tendency, such as the fragility of a glass to shatter or crack if dropped, or the solubility of salt in water. It may be used to refer to a power to control or direct, as with a judge who has the disposition to determine the sentence of a criminal. The recent philosophical discussion has focused on dispositions as physical properties of things or individuals.

While dispositions appear to be real properties of things, they have a certain oddity about them in that they refer to an object's possible rather than actual behaviors. Thus, wine glasses and fine china may have the disposition to break if dropped, but they may never actually manifest those dispositions. How can dispositions be "real" properties of objects and serve to distinguish one kind of object from another, if they refer to how an object might behave in the future rather than how it actually behaves? In addition, how is the possibility or probability of a disposition manifesting itself related to whether an object has a disposition? Is the possibility or probability of the disposition manifesting itself irrelevant to whether an object has a disposition? Or must there be some possibility or degree of probability? If some possibility of manifestation is necessary, is logical possibility sufficient? Or must there be a more robust sense of physical possibility or probability?

The contemporary discussion of dispositions has aimed to provide an analysis or explanation of such properties and to address certain metaphysical questions about them. As Michael Fara explains,

> One group of questions concerns the "grounds" or "bases" of dispositions: my glass vase is fragile, it seems, in virtue of its irregular atomic structure, and in that sense the atomic structure of the vase *grounds* its fragility. What exactly is the relation between the dispositions, like fragility, and their grounds or bases, like my vase's atomic structure? And need there always be a ground or basis to a disposition: might there be "bare" dispositions, ones not grounded in anything at all? Another metaphysical question about dispositions is whether they are (all) intrinsic properties, or whether instead they can be acquired and lost without any change in their bearers? Finally, there is the question about the role of dispositions in causation: are dispositions causally efficacious properties, or are they instead epiphenomenal? (Fara 2006)

Fara points out that the standard approach to distinguishing dispositional properties, such as the fragility of the glass vase, from "categorical" properties, such as the atomic structure of the vase, is that ascriptions of dispositional properties entail certain subjunctive conditionals, whereas ascriptions of categorical properties do not. Thus, the fragility of the glass vase requires that the vase would shatter or crack, if it were dropped. Although some commentators (Mellor 1974, Mumford 1998) have persuasively argued that categorical properties also entail subjunctive conditionals, most seem to agree that any account of dispositions will involve some sort of conditional analysis. Fara dubs the simplest form of conditional analysis, "Simple Conditional Analysis":

> SCA: an object is disposed to M when C, if and only if it would M if it were the case that C. (Fara 2006)

There are some important similarities between dispositions, as so far characterized, and potentiality. Indeed, potentiality shares some of the oddities found in dispositions and similar metaphysical questions arise. When people argue that abortion is wrong because a human fetus has the potential to become a rational, self-conscious being, "potentiality" refers to the fetus's power and possibility of developing into a rational, self-conscious being, assuming certain conditions obtain, for instance, the fetus is left alone to develop in a normal environment. Is the potential to develop rationality and self-consciousness grounded in the fetus's genetic matter (DNA)? Or might the potentiality be dependent on some nonphysical power, such as a soul? Is the potentiality intrinsic to the fetus or might it be affected or determined by factors extrinsic to the fetus? Is the potentiality appealed to causally efficacious in the fetus's realizing rationality and self-consciousness? Finally, an approach to understanding potentiality may also be in terms of subjunctive conditionals as expressed in SCA. For example, a fetus may have the potential to develop rationality and self-consciousness when left alone in a normal environment, if and only if it would develop rationality and self-consciousness when left alone in a normal environment. If some analysis like SCA is correct for potentiality, it would make sense to attribute a potentiality for rationality and self-consciousness to a fetus only if SCA were true of it.

Many questions have been raised about whether SCA or modified versions of it can adequately account for dispositions. In particular, problems involving "finks" and "masking" have challenged whether dispositions can be understood as entirely intrinsic to the things that have them or whether they are defined in part by extrinsic factors.[8] In her essay in this volume, Jennifer McKitrick suggests the following test for a disposition being extrinsic:

> If F is an extrinsic property of x, then it is possible that x could be not F without changing intrinsically, and possibly, a perfect duplicate of x is not F.

If certain dispositions are extrinsic, then it becomes critically important to identify the extrinsic factors. Moreover, whether a disposition should exist could not be addressed without addressing the issue of whether the extrinsic factors should exist. Problems analogous to those raised about dispositions arise for potentiality in the bioethical context. If the fetus's potentiality to develop in certain ways is a kind of disposition, is it intrinsic to the fetus or dependent on extrinsic factors? If intrinsic, what categorical properties must the fetus have to have the potentiality? If extrinsic, what extrinsic factors affect the potentiality?

Because the problems for an account of dispositions are similar to the problems for an account of potentiality, the most promising account of dispositions to emerge from the debate may be useful in formulating an account of potentiality in the bioethical context. In addition, since the most promising account of dispositions will be one that best responds to the difficulties raised in that context, the most promising account of potentiality may similarly be the one that best responds to similar difficulties that arise in the bioethical context. In short, the best theory of dispositions may help shed light on when it is correct to ascribe certain potentialities to various beings and therefore guide our bioethical deliberations.

Potentiality and Possibility

As noted above, it is generally assumed that, if *X* has the potential to become *Y*, in some sense it must be possible for *X* to become *Y*. However, there is a need to clarify the sense of possibility invoked in statements about potentiality. For example, in "The Paradoxes of Potentiality" (reprinted in this volume), Joel Feinberg raises challenging problems for any account of potentiality—problems that have not been adequately addressed in the literature and that require much more serious consideration (Feinberg 1974). He asks us to consider the potential of a pile of dehydrated orange juice. The powder is potentially orange juice (just add water). However, it is potentially many other things as well. All that we have to do is adjust the conditions. Since we could add water and arsenic, it is potentially poison. Since we could add flour, eggs, and yeast, and then bake, it is potentially orange cake. Feinberg observes that this sense of "potentiality" is so "promiscuous" as to be practically useless. We therefore need to distinguish direct or proximate potentialities from indirect or remote ones. Feinberg suggests that we draw this distinction by appealing to criteria like causal importance, the degree or ease or difficulty of supplying the missing elements to realize the potential, or what occurs in the "normal course of events." However, he notes that "words like *important, easy,* and *normal* have sense only in relation to human experiences, purposes, and techniques." They are normative and may change with advances in technology and our interests. If Feinberg is right, then potentiality itself cannot be understood in a value-neutral way, as any useful notion of potentiality is made against a background of normative assumptions. Disagreement over ascriptions of potentiality may therefore stem from dis-agreement over the normative assumptions behind those ascriptions.

Moreover, if the sense of possibility assumed in an understanding of potentiality cannot be a logical possibility but must be some actual or realistic possibility, the issue then arises as to what kind of factors (intrinsic or extrinsic) may affect this sense of possibility. For example, does the fact that a fertilized ovum may be frozen or implanted in a womb unable to sustain it affect its potential to develop rational-ity and self-consciousness? Or is potentiality only affected by intrinsic factors that would prevent the possibility of the fetus developing, such as a defective or absent gene? How might advances in technology affect potentialities? Does the availability of cloning technology now make it the case that every somatic cell has the potential to develop intellect and will? Do advances in resuscitative techniques change whether a condition is considered irreversible? Finally, if individual and societal decisions can restrict actual possibilities, do they thereby affect potentialities?

Potentiality and Bioethics

The above considerations suggest that debate over potentiality and its ethical signifi-cance is inextricably bound up with debate over the nature of persons, an account of dispositions, and the sense of possibility assumed in ascriptions of potentiality. There is a further difficulty. Ascriptions of potentialities are made against a back-ground set of assumptions about the world, often with reference to a "natural" course of events or suitable environment. The fact that human beings are not simply biological beings but also social and cultural beings complicates matters. When it comes to human beings, it is unclear how any account of what a "normal" or "suit-able" environment is can be given independently of social and cultural consider-ations. To do so would involve a distortion of our nature. In contrast to other biological beings, we can shape our environment based on rational consideration of the good and how to best realize it. Thus, it is hard to see how the attribution of potentialities to human beings or persons can be given without considering at the same time the nature of a good or suitable environment. However, such consider-ations take us beyond strictly biological considerations of potentiality in the "natu-ral" world. Accordingly, future discussion of potentiality in the bioethical context must take into consideration how such ethical, social, and cultural conditions may be part of the background conditions assumed in ascriptions of potentiality. This last problem may be the most challenging one, as it may underlie the first three problems. Ethical, social, and cultural factors may be among the factors that at least in part determine the nature of persons, relevant dispositions or potentialities, and actual or realistic possibilities.

The Readings

The readings in this collection reflect how considerations of "potentiality" complicate the analysis of the moral standing of persons at the beginning and end of life. The first part consists of more theoretical readings on the nature of potentiality and its application to issues in bioethics. The second part offers a selection of readings representative of how the concept of potentiality has been used to support different positions on the moral status of human fetuses, abortion, and the use of stem cells for research. They illustrate how different assumptions about the nature of a human being or person underlie consideration of the ethical significance of the potentiality of human fetuses. The third part focuses on potentiality at the end of life and its relevance to the definition and determination of death.

In Chapter 1, "Aristotle's Theory of Potentiality," Mohan Matthen provides background for understanding the concept of potentiality as developed by Aristotle in his account of change, or *kinēsis*. He explains that, according to Aristotle, change (kinēsis) is caused by an active potentiality in an agent and a matched passive potentiality in a patient, for example, a builder has the active potentiality to transform the passive potentiality of building materials into a house. However, when both active and passive potentialities belong to a single substance in virtue of the kind of substance it is, natural kinēsis, such as an organism's growth by metabolic activity, occurs. Matthen suggests that on an Aristotelian analysis life begins sometime after fertilization when "the embryo is able to metabolize nutriment on its own, without relying on the assistance of the mother's metabolic system." He identifies this causal power with Aristotle's "nutritive soul." However, according to Matthen, it is unclear exactly when this occurs. Moreover, it is unclear whether the genesis of a "nutritive soul" is sufficient for the embryo to be a "human" being and to have moral standing in Aristotle's view. Matthen argues that Aristotle goes on to define human life in terms of quite robust operations of reason, disqualifying, for example, fetuses and those deficient in rational ability, such as natural slaves, from being human.

It is worth noting that, according to Matthen's interpretation of Aristotle, once the fetus has the requisite potentiality to develop in certain ways, its potentiality is not affected by whether it is actually possible for it to develop and ultimately perform activities, such as self-conscious rational thought. The fact that external circumstances, for example, an illness preventing the mother from converting food into nutriment suitable for the fetus to metabolize, may make it impossible for the fetus to develop does not affect whether the fetus has that potentiality. Thus, Aristotle appears to treat at least certain potentialities as intrinsic properties.

In Chapter 2, "Dispositions and Potentialities," Jennifer McKitrick examines the connection between the concepts of dispositions and potentiality with an eye on some of the problems that have been raised for SCA as an analysis of dispositions. She also focuses on the issue of whether dispositions and potentialities are intrinsic or extrinsic to the things that have them. She explores how problems analogous to those raised in the discussion of dispositions have been raised in the discussion of potentiality in the bioethical context.

McKitrick treats potentialities as dispositions. Although she does not offer a complete account of dispositions or potentiality, she is critical of conditional analyses of these concepts and the categorical claim that dispositions and potentialities are intrinsic properties of the things that have them. If some dispositions and potentialities are extrinsic, that is, they are determined by internal and external factors, it becomes critically important in the bioethical context to consider whether certain potentials are intrinsic or extrinsic. For example, if a fetus's potential for intellect and will is extrinsic, then it may not ground an ethical claim about the moral standing of the fetus independently of consideration of the existence of the extrinsic conditions that make it possible or the ethical question of whether those extrinsic conditions should obtain. Indeed, McKitrick is skeptical about whether determining the intrinsic or extrinsic nature of such potentialities can be done in a value neutral way. Her article presents many interesting and challenging questions for future research.

The next three articles in Part I focus on the concept of possibility involved with potentiality and the ethical significance of possibilities and probabilities. As mentioned above, Joel Feinberg calls attention to how normative notions may be necessary to delineate any useful notion of potentiality. Attention to this normative dimension of potentiality is reflected in a number of other works later in this collection, perhaps most clearly in Chapter 7, by Agata Sagan and Peter Singer, who ask for grounds for saying that a fetus has the potential for intellect and will while denying this same potential to somatic cells that can be manipulated to develop intellect and will. It is also reflected in Jennifer McKitrick's skepticism about whether a theory of dispositions or potentiality can be done in a value neutral way, Jeff McMahan's discussion in Chapter 8 of the ethical significance of the distinction between intrinsic and extrinsic potentiality, Tom Tomlinson's claim in Chapter 12 that the meaning of *irreversibility* in the definition of death is an ethical one, and John Lizza's challenge to the ethical relevance of the distinction between active and passive potentiality in Chapter 13.

In Chapter 4, "Physical Possibility and Potentiality in Ethics," Edward Covey argues that the sense of possibility invoked in claims about potentiality must be actual physical possibility, not logical possibility. Moreover, even if something is absolutely physically possible, it may not be actually possible. According to Covey, absolute physical possibility does not yield actual possibility unless there are actually possible and not just absolutely possible intervening steps that can realize the possibility. Such consideration would rule out, for example, the potential for an anencephalic fetus to develop intellect and will. Covey also holds that our own decisions cannot form part of the intervening conditions for ruling out an actual possibility. According to Covey, "dispositional states which may determine our actual choices never count as criteria of physical necessity in our calculations of what we can and cannot do." Thus, while intrinsic and extrinsic conditions can affect actual possibilities and therefore potentialities, decisional factors are excluded from the criteria for what is actually physically possible and therefore from considerations of potentiality.

In Chapter 5, "Abortion: Listening to the Middle," Edward Langerak argues for a moderate position in the abortion debate that holds (1) there is something about the fetus itself that makes abortion morally problematic and (2) late-term abortions are more morally problematic than early abortions. He rejects the extreme positions that all abortions are equivalent to murder or that all abortions are no more morally problematic than elective surgery, as neither position can do justice to the beliefs of the moderate position. Langerak holds that potentiality entails realistic probability and argues that realistic probabilities are ethically relevant. Accordingly, he gives ethical weight to the probability of a fetus's developing into a person. In general, the further along the fetus develops and more likely it is to realize its potential, the greater its moral standing. Potentiality thus accounts for what it is about the fetus itself that makes abortion morally problematic. However, while the potentiality of the fetus gives it some moral standing, it does not have the same moral standing as an actual person. The crucial question is then how much moral standing does the fetus have or how strong a claim to life should be attributed to the fetus? Langerak adopts a "conferred claims" approach to rights to answer these questions. This approach takes into consideration the interests and sympathies of actual persons and the social consequences of different policies. He looks to such considerations to draw lines as to when abortions may be permissible and when not. While Langerak makes some suggestions as to where he thinks the lines should be drawn, much more empirical work about the interests and sympathies of actual persons and the social consequences of drawing lines at various points would be needed to follow up on his proposal. Nonetheless, Langerak's article is one of the few in the bioethical literature that tries to account for how probabilities involved with considerations of potentiality matter in our ethical deliberations.

Part II offers a selection of readings that show how different assumptions about the nature of human beings or persons affect the ethical evaluation of potentiality at the beginning of life. In "Persons with Potential," Chapter 6, Jason Eberl begins with an account of Aristotle's concept of potentiality and how it has been developed by the contemporary theorists Robert Pasnau (2002) and Norman Kretzmann (1999). Following Aquinas in holding that an active potentiality for self-conscious rational activity is sufficient for something to be a person, Eberl defends the moral status of human fetuses against objections raised by Michael Tooley (1983, 1998) and R. Alta Charo (2001), objections that appear in alternative form in the chapter by Sagan and Singer.

Tooley and Charo both contend that the appeal to the potentiality of the fetus as a basis for moral status has unacceptable implications. Tooley (1983) argues that, if it is wrong to destroy something with an unexercised capacity for rational awareness, it is equally wrong to refrain from producing something with the capacity for rational awareness. He then claims that if it is wrong to abort a human fetus, it is equally wrong to use contraceptives and to refrain from procreative activity. However, both consequences, according to Tooley, are clearly unacceptable. Charo raises a similar concern about the implications of the potentiality argument. She argues that since a person can be cloned from any somatic cell, any somatic cell is potentially a person and therefore, according to the potentiality argument, would have the same moral status, not only as human fetuses, but as any adult human person—a conclusion she thinks is clearly absurd.

Eberl challenges Tooley's "moral symmetry principle" and responds to both Tooley and Charo's objections by appealing to the "identity criterion" that is used in the potentiality argument to distinguish an individual's having an active as opposed to passive potentiality to develop in certain ways. Whereas the human fetus is a potential person insofar as it has the active potential to develop in certain ways, sperm, ova, and somatic cells are merely possible persons with only a passive potentiality to develop in certain ways. Whereas the fetus is the same person as the adult into which it has the active potentiality to develop, the gametes and somatic cells would need to be changed into a different kind of thing in order to have the active potentiality for personhood. Eberl in the end endorses Don Marquis's view (Marquis 1989) that it is *prima facie* wrong to kill human fetuses, in contrast to human sperm, ova, and somatic cells, because human fetuses have futures of value insofar as they are numerically identical to the later person who will have valuable experiences. Interestingly, although Mohan Matthen and Jason Eberl agree on many details of Aristotle's account of potentiality, they draw very different conclusions about when human life begins and which beings get classified as human on an Aristotelian account.

In Chapter 7, "The Moral Status of Stem Cells," Sagan and Singer challenge the standard potentiality argument. They treat personhood as a certain set of qualities and argue that the immediately exercisable (or previously exercised) capacity to reason and make free choices, and not just the potential for these capacities, is required for killing an individual to be gravely wrong. They maintain that, even if one grants the fetus has an intrinsic rational nature that distinguishes it from gametes and somatic cells that could be cloned, such a rational nature is not what matters when it comes to whether a being can be harmed, deserves moral respect, or can be a subject of rights.

Sagan and Singer also offer a serious challenge to the claim that the fetus can be distinguished from gametes and somatic cells in the way proponents of the standard potentiality argument claim. Sagan and Singer argue that, if the fetus deserves respect because it has the potential to develop into a being with intellect and will, then the same respect should be accorded to the billions of somatic cells in every human body that have the potential to develop similarly through somatic cell nuclear transfer technology. Sagan and Singer point out the absurd implication that such cells would then deserve the same respect and protection as proponents of the potentiality argument think should be accorded to fetuses. Moreover, we might then have an obligation to bring into existence many more billions of human beings. Sagan and Singer also argue that because we do not think it is morally tragic for these somatic cells to not realize their potential, there is no reason to think that it is morally tragic for fetuses to not realize their potential. Crucial to their argument is their claim that the human fetus does not have a rational nature in itself, but, like somatic cells, has "the genetic coding that may, under favorable circumstances, lead it to develop into a being with a rational nature." In short, by expanding the set of antecedent conditions that are assumed in the ascription of potentiality to include things like cloning technology, they argue that there is no difference between the potentiality in a fetus and that of a somatic cell.

In Chapter 8, a selection from his book *The Ethics of Killing* (2002), Jeff McMahan analyzes the potential for the fetus to become a person as involving the creation of a new kind of being. For McMahan, *person* refers to an embodied mind, a substantive entity with the capacity for consciousness. According to McMahan, the realization of the human fetus's potential for intellect and will thus involves the creation or coming into existence of an individual of a different kind. Human organisms, with which we are not identical, give rise to the existence of persons, with which we are identical. The moral significance of the fetus's potential for developing into a person thus has to do with its potential to bring a person into existence. Since McMahan does not identify the early fetus with the person that later develops, he concludes that early abortion is unproblematic, since it does not involve the killing of a person. Later-term abortions are more problematic for him, since later in gestation killing the fetus does involve killing a person. However, he then applies a theory of time-relative interests to argue that such persons have a weaker interest in continuing to live and thus are harmed to a lesser degree by being killed. This, he argues, affects the ethics of how they may be treated.

In Chapter 9, "Abortion and the Margins of Personhood," Margaret Olivia Little treats persons as emerging gradually in the context of material support from the mother. Although she does not explicitly invoke the concept of potentiality in her analysis, she explores how the ontological and moral status of the fetus develops across pregnancy. By treating the fetus's coming-to-be a person (or potentiality) as a relational phenomenon in this sense, her chapter addresses a central issue in the anthology: how external factors may affect an individual's potentiality and moral status.

In Chapter 10, "Revisiting the Argument from Fetal Potential," Bertha Manninen begins by defending the standard potentiality argument against the objection that the rights of actual persons should not be extended to potential persons and that the future prospects of a fetus cannot provide grounds for attributing interests and rights to the fetus.[9] However, she recognizes that a crucial premise in the standard argument is the assumption that the fetus is the same individual as the later person. She points out how this premise is challenged by those who accept a psychological criterion of personal identity and do not identify the later person with the fetus. She concludes by suggesting the disagreement over the ethical significance of potentiality is rooted in disagreement over the metaphysical question of personal identity.

As noted at the beginning of this introduction, *potentiality* has been less of an issue at the end of life. However, it has figured prominently in debate over the neurological criterion for determining death and the meaning of *irreversibility* of the loss of circulatory and respiratory functions in the context of determining death by the traditional circulatory and respiratory criterion in organ donation after cardiac death (DCD). As also noted earlier, irreversibility and potentiality are complementary concepts in this sense: to say that circulation and respiration have irreversibly ceased is to say that there is no potential for those functions to resume. This is the focus of Part III of this volume.

Successful organ donation requires well-preserved organs. In the case of transplantation of vital organs, such as the heart or liver, there is reason to remove the organs as soon after death as possible. However, the "dead donor" rule restricts the removal of vital organs from living persons. While most vital organ transplants come from donors who have been declared dead based on the neurological criterion of determining death, that is, total brain failure, some vital organs come from non-heart-beating donors that are thought to satisfy the traditional criteria for determining death, namely, the irreversible loss of circulation and respiration. Under current protocols involving such donors, the transplant team will wait anywhere from 75 seconds to five minutes of asystole before removing organs.[10] However, critics of such protocols, such as Joanne Lynn (1993), Robert Veatch (2008), and Don Marquis (2010; reprinted in this volume), question whether the cessation of circulation and respiration in these donors is truly "irreversible." In their view, because of the possibility of spontaneous auto-resuscitation and the fact that we could intervene to artificially resuscitate these donors, the potential for the resumption of their functions still exists. Consequently, these critics argue that the donors have not satisfied the "irreversibility" requirement in the circulatory and respiratory criterion for determining death and thus removing their vital organs violates the "dead donor" rule.

Don Marquis's Chapter 11, "Are DCD Donors Dead?" represents this criticism of the DCD protocols. Marquis treats reversibility as a dispositional property. Although he does not offer a complete account of dispositions, as it is beyond the scope of his paper, he accepts a conditional analysis of dispositions and understands them as intrinsic properties. As noted in McKitrick's contribution to this volume, if a disposition is intrinsic, its presence is not affected by factors external to it but "only depends on how the thing is in itself." Thus, Marquis claims that if two human organisms, for instance, someone in the emergency room and a prospective donor in a DCD protocol, are in the same physical state after, say, one minute of asystole, they must have the same dispositional property with respect to whether their condition is irreversible. He therefore treats the reversibility of the cessation of circulatory and respiratory functions as an intrinsic dispositional property of the human organism and as not dependent in any way on ethical considerations regarding how these two individuals should be treated. Since the cessation of circulatory and respiratory functions after two minutes of asystole is insufficient to conclude that those functions are irreversible in most human organisms, the fact that the human organism may be in a donor protocol does not alter the fact that the organism has the potential for the cessation of functions to be reversed.

Defenders of the DCD protocol, such as Tom Tomlinson (in this volume) and John Robertson (1999), argue that the donors are irreversibly dead, because they hold that the meaning of *irreversibility* in the definition and criteria of death is an ethical one, determined by the ethical context in which the determination of death is made. Tomlinson, for example, argues that advances in medical technology and resuscitative techniques have introduced a new meaning of irreversibility: *medical irreversibility*. Whereas *physiological irreversibility* refers to an organism's inability to revive itself, medical irreversibility considers how factors external to the organism, such as artificial resuscitation, can affect irreversibility. Medical irreversibility, in Tomlinson's view, would thus appear to be a relational or extrinsic property. Moreover, whereas physiological irreversibility was the only practical sense of irreversibility before modern resuscitative techniques, we now have a choice of which concept to apply in different contexts. According to Tomlinson, there is no univocal meaning of irreversibility in the definition of death. He argues that physiological irreversibility may be the appropriate meaning and criteria to use in DCD protocols, whereas it would be inappropriate to invoke this meaning and criteria in the context of an emergency room, when resuscitative measures should be applied. Thus, ethical considerations, rather than some intrinsic state of the organism, determine the sense of irreversibility for purposes of defining death. Marquis rejects this "appeal-to-a-norm" defense of DCD, because it is inconsistent with his treating reversibility as an intrinsic dispositional property of the organism.

It is worth noting that Marquis does not rely on physiological irreversibility in his analysis of the irreversibility involved in determining death. He is not claiming that donors in the DCD protocol have an active potentiality in an Aristotelian sense to reverse the cessation of circulation and respiration on their own. Instead, he relies on what Tomlinson defines as medical irreversibility. However, even if Marquis admits that the reversibility of a condition may change over time due to advances in medical knowledge and technology, this may not commit him to admitting that reversibility is an extrinsic disposition. Marquis may construe the impact of advances in medical knowledge and technology as a change in the conditions of the manifestation of an intrinsic property of the organism, rather than a change in whether the organism actually possesses the disposition of being in a reversible condition. Thus, advances in resuscitative techniques may not affect the reversibility of a physical state of an organism, such as the cessations of circulation and respiration; it merely affects whether that disposition is ever manifested. Thus, Marquis could hold that it is not possible for one human organism at one point in time to have a reversible condition and another organism in a duplicate internal biological state at another point in time to not have that same disposition.

Alternatively, Marquis could admit that the disposition for the resumption of circulatory and respiratory functions is an extrinsic disposition and hold that whether an organism is in a reversible state is affected by the state of knowledge and technology at the time. In this case, he would admit the possibility that a human organism at one point in time may have a reversible condition and another organism in a duplicate internal biological state at another point in time may not have that same disposition. Nonetheless, he could maintain that whether a human organism has that disposition at any point in time is an objective fact about the organism at that time and state of the world, and that any other human organism in that same biological state at the same time must have the same disposition. He thus would be admitting that the disposition of reversibility is extrinsic in one sense, that is, the state of knowledge and medical technology affects the possession, not just the manifestation, of the disposition. But it is not extrinsic in the sense that it is affected by the ethical context. He may still deny that ethical factors have any bearing on whether the organism has the disposition.

In the last article in this collection, John Lizza considers the issue of potentiality in the context of debate over the neurological criterion for determining death. Critics of the neurological criterion, such as D. Alan Shewmon (1997, 2004b, 2010), argue that because artificially sustained human organisms with total brain failure retain their organic integration, they are still alive. Moreover, because they are still living human organisms, they retain the active potentiality for intellect and will. Shewmon thus understands total brain failure as an impediment in the manifestation of intellect and will, but as not entailing the loss of the active potential for intellect and will. Relying on an Aristotelian-Thomistic understanding of potentiality in which active potentialities are determined by membership in a natural kind, Shewmon holds that the potentiality for intellect and will resides not in any particular organ like the brain, but in the living organism as a whole. Lizza contrasts Shewmon's view with that of Eberl (2008), who also accepts an Aristotelian-Thomistic understanding of potentiality but accepts total brain failure as a criterion for determining death. Lizza points out how both Shewmon and Eberl appeal to the distinction between active and passive potentiality to support their views. However, Lizza argues that there is no way to determine whether such artificially sustained individuals with total brain failure have an active or passive potentiality for intellect and will and thus no way to resolve the disagreement between Shewmon and Eberl. He concludes that the distinction between whether an individual has an active or passive potentiality is, in itself, ethically irrelevant to the determination of death and how individuals should be treated. Instead, Lizza proposes that realistic possibilities are what are ethically relevant, regardless of whether such possibilities are connected with an active or passive potentiality. Moreover, given that intrinsic and extrinsic factors may affect an individual's realistic possibilities and that decisional factors may be one type of extrinsic factor, Lizza argues that in some cases the meaning and ethical significance of certain potentialities cannot be assessed independently of an ethical assessment of the extrinsic factors. In closing, he suggests that the meaning of irreversibility in the determination of death in DCD protocols is one such case.

NOTES

1. The term *embryo* refers to an animal in the early stages of development, from conception to the eighth week, after which and until birth the term *fetus* then applies. However, to avoid having to repeatedly use the cumbersome phrase "embryo or fetus," I henceforth use

the term *fetus* in this introduction to apply to the animal from the zygote stage to birth. Direct quotes from other authors, of course, will retain their usage.

2. See, for example, Engelhardt (1975), Veatch (1975, 1988, 1993), Green and Wikler (1980), Gervais (1986), Zaner (1988), Lizza (1993, 2004, 2011), Machado (1995), McMahan (1995).

3. Other theorists, such as Norman Ford (1988) and Don Marquis (2007), hold that the individual substantive entity, i.e., the human being or person, is not formed until twinning is no longer possible. The zygote could not be identical with both twins, as the transitivity of identity would then falsely imply that the twins are identical. However, once the primitive streak is formed, there is no longer a possibility of twinning. It is at that point that these theorists believe that a substantive being with the potential to naturally develop characteristics, such as intellect and will, begins to exist. For Eberl's response to this view and defense of the claim that a person's life begins at conception, see Eberl (2007).

4. A good example of the use of potentiality in this sense is evident in the justification given by the President's Council on Bioethics (2002) in calling for a four-year moratorium on research on human fetuses. Most members of the council held that the developing fetus was a being worthy of "special respect" (xxxi) and claimed that those who deny the potentiality of the fetus to become a person lack an understanding of the meaning of potentiality. The majority stated that to treat the developing human fetus as nothing more than "mere cells"

> gravely mischaracterizes the meaning of potentiality–specifically, the difference between having the capacity to become anything at all (a pile of building materials, for example) and the capacity to become something in particular (an individuated human person or persons). (President's Council 2002, 139)

> It denies the continuous history of human individuals from zygote to fetus to infant to child; it misunderstands the meaning of potentiality–and, specifically, the difference between a "being-on-the-way" (such as a developing human embryo) and a "pile of raw materials," which has no definite potential and which might become anything at all. (President's Council 2002, 54)

Again, invoking the potentiality of the "embryo," the majority concluded,

> We are also not persuaded by the claim that in vitro embryos (whether created through IVF or cloning) have a lesser moral status than embryos that have been implanted into a woman's uterus, because they cannot develop without further human assistance. The suggestion that extra-corporeal embryos are not yet individual human organisms-on-the-way, but rather special human cells that acquire only through implantation the potential to become individual human organisms-on-the-way, rests on a misunderstanding of the meaning and significance of potentiality. An embryo is, by definition and by its nature, potentially a fully developed human person; its potential for maturation is a characteristic it *actually* has, and from the start. The fact that embryos have been created outside their natural environment–which is to say, outside the woman's body–and are therefore limited in their ability to realize their natural capacities, does not affect either the potential or the moral status of the beings themselves. A bird forced to live in a cage its entire life may never learn to fly. But this does not mean that it is less of a bird, or that it lacks the immanent potentiality to fly on feathered wings.

It means only that a caged bird–like an in vitro human embryo–has been deprived of its proper environment. There may, of course, be good human reasons to create embryos outside their natural environment–most obviously, to aid infertile couples. But doing so does not obliterate the moral status of the embryos themselves. (President's Council 2002, 156)

5. In this view, it may be thought that the natural potentialities that an individual has are determined by the kind of thing it is. Thus, even if a member of a certain kind may be defective in certain respects, it still has whatever potentialities normal members of the kind have. For example, human beings, in contrast to (say) clams, are the kind of beings with a natural potential for sight. Even though a particular human being may have cataracts or glaucoma, he or she may still have the potential for sight. The cataracts or glaucoma are understood as impediments in the actualization of the potential for sight. They do not negate the potential for sight: the individual has the potential in virtue of the kind of thing it is. However, two critical issues arise at this point. First, does it make sense to attribute potentialities to an individual simply in virtue of its being a member of a kind? If a human being suffers enucleation of both eyes and destruction of the entire neural system necessary for sight, does the individual still have the potential for sight? Second, if the individual is "defective" because he or she lacks internally some physical parts necessary for having any realistic possibility for the actualization of some essential characteristic of the kind, does that disqualify the individual from being a member of the kind? If the potential for intellect and will is essential to being human, does anencephaly preclude an individual from being human?

6. See, for example, Mead (1925, 1934), Sartre ([1942] 1994, [1945] 1955, [1946] 1970), Wittgenstein (1953), Geertz (1964, 1965, 1966), Harré (1984, 1989), Gergen (1991, 2011), Baier (1985), and Mackenzie and Stoljar (eds.) (2000).

7. See, for example, Peter Singer (1987) and John Harris (1985, 11–12).

8. Sungho Choi and Michael Fara (2012) explain "finks" and "masking":

Counterexamples to *SCA* first raised by Martin (1994) exploit the fact that some dispositions are "finkish" in the sense that the conditions for an object's acquiring or losing disposition *D* might be the same as *D*'s stimulus conditions. Suppose that an electrical wire is live just in case it has the canonical disposition to conduct electricity when touched by a conductor. (This is an artificial definition that might differ from a dictionary definition of "live.") *SCA* then entails that a wire is live if it would conduct electricity if touched by a conductor. Suppose now that a dead wire is connected to an electro-fink, a device which senses when the wire is about to be touched by a conductor, and which makes the wire live in every such circumstance. If the wire were touched by a conductor then, thanks to the work of the device, the wire would become live, and so would conduct electricity. Hence the wire would conduct electricity if touched by a conductor. Being dead, however, it is not disposed to conduct electricity if touched by a conductor. The device can also operate on a reverse cycle, attaching to a naturally live wire but removing its property of being live if ever it is touched by a conductor. In this case, although the wire is disposed to conduct electricity when touched by a conductor, the "reverse-cycle" fink ensures that the associated counterfactual conditional is false.

. . . Another kind of counterexample to *SCA*, due to Johnston (1992) and Bird (1998), involves a fragile glass that is carefully protected by packing material. It is claimed that the glass is disposed to break when struck but, if struck, it wouldn't break thanks to the work of the packing material. There is an important difference between this example and Martin's: the packing material would prevent the breaking of the glass not by *removing* its disposition to break when struck but by blocking the process that would otherwise lead from striking to breaking. . . . The packing material is called a masker (Johnston) or antidote (Bird) to the glass's disposition at issue.

9. For example, Bonnie Steinbock (1992, chap. 1) has questioned whether it is sensible to attribute rights to individuals without conscious interests.

10. The Society of Critical Care Medicine (Bernat 2006) recommends waiting a minimum of two minutes after cardiac arrest before declaring death and proceeding with organ transplantation in DCD protocols. Many hospitals with DCD protocols wait at least five minutes after cardiac arrest before procuring organs. However, Boucek et al. (2008) reported a waiting period of only seventy-five seconds in two cases involving pediatric heart transplantation.

REFERENCES

Baier, A. 1985. *Postures of the Mind: Essays on Mind and Morals*. Minneapolis: University of Minnesota Press.

Benn, S. 1973. Abortion, infanticide, and respect for persons. In J. Feinberg (ed.), *The Problem of Abortion*. Belmont, CA: Wadsworth.

Bernat, J. 2006. Report of a national conference on donation after cardiac death. *American Journal of Transplantation* 6:281–91.

Bird, A. 1998. Dispositions and antidotes. *Philosophical Quarterly* 48:227–34.

Boucek, M. M. et al. 2008. Pediatric heart transplantation after declaration of cardiocirculatory death. *New England Journal of Medicine* 359:709–14.

Buckle, S. 1988. Arguing from potential. *Bioethics* 2(3):227–53.

Charo, R. 2001. Every cell is sacred: Logical consequences of the argument from potential in the age of cloning. In P. Lauritzen (ed.), *Cloning and the Future of Human Embryo Research*. New York: Oxford University Press.

Choi, S., and Fara, M. 2012. Dispositions. In Edward N. Zalta (ed.), *Stanford Encyclopedia of Philosophy*. www.plato.stanford.edu/archives/spr2012/entries/dispositions.Rev.and rpr. from Fara 2006.

Eberl, J. 2007. A Thomistic perspective on the beginning of personhood: Redux. *Bioethics* 21(5):283–89.

————. 2008. Potentiality, possibility, and the irreversibility of death. *Review of Metaphysics* 62(1):61–77.

Engelhardt, T. 1975. Defining death: A philosophical problem for medicine and law. *American Review of Respiratory Diseases* 112:587–90.

Fara, M. 2006. Dispositions. In Edward N. Zalta (ed.), *Stanford Encyclopedia of Philosophy*. Rev. and rpr. in Choi, S., and Fara, M. 2012.

Feinberg, J. 1974. The rights of animals and unborn generations. In W. T. Blackstone (ed.), *Philosophy and Environmental Crisis*. Athens: University of Georgia Press.

Ford, N. 1988. *When Did I Begin? Conception of the Human Individual in History, Philosophy, and Science*. Cambridge: Cambridge University Press.

Geertz, C. 1964. The transition to humanity. In S. Tax (ed.), *Horizons of Anthropology*. Chicago: Aldine.

———. 1965. The impact of the concept of culture on the concept of man. In J. R. Platt (ed.), *New Views on the Nature of Man*. Chicago: University of Chicago Press.

———. 1966. Religion as a cultural system. In M. Banton (ed.), *Anthropological Approaches to the Study of Religion*. New York: Frederick A. Praeger.

Gergen, K. 1991. *The Saturated Self: Dilemmas of Identity in Contemporary Life*. New York: Basic Books.

———. 2011. The social construction of self. In S. Gallagher (ed.), *The Oxford Handbook of the Self*. Oxford: Oxford University Press.

Gervais, K. 1986. *Redefining Death*. New Haven: Yale University Press.

Green, M., and Wikler, D. 1980. Brain death and personal identity. *Philosophy and Public Affairs* 9:105–33.

Guérit, J.-M. 2004. The concept of brain death. In C. Machado and D. A. Shewmon (eds.), *Brain Death and Disorders of Consciousness*. New York: Kluwer.

Harré, R. 1984. *Personal Being: A Theory for Individual Psychology*. Cambridge: Harvard University Press.

———. 1989. The "self" as a theoretical concept. In M. Krausz (ed.), *Relativism, Interpretation and Confrontation*. Notre Dame, IN: University of Notre Dame Press.

Harris, J. 1985. *The Value of Life*. London: Routledge and Kegan Paul.

Johnston, M. 1992. How to speak of the colors. *Philosophical Studies* 68:221–63.

Kretzmann, N. 1999. *The Metaphysics of Creation: Aquinas's Natural Theology in* Summa contra Gentiles II. Oxford: Clarendon Press.

Lizza, J. 1993. Persons and death: What's metaphysically wrong with our current statutory definition of death? *Journal of Medicine and Philosophy* 18:351–74.

———. 2004. The conceptual basis for brain death revisited: Loss of organic integration or loss of consciousness? In C. Machado and D. A. Shewmon (eds.), *Brain Death and Disorders of Consciousness*. New York: Kluwer.

———. 2011. Where's Waldo: The "decapitation gambit" and the definition of death. *Journal of Medical Ethics* 37(12):743–46.

Locke, J. [1694] 1975. *An Essay Concerning Human Understanding*. 2nd ed. P. H. Nidditch (ed.). Oxford: Clarendon Press.

Lynn, J. 1993. Are the patients who become organ donors under the Pittsburgh protocol for "non-heart-beating donors" really dead? *Kennedy Institute of Ethics Journal* 3:167–78.

Machado, C. 1995. A new definition of death based on the basic mechanism of consciousness generation in human beings. In C. Machado and D. A. Shewmon (eds.), *Brain Death and Disorders of Consciousness*. New York: Kluwer.

Mackenzie, C., and Stoljar, N. (eds.). 2000. *Relational Autonomy*. Oxford: Oxford University Press.

Marquis, D. 1989. Why abortion is immoral. *Journal of Philosophy* 76(4):183–202.

————. 2007. The moral principle objection to human embryonic stem cell research. In L. Gruen, L. Grabel, and P. Singer (eds.), *Stem Cell Research: The Ethical Issues*. Malden, MA: Blackwell.

————. 2008. Abortion and human nature. *Journal of Medical Ethics* 34(6):422–26.

————. 2010. Are DCD donors dead? *Hastings Center Report* 40(3):24–31.

Martin, C. B. 1994. Dispositions and conditionals. *Philosophical Quarterly* 44:1–8.

McMahan, J. 1995. The metaphysics of brain death. *Bioethics* 9:91–126.

————. 2002. *The Ethics of Killing*. New York: Oxford University Press.

Mead, G. H. 1925. The genesis of self and social control. *International Journal of Ethics* 35:251-73.

————. 1934. *Mind, Self and Society from the Standpoint of a Social Behaviorist*. Chicago: University of Chicago Press.

Mellor, D. H. 1974. In defense of dispositions. *Philosophical Review* 83:157–81.

Mumford, S. 1998. *Dispositions*. Oxford: Oxford University Press.

Parfit, D. 1986. *Reasons and Persons*. Oxford: Oxford University Press.

Pasnau, R. 2002. *Thomas Aquinas on Human Nature*. New York: Cambridge University Press.

President's Council on Bioethics. 2002. *Human Cloning and Human Dignity: An Ethical Inquiry*. Washington, DC: U.S. Government Printing Office.

Robertson, J. 1999. The dead donor rule. *Hastings Center Report* 29(6):6–14.

Sartre, J-P. [1942] 1994. *Being and Nothingness*. Trans. H. E. Barnes. New York: Gramercy Books.

————. [1945] 1955. *No Exit*. Trans. S. Gilbert. New York: Vintage Books.

————. [1946] 1970. *L'existentialisme est un humanisme*. Rpr. Paris: Les Editions Nagel.

Shewmon, D. A. 1988. Anencephaly: Selected medical aspects. *Hastings Center Report* 18(5):11–18.

————. 1992. Brain death: A valid theme with invalid variations, blurred by semantic ambiguity. In H. Angstwurm and I. Carrasco de Paula (eds.), *Working Group on the Determination of Brain Death and Its Relationship to Human Death*. Vatican City: Pontificia Academia Scientiarum.

————. 1997. Recovery from "brain death": A neurologist's apologia. *Linacre Quarterly* 64(1):31–96.

————. 2004a. The ABC of PVS. In C. Machado and D. A. Shewmon (eds.), *Brain Death and Disorders of Consciousness*. New York: Kluwer.

————. 2004b. The "critical organism" for the "organism as a whole": Lessons from the lowly spinal cord. In C. Machado and D. A. Shewmon (eds.), *Brain Death and Disorders of Consciousness*, 23–41. New York: Kluwer.

————. 2010. Constructing the death elephant: A synthetic paradigm shift for the definition, criteria, and tests for death. *Journal of Medicine and Philosophy* 35:256–98.

Shinnar, S., and Arras, J. 1989. Ethical issues in the use of anencephalic infants as organ donors. *Neurologic Clinics* 7:729–43.

Singer, P. 1987. Creating embryos. In W. B. Weil, Jr., and M. Benjamin (eds.), *Ethical Issues at the Outset of Life*, 43–51. New York: Macmillan.

————. 1993. *Practical Ethics*. New York: Cambridge University Press.

Singer, P., and Dawson, K. 1988. IVF technology and the argument from potential. *Philosophy and Public Affairs* 17(2):87–104.

Steinbock, B. 1992. *Life before Birth: The Moral and Legal Status of Embryos and Fetuses*. New York: Oxford University Press.

Tooley, M. 1983. *Abortion and Infanticide*. New York: Oxford University Press.

———. 1998. In defense of abortion and infanticide. In L. Pojman and F. J. Beckwith (eds.), *The Abortion Controversy Twenty-Five Years after* Roe v. Wade*: A Reader*. Belmont, CA: Wadsworth.

Veatch, R. M. 1975. The whole-brain oriented concept of death: An outmoded philosophical formulation. *Journal of Thanatology* 3:13–30.

———. 1988. Whole-brain, neocortical, and higher brain related concepts. In R. M. Zaner (ed.), *Death: Beyond Whole-Brain Criteria*. Dordrecht: Kluwer.

———. 1993. The impending collapse of the whole-brain definition of death. *Hastings Center Report* 23(4):18–24.

———. 2008. Donating hearts after cardiac death—reversing the irreversible. *New England Journal of Medicine* 359:672–73.

Warren, M. 1981. Do potential persons have rights? In E. Partridge (ed.), *Responsibilities to Future Generations*. New York: Prometheus Books.

Wittgenstein, L. 1953. *Philosophical Investigations*, trans. G. E. M. Anscombe. Oxford: Blackwell.

Zaner, R. M. (ed.). 1988. *Death: Beyond Whole-Brain Criteria*. Dordrecht: Kluwer.

PART ONE

THE NATURE OF POTENTIALITY

CHAPTER ONE

Aristotle's Theory of Potentiality

MOHAN MATTHEN

Aristotle's theory of potentiality plays a large role in his metaphysics and philosophy of science. In some ways, it is insightful and prophetic, for it introduces a model of explanation by functional analysis, which is still standard in some of the cognitive and (arguably) life sciences. In other ways, it is outmoded, for explanation by functional analysis is not, as Aristotle thought, applicable to *all* the sciences.[1] In this essay, I review some major features of the theory. My aim is to explore how an Aristotelian should think about questions concerning the beginning and end of life.

I want to make it clear at the outset that since I am interested (here) in how Aristotle's ideas impact contemporary controversies, historical accuracy is not my only concern. It is of no special interest to be told that Aristotle's theory has such and such a consequence for the question of when life begins, if one is inclined to reject the theory out of hand. It serves both history and philosophy to make a plausible argument using Aristotelian ideas, even if in order to do so, one is obliged to interpret these ideas with one's eyes somewhat more fixed on contemporary philosophical applications than historians generally find appropriate. I shall be concerned, therefore, to advance an interpretation that is flexible enough to accommodate contemporary questions and concerns.

How does a suitably reconstructed version of Aristotle's theory apply to issues concerning the beginning and end of life? Here, it is even more urgent to distinguish this question from the one about how Aristotle himself would have spoken about life. As we shall see, Aristotle had some morally objectionable beliefs about how to assess the moral entitlements of humans with regard to life. So we should ask how an Aristotelian theory of *potentiality* affects issues concerning the beginning and end of life, given a more acceptable position on the moral entitlements of humans.

I. Potentiality and Nature in Aristotle's *Physics*
a. Kinēsis and Potentiality

In Aristotle's system (*Physics* III 1–3), a *kinēsis* is an agent-initiated change that has well-defined starting and ending termini. (The term *kinēsis* [plural *kinēseis*] is sometimes translated as "motion," sometimes "change": both are sometimes misleading. Here, I leave it transliterated as a term of art.) Standard examples are building a house and teaching a lesson. These *kinēseis* begin, respectively, when an agent—a builder or a teacher—begins to act purposefully upon materials from which the house is to be constructed or upon an ignorant student who is to be taught. They *must* end—there is not a way for them to be extended—when the house has been built and when the student has learned the lesson. These changes contrast with activities such as hammering or sawing, or speaking to students. There is no natural point at which these activities end, no point at which it is impossible for them to be extended further.

Kinēsis always has an agent and a patient (or thing acted upon)—the builder acts upon building materials or unfinished houses; the teacher acts upon ignorant students. This is where potentiality comes in. The causes of kinēsis are not properly the agent and patient themselves, but an active potentiality in the agent and a matched passive potentiality in the patient. The builder has a capacity to turn the building materials into a house; a house comes to be because she comes into contact with building materials that can be made into a house, and having come into contact with them, exercises her capacity on them. Analogously with teacher and student—a student comes to know something because a teacher comes into contact with something able to be taught.[2]

As said before, the agent initiates the kinēsis. When the house has been built, or the student has learned the lesson, the passive potentiality in that thing has disappeared, for then there is nothing further for the builder or teacher to do. Both potentialities are essentially self-limiting, though in different ways. The patient changes, and thereby loses its passive potentiality. Once the student learns his lesson, he is no longer ignorant and cannot be instructed (in this lesson). The teacher, however, does not change. Her teaching potential has done its job, and stops, but she retains the active potentiality.

b. Nature and Self-Initiated Change

A kinēsis occurs *by nature* when both active and passive potentials belong to a single substance in virtue of the kind of substance it is. Growth is natural kinēsis. Over the period of a year, a newborn infant might triple its birth weight. (Of course, this is just part of a larger natural kinēsis, which terminates naturally when the individual is full-grown.) Though growth requires feeding by the mother, an outside source, the potentiality to convert food into bodily mass is intrinsic to the infant. (More about this in a moment.) That is, some part or aspect of the infant (its "nutritive soul") carries an active potential to transform another part or aspect (its body) by metabolizing nutriment. (Note that even self-initiated self-directed kinēseis—i.e., natural changes such as growth by metabolism—conform to the apparatus of active and passive potentialities. This will be important in what follows.)

Sometimes, it is tricky to identify the substance that contains these matched capacities. Penelope and Odysseus had a bed that was shaped from a live olive tree. The bed and the olive tree are not one and the same—the tree predates the bed, and the bed could be destroyed without the olive tree being destroyed. So there are two substances here. Now, what should we say when the olive tree sprouts? Is it the bed or the tree that is naturally changing? The obvious answer is that it is the olive tree that sprouts by nature, not the bed. It is the tree, and not the bed, that has a nutritive soul matched to its body in virtue of the kind of thing it is. The bed sprouts, but only because it coincides with the tree.

It is crucial here that the active and passive potential responsible for growth by metabolism are *essential* parts of the baby—parts of the baby by virtue of the kind of thing it is. A doctor too can act upon herself. That is, she can heal herself—her medical skill is the active potentiality, and her ailment constitutes a passive potentiality in her body; both are in her, and she acts on herself by virtue of them. However, this is not a natural change, for medical knowledge does not inhere in her as a consequence of the kind of thing (i.e., substance) she is (namely, a human).

Life consists (among other things) in the capacity to metabolize *naturally*, i.e., by means of active and passive potentialities that belong to a thing because of the kind of thing it is. This indicates the difference between the mother's act of feeding and the baby's act of metabolizing. The first is other-directed and hence *non-natural*; the second self-directed by nature. The second defines the baby as living; the first is merely made possible by the life of the baby, but not constituted by it. (Note that "non-natural" here means "not by nature"; it does *not* mean "against nature.")

It should now be clear why the self-contained agent-*patient* kinēsis that constitutes an embryo's nutritive soul is different from the mother's potentiality to nourish it in utero. The former is constitutive of the embryo's capacity to act on itself; the latter is not an exercise of the mother's self-acting capacity. The embryo's dependence on the mother as a source of nutriment does not gainsay its standing as a self-acting metabolizer. At least as far as Aristotle is concerned, Jason Eberl is right, elsewhere in this volume, to write, "The form of external assistance a uterus provides is analogous to an astronaut's spacesuit or an underwater explorer's submarine" (Eberl 2014).

Modern science does not, however, support the position that from the moment of fertilization onward, the embryo possesses a natural potential for metabolism. (Actually, it's not clear that Aristotle believes this either.) Early in its development, an embryo is dependent on the mother for metabolism. For in the moments after fertilization, the embryo is nothing more than a fertilized ovum. It does not, at this point, possess a metabolic system. Or to put it in Aristotelian terms, it does not, immediately upon fertilization, possess a "nutritive soul." When exactly it comes to possess a nutritive soul cannot be decided *a priori*. The best way to look at the matter is that Aristotle provides us with a criterion for the beginning of life—life begins when the embryo is able to metabolize nutriment on its own, without relying on the assistance of the mother's metabolic system.

This criterion is evidently very difficult to apply. For one thing, an embryo cannot be simply given adult food; it cannot, for instance, metabolize milk or eggs. So the mother needs to convert what she eats into a form suitable for the embryo to metabolize. What counts as merely providing nutrition fit for an embryo to metabolize for itself, and what counts as metabolizing by the mother for the embryo? That is, with respect to what kind of nutriment is it appropriate to regard the embryo as a self-acting metabolizer? Again, only science can answer such questions, or even decide whether they have a definite answer. For what it is worth, it seems that there *is* a distinction. For metabolism consists of producing energy for one's own activities, and matter for one's own growth. Regardless of what nutriment is used for producing these things, one can ask whether it is the embryo's body that performs the relevant transformation or the mother's that does so. And there is clearly a point (or interval) of time at which the embryo's body has begun to do so. This is the point at which the embryo has begun to be alive.

One important point that comes out of this discussion is that the crucial question for Aristotle is when the embryo is able to sustain its own metabolic activities. The question is *not* when it is possible for it to grow into an organism capable of performing characteristically human activities. This distinction cuts two ways. The crucial determinant is *not* whether a fertilized ovum can ultimately perform human activities. The question is rather whether it can sustain its own metabolic processes. And clearly there is a period of time during which it is capable ultimately of performing human activities but not capable of sustaining its own metabolism.

And yet, it is also irrelevant whether or not it is *possible* for it to develop. It could be that unfavorable circumstances make it impossible for the embryo to get nutrition, though it has already developed the capacity to metabolize this nutrition. For instance, the mother might have developed some kind of illness that makes it impossible for her body to convert the food she eats into nutriment suitable for the embryo to metabolize. This situation is, as Eberl (2014) rightly suggests, analogous to that of an astronaut in a malfunctioning spacesuit. The astronaut is self-sustaining despite the fact that the malfunction makes it impossible for her to get the external materials needed to sustain herself. Nonetheless, the astronaut is still alive.

We should keep in mind that the genesis of a nutritive soul may not constitute the right kind of life to be worthy of moral standing. (I'll return to this question in section IV.) But *if* possessing a nutritive soul is regarded as constituting moral worth, then unfavorable external circumstances would not abrogate its rights. Abandoned and exposed by its parents, a baby cannot find food for itself, and would die without external intervention. Though it is not, in this sense, self-sustaining, it retains its natural capacity to metabolize and whatever moral standing it has in virtue of (this form of) life. Like the astronaut in the tragically malfunctioning spacesuit, it is still alive.

II. Potentiality and Functional Analysis
a. Coincident versus Proper Potentialities

The potentiality theory is sometimes attacked for being vacuous. Molière's character Tartuffe pretends to wisdom by saying that opium puts people to sleep in virtue of its "dormative power." Yet, he sheds no light on the matter by so saying: dormative power is trivially the cause of sleep. At times Aristotle sounds like Tartuffe, but there is a more fruitful line of explanation behind the appearance of vacuity.

In *Physics* II 3, Aristotle says:

> In investigating the cause of each thing it is always necessary to seek what is most precise . . . thus man builds because he is a builder, and a builder builds in virtue of his art of building. (195b21–24)

And, a little earlier:

> All causes, both proper and coincident, may be spoken of either as potential or as actual; e.g. the cause of a house being built is either *house-builder* or *house-builder building.* (195b4–6)

These passages seem to describe explanatory potentialities in the same words as the effect that is being explained. They appear to echo the vacuity of Tartuffe's *vis dormativa*: this house came into being because a house-builder actualized his house-building skills on materials that could be turned into a house. This suggests that Aristotle had no more to say than that if a house came into being at a certain time, there was, earlier, the possibility of there being a house. The contemporary philosopher of science will object: this possibility is implied by but does not imply the actuality. How then can it *explain* the actuality?

This impression of vacuity is incorrect. Throughout this chapter, Aristotle talks about "coincident" causes. Here is what he says:

> Another mode of causation is the coincident and its genera, e.g., in one way *Poly-cleitus*, in another *sculptor* is the cause of a statue, because *being Polycleitus* and *sculptor* are coincident. (195a33–36)

To understand some of the implications of this passage, imagine an interlocutor who says:

> The statue was made by the action of the chisel on the stone. The sculptor's action was not necessary, since the very same chisel movements coincidentally applied would have had the same result.

To this interlocutor, Aristotle would reply first that without the skill of the sculptor, the sequence of chisel motions would have been a massively improbable random sequence without any explanation.[3] There is nothing *impossible* in a nonsculptor executing the sequence by throwing a bucket of chisels at some marble, but he could do so only by virtue of an extremely improbable *accident*, as when a monkey banging away randomly at a typewriter manages to produce a coherent sentence. But there are many statues in the world—they cannot all have come to be by accident. According to Aristotle, the frequency of statues can only be explained if in most of them, there is an overarching coordinating cause—something that ensures that the chisel strokes are executed rightly and in proper order. (See Matthen 1989 for an account of this argument.) The skill of the sculptor is canonically this cause. The sculptor ensures the correctness of the sequence by coordinating it in accordance with her skill. So, to say that the skill of the sculptor is responsible for the statue is *not* vacuous; minimally, it is to say that there is something that so coordinates chisel strokes as to bring about the genesis of the statue non-accidentally. Obviously, the sculptor's skill serves this role in the production of statues.

The "coincident" causes are bearers of these and other necessary conditions of production. Nonvacuous explanation resides in them. In the particular case of Poly-cleitus's statue, the sculpting skill was coincident with being-Polycleitus—which is to say that the sculpting skill has come to reside in the person who is Polycleitus (though not in virtue of the sort of thing he intrinsically is, which is why it is merely coincident). The consequence is that this person is able reliably to execute the right chiseling actions in the right way. By identifying "the being of Polycleitus" as coincident with the sculptor's skill, we identify the efficient cause of the statue. It was by being coincident with the being of Polycleitus that the sculpting skill had its effect.

b. Functional Analysis

Aristotle's strategy of proper and coincident causes is reminiscent of "functional analysis" (Cummins 1975). Suppose you want to explain how an adding machine adds. First, you specify what "adding power" (or *vis addens*) is: it is the potentiality in the adding machine that ensures that when you sequentially press the keys 'x', '+', 'y', and '=' (for any numerical values of x and y), you get a display of the numerical expression that stands for the sum of x and y. To explain this power of the machine, you need to cite the physical properties of the electronic circuit buried inside the adding machine; you have to show how these properties yield the correct output when a given input is entered. The crucial success condition of your explanation is that the sequence of events set off in the machine by the key presses should be provably equivalent to *adding*. In short, you must show how the power to add decomposes into simpler powers, and you must show how these simpler powers transform the key-presses '7', '+', '4', and '=' and lead to the display '11' (and similarly, for all values of x and y). This is the sine qua non of functional analysis.

Plausibly, this is the kind of analysis Aristotle had in mind when he spoke of coincident causes. The "proper cause" is identified in terms that are logically proximate to the description of the target phenomenon: *house-building* for houses built, *teaching* for learning, *sculpting* for statues, etc. But then you produce another logically more distant description to show how the logically proximate cause comes to be instantiated in the case under consideration. Thus consider what he says about a wall in *Physics* II 9:

> [One should not] suppose that the wall of a house comes to be because what is heavy is naturally carried downwards and what is light to the top, wherefore the stones and foundations take the lowest place, with earth above because it is lighter, and wood at the top of all as being the lightest. Whereas, though the wall does not come to be *without* these, it is not *due* to these, except as its material cause: it comes to be for the sake of sheltering and guarding certain things. (200a1–7)

This suggests a functional analysis of wall-building.

Thus, the art of house-building will seek stone for the lower part of the wall, and the potentiality to stand stably will be actualized by the stone below.

TABLE 1

Goal	Definition	What is needed
To build a house	House = stable shelter-providing structure	Weight-bearing walls to support sheltering roof
To build a wall	Wall = stable weight-bearing structure	Upper parts of wall should be supported stably by lower parts
To build structure in which lower parts stably support upper parts	Stable support → upper parts should not disturb position of lower parts on which they rest	Upper parts light in order to exert less pressure on lower parts; lower parts strong and heavy to support upper parts
Strong and heavy lower part of wall	← coincides with →	stone

> The arts that govern the matter and have knowledge are two, namely the art that uses the product and the art that directs the production of it. That is why the using art also is in a sense directive; but it differs in that it knows the form, whereas the art which is directive as being concerned with production knows the matter. For the helmsman knows and prescribes what sort of form a helm should have, the other from what wood it should be made and by means of what operations. (*Physics* II 2.194b1–6)

The success condition of a more distant description being the correct explanation is that the "proper cause" should "coincide" with it. The capacity to provide stable shelter coincides with structures that have stone below. Similarly, the adding potential coincides with the underlying electronic operations, not with the whine of the machine. And sculpting capacity explains the sequence of chisel strokes, and it coincides with Polycleitus, not the chisel he wields.

Bringing this back to natural kinēsis, it is relatively vacuous to be told that a baby grows because it has within it an active potential to convert nutriment into bodily mass. To provide a more explanatory theory, Aristotle must cash this out in terms of coincident causes. He must, in other words, show how the baby is so put together that it is able to metabolize food. There are places where he takes a stab at doing something like this, but obviously his science was not up to this task. However, Max Delbrück (1971), a Nobel laureate and James Watson's teacher at Caltech, provides a brief appreciation of the progress Aristotle made toward delineating the parameters of such a functional analysis. According to Delbrück, Aristotle realized that:

> The form principle is the information stored in the semen. After fertilization, it is read out in a preprogrammed way; the readout alters the matter on which it acts,

but does not alter the stored information, which is not, properly speaking, part of the finished product. (54)

There is a long distance, and many centuries, to go before this analysis could be taken to its ultimate conclusion; nevertheless, Delbrück suggested that "if that committee in Stockholm, which has the unenviable task of pointing out the most creative scientists, had the liberty of giving awards posthumously, I think they should consider Aristotle, for the discovery of the principle implied in DNA."

III. Potentiality and Possibility
a. Possibility Insufficient for Potentiality

I have gone into some detail concerning Aristotelian potentialities in order to make three points about them.

First, Aristotle's attributions of potentialities are tied to functional analysis. Thus, the potentialities are not merely vacuous verbal re-descriptions. In fact, Aristotle here anticipates an important explanatory tool in modern cognitive science—functional analysis. One should not, however, exaggerate his prescience here. Aristotle's use of functional analysis is ubiquitous—he defines the elementary building blocks of the Universe functionally. For example, in the *De Caelo* I, he defines earth, which is an element in his system, in terms of its power to actualize itself at the center of the Universe. But we have seen that functional analysis is ultimately dependent on an analysis of powers in terms of other kinds of properties. Aristotle's over-use of functional analysis robs his system of the causal foundation it requires.

Second, Aristotelian potentialities are *causes*, not merely earlier possibilities of later realities. When Aristotle says that this building material has a potential to be made into a house, he is not merely saying that it is *possible* for the material to be worked on so as to yield a structure that affords shelter to people. In the first place, even if the possibility of p is materially equivalent to the potentiality in something of p, potentialities are causally efficacious attributes and reside in substances; possibilities are not.

Third, and crucially for my argument, the possibility is *not* even materially equivalent to the potentiality. Consider water and cement powder. It is possible for this stuff first to be made into cement blocks and then to be made into a house, so it is possible for the water and cement powder to be worked into a house. However, water and cement powder do not have the potentiality to be made into a house. This is, first, because water and cement powder do not have the appropriate potentialities—they do not, for instance, keep their shape when subjected to pressure. In order to get

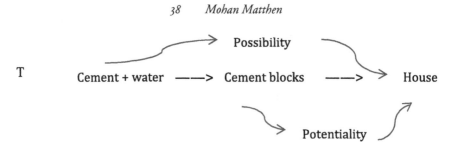

Figure 1: Possibility Unnecessary for Potentiality

things with the appropriate potentialities from cement powder and water, these things must be mixed together and allowed to set. (This supplements the point I made toward the end of section I, namely that the point of interest is when an embryo comes to acquire the potentiality to metabolize. This potentiality is more than a possibility.)

Plausibly, the *new* potentials that mixed-and-set concrete blocks possess indicate that some new thing has come to be from cement powder and water. This would suggest that these materials must first go out of existence and cement blocks must come to be from them. If this is correct, the house-building potentiality cannot be exerted on cement powder and water as such. It must be exerted on cement blocks.

This makes for a complicated link between x's potentialities (where x is a substance) and possibilities *for x* (Krizan 2006). Aristotle says: "a thing is capable of doing something if there is nothing impossible in it having the actuality of that which it is said to have the capacity" (*Met.* 1047a24–26). Water and cement are not actually present in the material of a house. Hence, *they* do not have the relevant potentiality. (Remember, though, that even if water and cement *were* present in the house, as modern chemistry would have it, they do not have the potentiality to support weight except when thoroughly mixed together.) On the other hand, it is possible for the cement blocks to have the actuality of being parts of a house. So, it is a possibility for them. It is on the basis of similar reasoning that Aristotle says that the possibility *for x* to be made into a house implies the potentiality to be made into the house.

b. Possibility Unnecessary for Potentiality

Possibility is not *necessary* for potentiality either. (Here I am indebted to John Lizza for probing questions.) Consider an embryo whose mother dies during pregnancy. This embryo possesses a natural capacity to metabolize nutriment and develop into an adult. However, it is now not possible for this embryo to develop into an adult, because it cannot get nourishment. For at least a short time after the mother dies, the embryo retains the natural *potentiality* for development, though there is, in fact, no possibility of it developing any further.

This situation contrasts with that of a genetically or developmentally defective embryo. Embryos sometimes suffer a catastrophic developmental event, which causes them to be born without a skull, or even a brain. (This is known as *anencephaly*.) Such embryos lack the innate potentiality to develop into intellectually functioning adults. In Aristotle's way of looking at things, this is very different from the situation where the embryo *has* the potential but lacks the possibility for development because of the absence of external sources of nutriment.

If *natural* (i.e., self-acting) potentiality is the basis for moral standing, then the embryo whose mother has died has moral standing, and the anencephalic baby lacks it.

c. Genesis and Nature

In the case of the arts, it is, to some extent, arbitrary how potentialities are assigned. Consider a stone quarry. It is not a builder's job—not part of his art—to cut stone from a quarry and make it into blocks suitable for building. Consequently, the stone in the quarry does not have the potential to be made into a building; a builder could not work on it (though he would have a say, as the last quotation above shows, in the form that the cut stone would take). But (whether Aristotle took this into account or not) the division of labour between the quarry-man and the builder is contingent. If it had been considered part of the builder's job to excavate and cut stone, then the rock in the quarry would have had the potential to be fashioned into a house.

Things are different with natural substances. The *kuēma*, or fertilized union of male and female genetic material, develops more or less spontaneously into a mature organism. But this does not mean that either the male or the female genetic material has the potential to become a mature human being all by itself. Left alone, neither will develop. First they must be made into a kuēma (see below) and then this spontaneously develops. There are (at least) two kinēseis here, the second one of which is natural.

This is an important point, for as Alfonso Gómez-Lobo (2004) reports, some have argued as follows:

> The potentiality argument is understood as moving backwards in the following way: if a human person deserves respect, then a potential human person . . . also deserves respect. But . . . by virtue of the transitivity of potentiality, . . . the sperm and ovum also deserve respect. [But this is] "a position almost no one finds plausible," to quote an elegant understatement by Professor [R. M.] Veatch. (200)

Of course, Gómez-Lobo is right. Nothing of the sort follows. Potentials are not transitive in the way that the "moving backwards" argument assumes. The ovum is not a potential human being *at least* until fertilized. And in Aristotelian science, similarly, the genetic material of each parent does not have the potential to develop naturally into a mature human by itself.

IV. Soul: The Capacities That Define Human Life

We are now ready to consider some questions about the beginning of life. According to Aristotle, sexual intercourse leads to pregnancy when male and female genetic material intermingle and join in such a way that the form of the male can work on the matter provided by the female. At this point, we have a kuēma, the very first stage of the embryo. Embryonic development, or ontogenesis, is the natural kinēsis that results in the baby born nearly forty weeks later. (It is possible to regard this kinēsis as terminating a couple of decades later, when the child becomes an adult.) Aristotle's account of ontogenesis is thus an application of his theory of kinēsis.

Three questions can now be posed:

1. At what stage does the embryo become a human being?
2. At what stage is the embryo a potential human being?
3. At what stage is the embryo alive?

First, in agreement with Gómez-Lobo above, fertilization is, on anybody's account but especially Aristotle's, the very earliest point at which there could be said to be a new life or new being. (As I argued earlier, the Aristotelian account probably implies that life, or natural metabolism, starts later.) Prior to fertilization, the active potential of ontogenesis, the human form provided by the father is not in contact with the matter provided by the mother. Consequently, though there is the *possibility* of the female matter being part of a continuous process that culminates in a mature human being, this genetic material lacks the potentiality to become a mature human being *naturally*.[4] And as we have seen, possibilities and potentialities are quite different conditions.

Of course, Aristotle would allow that both the female and the male genetic material had the potentiality to interact with one another to become first a fertilized ovum and ultimately a mature human being, in the way that stone and builder have potentialities to interact with one another to produce a house. There are two reasons why this is irrelevant. First, there is no *particular human being* it will produce: both male and female genetic material require something of the other kind, but prior to fertilization, there is no particular thing of the complementary kind that provides the potentiality to produce the offspring.[5] Thus, there is, before fertilization, no substance that is potentially human or potentially alive. Second, and perhaps more importantly, there is not, prior to fertilization, anything that can initiate change within itself—and as we have seen, this is the hallmark of life. Thus, alluding to a more modern notion of "respect" or "regard," there is, as Gómez-Lobo says, no plausibility in thinking that sperm and ovum deserve respect. In answering questions 1–3, we should, therefore, consider only stages of the embryo, and nothing earlier.

Embryonic development is the acquisition of some *capacity* that defines life. (We'll come in a moment to what capacity this might be. I am assuming for now that "capacity" and "potentiality" are interchangeable, though as we'll see this is too simple.) The acquisition of the life-defining capacity takes place in something, X, that did not possess it at the start of the process. Does this mean that X (whatever it is) has the potentiality to be alive? Or is some new thing, Y, created in the process (in the way that cement blocks were created out of cement powder and water), such that Y is alive—but is not the same as X? If Y is a new thing, it would be wrong to say that X is potentially alive simply in virtue of the fact that X becomes, or becomes a constituent of Y. Thus:

- If X did not initially have the life-defining capacity, but only later came to have it, is X potentially alive at the start of the process (in virtue, perhaps, of potentially possessing the life-defining capacity)?
- If a thing that has life (e.g., X above) is necessarily distinct from that which does not have life (Y), then could X be one and the same as Y?

These difficult questions are crucial to any determination of the starting point (and endpoint) of life for a human. They are not explicitly dealt with by Aristotle, but one can speculate as to what his answers might be.

In order to answer these questions, I turn now to Aristotle's conception of life. In Aristotle's system, as in most modern ones, life is defined by certain capacities: that is, a living thing is defined as one that is capable of certain activities (e.g., metabolism). As we have noted, capacities or potentialities inhere in substance. So the capacities that define life inhere in living things. This thing lives in virtue of having certain capacities. It does *not* live in virtue of the presence in it of a separable soul (as Plato had it in the *Phaedo*). In Aristotle's ontology, souls depend for their existence on the living substances in which they reside, not the other way around. Soul is a capacity in virtue of which its possessor is alive; but this capacity would not exist but for the thing in which it inheres.

Aristotle's conception of soul is of particular interest because he defines *three kinds* of living. All living things, including plants, are capable (1) of metabolizing nutriment and growing. This capacity is sometimes known as the "nutritive" soul.

Animals have a nutritive soul, but in addition they are capable (2) of perception and self-movement; this is the "sensitive" soul. Finally, humans have both a nutritive and a sensitive soul, but are, in addition, capable (3) of thought and reason. This is the rational soul.

Now, in modern ways of thinking about life, the emphasis is on what is common to *all* living things. If Aristotle had followed this line of thought, he would have identified life (hence, soul, which is the principle of life) with the nutritive soul. This, however, is *not* how he proceeds. He says:

> Living is *spoken about in different ways.* And should even one of these belong to something, we say it is alive: reason, perception, motion and rest with respect to place, and further the *kinesis* of nourishment, decay, and growth. (*De Anima* II 413a22–25)

Here, Aristotle acknowledges that we *say* of anything at all that it is alive if it merely nourishes itself. However, he says that life is spoken about in different ways. The same word is used, but it is used to describe different kinds of thing. Plants, which have only a nutritive soul, have a different kind of life than animals, which have a nutritive as well as a sensitive soul. (Notice that this kind of position would support subsuming respect for animals to respect for the kind of life that animals possess. Respect for animal life would not automatically imply that respect be paid to plants.)

Aristotle's idea here is, I believe, something like this. Plants nourish themselves statically: they stand still and draw up nutriment from the earth and air around them. Animals can sense and move, and they use these capacities to find food. The very activity of self-nourishment is modified by the manner in which animals engage in it. Thus, it is (according to Aristotle) in a way true, and in a way false, to say that plants and animals share a life-defining capacity. Plant and animal self-nourishment are different in kind. In a similar vein, one might note that humans use reason (among other things) to get food. This fundamentally modifies their way of going about an activity that, viewed from a certain perspective, they share with plants and animals.

Christopher Shields (2009) puts this point well. He contrasts two models of the human soul. There is first the "layer cake" model, with the nutritive soul forming a distinct layer under the sensitive soul, which in turn is separate and distinct from the rational soul. The second model emphasizes the unity of life-activities:

> A being with a rational soul has a perceptual capacity neither more nor less than a being with a perceptual soul. Still, the manner in which the perceptual faculty is present is distinct. A rational soul is not formed by the layering of a rational

faculty upon the top of *an actually existing perceptual faculty.* Rather, a rational soul subordinates a perceptual faculty to its own ends, thereby integrating it into a unified, single soul. (2009, 306; emphasis added)

The italicized words above are significant: the point is that the "perceptual faculty" is not, as such, sitting there deep in our souls, a separate entity that is the same as what animals possess. Rather, we have faculties that, *but for their integration with reason*, would be an animal perceptual faculty, pure and simple. Given this integration, our perceptual faculties do not constitute a separable animal soul.

This explains Aristotle's words:

What holds in the case of the soul is similar to what holds concerning figures: for both figures and the ensouled, what is prior is present as a capacity in what follows in the series, for example, the triangle in the square, and the nutritive in the perceptive. We must investigate the reason why they are thus in a series. For the perceptive faculty is not without the nutritive, though the nutritive is separated from the perceptive in plants. (414b28–415a3)

Triangles are present in squares, but not as actual triangles—they are only *potentially* present awaiting their generation from the square by the division of the latter. Similarly, the plant soul is present in us, but not as actual. We say that things are alive because they engage in "nourishment, decay, and growth": nevertheless, we speak of life in different ways when we do so.

Aristotle's notion of the human soul, then, is something like this: it is the capacity to self-nourish and to perceive in ways that are subordinate to reason. Now, God has reason but does *not* have self-nourishment or motion and, therefore, does not have a human soul. It is not very much noticed in the literature that because humans are unique with respect to the kind of soul they possess, Aristotle's discussion of soul in the early parts of *De Anima* II actually provide a definition of our species. This is a bit of a surprise, and it is germane to question 1, above. The question is: "At what stage does the embryo become a human being?" The answer is: "When it becomes capable of rational thought."

When is something *capable* of rational thought? Is an embryo capable of rational thought when it is at its very earliest stage of male genetic form united with the female genetic matter? To understand this, we have to take Aristotle's notion of a *first actuality* into account. Consider a sleeping adult. She is capable of thought and speech, but is not exercising this capacity. This is a *first* actuality; the *second* or complete actuality is present in somebody only when they are *actually* speaking. Now, Aristotle posits a potentiality that is prior to the first actuality. Babies are in this stage with respect to speech. That is, babies are *not* like sleeping adults who are capable of

TABLE 2

First potentiality	Second Potentiality/ First Actuality	Second Actuality
Baby (to speak): must learn language to move to second potentiality	Asleep adult (to speak)	Adult giving a speech
HYPOTHETICALLY: Embryo (to think): what must happen to move to second potentiality? Is a new entity created?	Asleep adult (to think)	Adult actively thinking

speaking when they awake. There is something they have to acquire in order to be capable of speaking. Babies, however, are unlike puppies because they will (in quite short order) acquire the capacity to speak. They have a "first potentiality." The first potentiality to speak and think marks them as human, even though they are still not, in the sense of the sleeping adult, capable of speaking and thinking.

The question remains. Is it the first potentiality or the first actuality that bestows upon an embryo the status of a human? Or to put it another way, when does *human* life begin, this being conceived as a different question than that concerning life as such. Here it should be noted that Aristotle's notion of human rationality is even more demanding than we have encountered so far. When a person reasons something out—for example, the solution to a math problem or a difficult course of action—she is not engaging in the highest form of rationality. Reasoning something out, whether in the practical or the theoretical realm, is a kinēsis. One starts with some premises, and arrives at a conclusion. Once one has arrived at the conclusion, the reasoning terminates. God, however, does not engage in kinēsis; God simply thinks. This is a so-called *energeia*, a non-goal-oriented activity without a natural terminus. God thinks in a non-goal-oriented way; the potential to think does not disappear when the goal is achieved. (This is the reason I said earlier that potentiality and capacity might not be exactly the same: we have a capacity for non-goal-oriented thought but not a potentiality, as I have explained the latter, i.e., relative to kinēsis.)

Now, according to Aristotle, it is part of human essence to emulate God in this form of non-goal-oriented, non-terminating thinking, and *though (of course) humans cannot achieve it,* it is (as we learn in Nicomachean Ethics X), the highest good for them. Here, it is perhaps helpful to contrast the rotational movement of the stars with the movement of the sublunary elements to their natural places. The latter kind of motion is kinēsis: it terminates when an element such as earth reaches its natural place at the center of the universe. Similarly, solving a problem has a natural terminus, but thinking per se does not.

This throws some doubt on Jason Eberl's approach elsewhere in this volume. Eberl writes:

> I follow Aquinas in contending that *all that is required for something to be a person is for it to have <u>at least an active potentiality</u> to perform self-conscious rational operations*. The actual performance of such operations is accidental to a person's existence. (Eberl, 2014)

This would be correct if human life was defined as the first actuality of thinking. My point here is that there are places in the corpus, notably in *Nicomachean Ethics* X and *Metaphysics* XIII, where Aristotle suggests that it is a failing not to be actually in a state of thinking.

This is an extremely powerful and telling result. It implies that human life is defined by an activity that the apparatus of potentiality and actuality does not perfectly fit. Eberl (2014, n.5) helpfully lists a number of attempts to say what activities define human life, and concludes "they all include the criterion of either *rationality* or *self-consciousness*." He goes on to say: "any being who possesses the capacity for both would undoubtedly qualify as a person." This is dubious. It could be argued that it is essential to humans that they are always *actually* self-conscious, and that a cessation of such self-consciousness was a cessation of life itself. Of course, much depends on how self-consciousness is defined—for example, whether it is to be understood in such a way as to include sleep. I do not want to deny that Eberl has strong considerations on his side. My point here is merely that Aristotle may well not agree. The cessation of self-conscious thought is *eo ipso* a failing with regard to human essence.

Put nonkinetic reason, that is, non-goal-oriented thinking, to one side. There is another reason Eberl's position is too undemanding. Aristotle defines *full* reason as the capacity to set goals, not merely work toward them. (Thus understood, full reason is kinetic.) If humans lack full reason, he says, they are deficient. And in his most explicit consideration of moral standing, he asserts that deficiencies in this regard *rob humans of their right* to autonomy. To illustrate the point, think of the morally repugnant conclusions he draws about slaves in *Politics* I 5:

> For he who can belong to another (and that is why he *does* belong to another), and he who participates in reason so far as to apprehend it but not so far as to possess (for the other animals obey not reason but feelings), is a slave by nature. The use made of them differs little; for from both—slaves and tame animals—comes bodily help in the supply of essentials. (1254b20–26)

The passage occurs in the context of a justification of slavery. Slaves are deficient in reason, Aristotle says, and this is why it is right to treat them as instruments, or tools. Further:

> Tame animals are by nature better than wild, and it is better for all of them to be ruled by men, because it secures their safety. Again, the relationship of male to female is that the one is by nature superior, the other inferior, and the one is ruler, the other ruled. And this must hold good of all mankind. (1254b10–15)

It is reasonably clear, then, that Aristotle identifies human living with some quite demanding conceptions of reason, and argues that those who (as he thinks) are deficient with respect to reason are also deficient with respect to being human. Such deficient humans lose their moral entitlements, for they are subject to being used, ruled, and owned by others. Inasmuch as embryos are similarly deficient with respect to the activity that defines human life, they too do not have a right to respect. Very much the same holds for those who suffer irreversible loss of cognitive faculties.

Apparently, then, Aristotle's notion of potentiality and natural change combined with his own notion of the human soul leads to a very negative answer concerning the beginning of human life, at least in its full form. His answer sanctions infanticide and euthanasia for people with irreversible senile dementia (and not just for those in a persistently vegetative state). And this is not merely a projection of his arguments. Given his position on slavery and the position of women, there is no good reason to think he would have rejected the position that I have attributed to him.

V. Pulling Back

Let me now briefly consider some ways of pulling back from the harsh consequences of Aristotle's position.

One might drop the idea that rationality is the threshold for moral regard. I offer two very brief comments.

1. First, one must do this in a way that preserves a reason for moral regard. That is, we should not be content simply to identify some beings as worthy of moral regard and others as not. This identification should, in addition, rest on some relevant difference between beings of the first sort and those of the second. We do not accord animals the same moral regard as we accord humans. One might ask: what do *arational* humans possess that is deserving of moral regard? How are they different from the animals from which we withhold regard? I am not suggesting that this question be answered by saying, "Noth-

ing." I simply observe that it poses a problem. Second, this is an utterly un-Aristotelian path and lies beyond the scope of my remit.

2. One might drop the idea that rationality defines the human species. In general, the idea that any intrinsic characteristic defines a species is suspect today. (See Ereshefsky and Matthen 2005 for an up-to-date version of the argument.) The quick reason is that according to contemporary Darwinian biology, species display variety, both synchronic and diachronic. Consequently, many have adopted a relational notion of species. One example of such a notion is the Biological Species Concept, which (to simplify greatly) implies that the offspring of two members of any species belongs to that species regardless of what characteristic it might have. This conception pulls us back from the worst in Aristotle's theory: it accords human status to slaves and women, and pushes back against the idea that being a human is a matter of degree. However, because such species concepts undermine the idea that certain capacities define the human species, it also casts doubt on the idea that humans are worthy of moral respect because they have certain potentialities. Thus, it gives us no help with the questions posed at the start of the last section. We are left in the dark with regard to when an embryo deserves moral respect.

To sum up, Aristotle's notion of natural kinēsis implies that we should not treat the entity at the beginning of embryonic development as human, or indeed as the same as the one that is born. This leads us to ask: When does the embryo turn into a human? Aristotle's own answer to this question is very harsh. Bracketing the views that lead to this harsh answer, his theory of kinēsis still gives us reason for searching for a replacement answer. Aristotle's own work unfortunately gives us no help in finding this answer.

NOTES

1. It goes seriously wrong in physics, for example, where it requires the motion of the sublunary elements to be defined by reference to a fixed point in space, namely the center of the Universe. (See Matthen and Hankinson 1993 for discussion.)

2. In this case, too, something comes to be, namely the student's knowledge. But this thing is not a substance (see Matthen 1983). Thus, the house-building *kinēsis* is a coming-to-be *proper*, the coming-to-be of a substance, but the teaching is not.

3. In *Physics* II, 8, he says that a rainstorm during the "dog days" might, but frequent rain in winter cannot, be the result of "chance and spontaneity." This looks like a response to an interlocutor who argues along the lines indicated in the text—perhaps Empedocles, who is referred to a few lines earlier as holding (what strikes the modern reader as) a well worked out theory of chance generation and natural selection.

4. Sagan and Singer suggest, elsewhere in this volume, that in vitro embryos are different from naturally produced ones because the former have to be sustained in certain ways from the outside. On my interpretation of Aristotle, this is not the crucial difference. Rather, we must ask whether the embryo is able to perform the activities characteristic of life by nature—whether it requires outside intervention to acquire the materials for self-sustenance is not important. (See my comments on Eberl's astronaut-and-spacesuit analogy.)

5. John Lizza asks whether intracytoplasmic sperm injection (ICSI) would challenge this point. After ICSI, as he points out, it is already determined which sperm conjoined with which egg produced the embryo. My position on ICSI is of a piece with what I say at the end of section I and in note 3. In Aristotle's theory, the *origin* of the embryo, and the source of its nutriment, are not the important points. Rather its current status determines its status. Are its life-functions performed by nature? If they are, then it has whatever moral standing is concomitant upon this kind of life.

REFERENCES

Cummins, R. 1975. Functional analysis. *Journal of Philosophy* 72:641–75.

Delbrück, M. 1971. Aristotle-totle-totle. In J. Monod and E. Borek (eds.), *On Microbes and Life*, 50–55. New York: Columbia University Press.

Eberl, J. 2014. Persons with potential. In J. Lizza (ed.), *Potentiality: Metaphysical and Bioethical Dimensions*. Baltimore: Johns Hopkins University Press.

Ereshefsky, M., and Matthen, M. 2005. Taxonomy, polymorphism, and history: An introduction to population structure theory. *Philosophy of Science* 72:1–21.

Gómez-Lobo, A. 2004. Does respect for embryos entail respect for gametes? *Theoretical Medicine and Bioethics* 25(3):199–208.

Krizan, M. K. 2006. Corpses, seeds, and statues: The relation between potentiality and possibility in Aristotle's *Metaphysics* and *De Interpretatione. Newsletters for the Society for Ancient Greek Philosophy* 7:27–31.

Matthen, M. 1983. Greek ontology and the "is" of truth. *Phronesis* 28:113–35.

———. 1989. The four causes in Aristotle's embryology. In R. Kraut and T. Penner (eds.), "Nature, Knowledge and Virtue," special issue, *Apeiron* 22(4):159–79.

———, and Hankinson, R. J. 1993. Aristotle's universe: Its form and matter. *Synthese* 96:417–35.

Sagan, A., and Singer, P. 2007. The moral status of stem cells. *Metaphilosophy* 38(2–3):264–84.

Shields, C. 2009. The Aristotelian psychê. In G. Anagnostopoulos (ed.), *A Companion to Aristotle*, 292–309. Oxford: Blackwell.

CHAPTER TWO

Dispositions and Potentialities

JENNIFER McKITRICK

Dispositions and potentialities seem importantly similar. To talk about what something has the potential or disposition to do is to make a claim about a future possibility—the "threats and promises" that fill the world (Goodman 1983, 41). In recent years, dispositions have been the subject of much conceptual analysis and metaphysical speculation. The inspiration for this essay is the hope that that work can shed some light on discussions of potentiality. I compare the concepts of *disposition* and *potentiality*, consider whether accounts of these concepts are subject to similar difficulties, and whether having a disposition or a potentiality can depend on extrinsic factors. The concept of a disposition I am working with is drawn from the recent literature in metaphysics and philosophy of science that focuses on the analysis of dispositional concepts and their role in a broader ontology. The concept of a potentiality is drawn from the bioethics literature that focuses on the moral relevance of potentialities that subjects of medical decisions may or may not possess. Some preliminary conclusions I draw are the following:

1. Potentialities are dispositions;
2. Due to problematic cases, potentiality ascriptions, like disposition ascriptions, are not reducible to counterfactual statements; and
3. Like dispositions, some potentialities can be extrinsic.

Here I do not aim to draw any conclusions about the moral relevance of potentialities but rather to outline conceptual and metaphysical options available to those who seek to employ this concept. However, to the extent that these options are relevant to answering moral questions, I am skeptical about the prospects of finding a value-neutral way to choose between them.

Dispositions

The following is a fairly common philosophical characterization of a disposition: A fragile glass will shatter if you strike it hard enough. Fragility is the glass's *disposition*, shattering is the *manifestation* of the disposition, and being struck is the *circumstance of manifestation*. The underlying cause of the glass's shattering constitutes the *causal basis* of the glass's fragility. The glass can remain fragile even if it never shatters. One can say of the fragile glass, with certain qualifications, that if it were struck, it would shatter. This characterization suggests certain "marks of dispositionality," according to which a property is a disposition if it meets the following conditions:

1. has a characteristic manifestation;
2. is such that certain circumstances can trigger that manifestation;
3. can be possessed without the manifestation occurring;
4. is instantiated by things of which a counterfactual of the form "if it were subject to the circumstances, it would exhibit the manifestation" is generally true; and
5. can be accurately characterized with an expression of the form "the disposition to produce the manifestation in the circumstances." (McKitrick 2003, 156)

I take it that these conditions are jointly sufficient for dispositionality, but I am not committed to their being individually necessary.

Dispositional terms and concepts are ubiquitous in human languages and conceptual schemes. This stands to reason, as humans frequently have pressing reasons to be concerned about predicting what things will do in various circumstances. It is important to know what is poisonous and what is nutritious, which animals are aggressive, and which situations are dangerous. As we investigate the natural world, we characterize substances as soluble, conductive, explosive, corrosive, and so on. We are interested to predict the behavior of our fellow human beings, and so describe them as *friendly, hostile, irritable, shy, ambitious, trustworthy,* and so on. Disposition ascriptions are the primary means of communicating our understanding of the causal structure of every aspect of our world.

Various accounts of dispositions have been offered. According to some accounts, to ascribe a disposition to something is tantamount to asserting a certain counterfactual conditional. For example, "x is fragile" is said to be true if and only if a counterfactual such as "if x were dropped, x would break" is true (Gundersen 2002; Choi 2006). According to other accounts, dispositions are second-order properties, and to have a disposition is to have some causal basis that would have a certain effect in certain circumstances (Johnston 1992). Another approach is to equate dispositions with fundamental, irreducible powers (Molnar 2003). While such powers cannot be analyzed in terms of anything more basic, proponents of such views argue, contrary to Hume, that it is a concept we acquire by experience that we can characterize roughly as outlined above. In this essay I do not take a stand on which account of dispositions is correct, other than to cast doubt on counterfactual analyses.

Problems for Counterfactual Accounts of Dispositions

Some philosophers claim that simple conditional analyses of dispositions have been conclusively refuted by a number of counterexamples (Martin 1994; Johnston 1992; Lewis 1997). One initial problem for a counterfactual analysis is trying to accurately specify the appropriate counterfactual. A few moments of reflection is enough to realize that "if you drop it, it will break" is a woefully inadequate and overly simplistic analysis of fragility. Such a counterfactual will not be true of a fragile glass if you drop it a fraction of an inch, drop it on to a fluffy cushion, or drop it in a low gravity environment. Dropping is not even necessary for a fragile glass to break— you can strike it where it sits. But if you strike it softly with a feather, it will not break. However, a very powerful blow could break even nonfragile things. In order to state a counterfactual that is true of a thing if and only if it is fragile, you would have to figure out the precise conditions under which fragile and only fragile things break—no easy task.

Even if you figure out the right counterfactual, a counterfactual analysis is still challenged by a number of counterexamples. One such counterexample is "masking," which challenges the necessity of the analysis (Johnston 1992). Imagine a fragile glass that is packed with internal supports to prevent the glass from warping and therefore from shattering when struck. If you struck the packed glass, it would not shatter. The ascription of the disposition is true (the glass is fragile) but the counterfactual claim is false.

A counterexample to the sufficiency of a conditional analysis of dispositions is the case of so-called "mimics" (Smith 1977). A mimic is something that lacks a certain disposition but, for idiosyncratic reasons, acts as if it does. Odd circumstances result in a certain counterfactual being true of something that nevertheless fails to instantiate the requisite disposition. For example, suppose that a wooden block is brought to Neptune and that something about the strange atmosphere results in the block shattering when it is dropped. The counterfactual "if you had dropped it, it would have broken" is true of the block, but intuitively, the block is not fragile.

Another purported counterexample to the conditional analysis is the case of "finkish" dispositions (Martin 1994; Lewis 1997). Once we note that things can acquire or lose dispositions, we can generate counterexamples to a conditional analysis by supposing that dispositional changes occur at inopportune times and ways. An example of a finkish disposition is the fragility of a glass protected by a wizard who will immediately render it nonfragile if it is ever struck. A less fantastical example of a finkish disposition is the instability of the DNA molecule. DNA is susceptible to breaking up due to certain forces, such as radiation and heat. However, forces which would break the molecule also trigger mechanisms within the cell nucleus that maintain the molecule's structure (Tornaletti and Pfeiffer 1996). An object has a *finkish disposition* if that object has a disposition that it loses in what would otherwise be the circumstances of manifestation. Consider the following conditional analysis:

(A) *x* is disposed to exhibit manifestation *M* in circumstance *C* iff
(B) if *x* were to be subject to *C*, *x* would exhibit *M*.

If the disposition *D* is finkish, the same *C* that would cause *x* to exhibit *M* instead causes *x* to lose *D* before it can exhibit *M*. In this case, (A) is true: *x* does have the disposition. But (B) is false: If *x* were subject to *C*, it would not exhibit *M*. So, the analysis fails to state a necessary condition for *x*'s having a disposition.

A similar type of counterexample is called "altering" (Johnston 1992). A glass swan is fragile, but a vigilant monitor equipped with a laser beam will rapidly melt the swan the moment it is struck. The conditional is false, but the swan is fragile. Another example is the shy but intuitive chameleon (Johnston 1992). A chameleon is green and thus disposed to look green, but before anyone can turn on the light and look at it, it blushes red. In both these cases, the conditions of manifestation are such that, if they were realized, the object would "alter" and lose its disposition.

A thing can also finkishly lack a disposition. When green, the chameleon does not have the disposition to appear red, but when the circumstances of manifestation occur, it acquires that disposition. In this case, an object *x* that does not have disposition *D* gains *D* when exposed to circumstance *C*, and subsequently exhibits manifestation *M*. Arguably, (A) is false: *x* does not have the disposition. However, (B) is true: if *x* were to be subject to *C*, *x* would exhibit *M*. This shows that the analysis fails to state a sufficient condition for *x*'s having a disposition.

Masks, mimics, finks, and many other clever counterexamples that may be devised suggest that analyzing a disposition ascription in terms of a counterfactual statement will always be fraught with difficulties. More sophisticated counterfactual accounts have been suggested, the prospects of which are an ongoing source of debate (Lewis 1997; Choi 2006).

Marks of Dispositionality as an Alternative?

Note that the fourth mark of dispositionality mentions counterfactuals but is carefully hedged. I claim that if a property is a disposition, then it is instantiated by things of which a counterfactual of the form "if it is subject to the circumstances, it exhibits the manifestation" is *generally true*, allowing for exceptions. That is to say, a thing might have the disposition in question even if the relevant counterfactual is not true of it. For example, "if you drop it, it will break" is not true of the carefully packed glass, but nevertheless, the glass is still fragile. Furthermore, it is not claimed that even this general truth of the counterfactual is necessary or sufficient for a property to be a disposition. Marks of dispositionality provide evidence that a property is a disposition, but do not constitute a reductive analysis of disposition ascriptions.

Since the marks of dispositionality are like rules of thumb, not necessary and sufficient conditions, there are limitations to the work that they can do. If a property bears most of the marks, I claim that that is some evidence that the property in question is a disposition. As an example of a disposition that lacks one of the marks, I suggest stability. Stability has most of the marks of dispositionality; however, it is not a property that can be possessed without being manifest—a structure that is not manifesting stability is not stable. Others argue that dispositions like radioactivity lack stimulus conditions (Vetter 2010). Like other rules of thumb, the marks of dispositionality are not decisive and will occasionally fail to deliver a conclusive verdict on particular problematic cases, where some of the marks are evident but others are missing or in question. This may be worrisome if the cases that interest us most in the bioethical context are borderline cases, where it is not clear whether a potentiality is present.

However, the marks of dispositionality are, I claim, still useful for deciding whether a general property is a dispositional property. This is the use that I put them to in this chapter, to argue that potentialities are dispositions. Note that the marks of dispositionality apply to property types, while the masking, mimicking, and finking cases feature particular property tokens. While there may be particular tokens or instantiations of a dispositional property that are finked or masked, that does not show that the general property does not bear the marks. So, even though a particular glass swan may be finkishly fragile, or have its fragility masked by careful packing, the general property *fragility* still (1) has a characteristic manifestation—breaking; (2) is such that certain impacts can trigger that manifestation; (3) can be possessed without breaking; (4) is instantiated by things of which a counterfactual of the form "if it were struck, it would break" is generally true; and (5) can be accurately characterized with an expression of the form "the disposition to break when struck." If a property was never instantiated by anything of which the relevant counterfactual were true, that would not be a clear case of a dispositional property.

So, the marks of dispositionality primarily show that a general property is a disposition, not whether a certain object tokens a particular disposition. Other accounts may be more helpful in this regard. Proponents of powers defend the view that perception can determine when and where a power is instantiated (Mumford and Anjum 2011). A second-order property account (Johnston 1992) helps to determine that something has a disposition, given that one can determine that something has a causal basis that would produce a certain effect in certain circumstances. A counterfactual analysis of dispositions (Gundersen 2002) offers a decision procedure, assuming one can determine which counterfactuals are true of an object. However, the many counterexamples to the counterfactual analysis show that the verdicts of that decision procedure are often counterintuitive: our judgments about what counterfactuals are true of an object are not decisive with respect to determining what dispositions the object has.

Extrinsic Dispositions

It is a common assumption that dispositions are intrinsic (Lewis 1997; Johnston 1992; Molnar 2003). If a property is intrinsic, then whether something has that property does not depend on how things are with anything else, but only depends on how the thing is, in itself. If a property is *extrinsic*, then whether a thing has that property *does* depend on how things are with something other than itself. The following is an intuitive test for extrinsicness (though not reductive analysis): If F is an extrinsic property of x, then it is possible that x could be not-F without changing intrinsically, and possibly, a perfect duplicate of x is not-F.

Intuitively, when two qualitatively identical glasses roll off an assembly line, they are equally fragile, reflective, thermally conductive, and alike in any other disposition they may have. However, as I have argued elsewhere, some dispositions are not intrinsic to the objects that have them (McKitrick 2003). Perfect duplicates could differ with respect to having certain dispositions; a thing can lose or acquire dispositions without changing intrinsically. Weight may be dispositional, but it is not intrinsic. The weight of an object is relative to the object's gravitational field. Such extrinsic dispositions present yet another challenge for counterfactual analyses. On a counterfactual analysis, weight could be defined as follows:

> An object weighs 100 pounds, that is, has a disposition to yield a reading of 100 pounds in circumstances of sitting on a standard scale; if it were sitting on a standard scale, then the scale would exhibit a reading of 100 pounds.

However, if the object were on the moon, sitting on the scale would not cause a 100-pound reading. One might object that being subject to a certain gravitational field is part of the circumstances of manifestation of weighing 100 pounds. However, this is not in accord with the meaning of *weight*, if ordinary usage is any guide. It is meaningful to ask what you might weigh on Mars or the moon (Exploratorium

1997). If the circumstances of manifestation of your weight included being in the Earth's gravitational field, there would be no cause to wonder what you weigh on the moon.

Other examples of extrinsic dispositions include vulnerability, visibility, recognizability, and marketability. Generally, when a certain counterfactual is true of something in some environments but not others, there is prima facie reason to think that that thing has a certain extrinsic disposition. If a property P (a) bears the marks of dispositionality and (b) is such that an object can have P while its perfect duplicate does not, then there is reason to think that P is an extrinsic disposition.

Potentiality

The paradigm examples of potentiality claims in the context of this volume are statements such as: An embryo is potentially a person, or is potentially capable of rationality and agency; a patient has (or lacks) the potential to regain consciousness, or recover life-sustaining bodily functions. Similarly, a caterpillar is potentially a butterfly, an acorn is potentially an oak tree, and some students have the potential to be philosophers.[1]

In general, it seems that when one says "x is potentially F," "F" refers to either (a) a property that x can have, or (b) a class or kind of which x can be a member. The occurrence or state of affairs, "x being F," is the actualization of x's potential to be F. One way for a thing to become a member of a kind is by acquiring certain properties that are characteristic of that kind. In that case, the two ways of being potentially F (where F is either [a] a property that one can have, or [b] a kind of which one can be a member) come to essentially the same thing (slightly complicated by the fact that kind membership may require having more than one simple property).

Another way one might become a member of a class is in virtue of decisions about group membership. This suggests that the possibility of future inclusion in a class would give one the potential to be a member of that class. For example, some astronomical body might potentially be a planet, or a college student might potentially be a sorority sister. These potentialities (if indeed they are potentialities) may seem to be different than the potentialities medical ethicists talk about. Arguably, the potentialities of an acorn or an embryo to develop involve intrinsic change of the individual with the potential, while the astronomical body or the student could become a member of the requisite class without developing or undergoing any intrinsic change. But, as I will later suggest, this might be a way in which some potentialities are extrinsic.

Another common use of the term *potentiality* that we should keep in mind is what might be called *epistemic potentiality*. When you think there is some chance that something has a certain property, you might say that it "potentially" has that property. For example, suppose your perfectly healthy friend, John, is in the next room and you are not sure whether he is asleep or awake. You might express your judgment about John by saying "John is potentially awake." Presumably, you are not making a claim that you would take for granted, that John, who is now sleeping, has the potential to be awake in the future. Rather, you are saying that, as far as you know, John is awake right now.

This sense of potentiality would seem to have little to do with the relevant potentialities of an embryo or a patient. However, it may be important to keep it in mind, lest we confuse our uncertainty as to whether something already has a certain property with the judgment that it could possibly acquire that property in the future. Perhaps this conflation is going on in Noonan's "An Almost Absolute Value in History," where he compares aborting a fetus with a hunter shooting into some bushes where a fellow hunter might be (Noonan 1970). In both cases, you could say "there is a potential person there." However, in the case of the hunter, the potentiality is epistemic, whereas in the case of the fetus, arguably on the most plausible interpretation of the claim "there is a potential person there," the potentiality is metaphysical (or at least not merely epistemic).

Potentiality as a (Type of) Disposition

Potentiality-talk and dispositions-talk seem virtually interchangeable. When x is potentially F, one can say that x is *disposed* to be F, where "being F" is the manifestation of x's disposition. Disposition ascriptions can likewise be put in terms of potentiality: If the bomb is explosive, it has the potential to explode; the fragile glass has the potential to break. Granted, potentiality-talk and dispositions-talk are not perfectly interchangeable. It might be the case that an oak tree is potentially a table, but that is not to say that it is disposed to be a table. And you might have the potential to be a drug dealer, even if you would not say that you are disposed to be a drug dealer. Many disposition ascriptions in ordinary language suggest a stronger tendency, a higher probability of the manifestation occurring, than do the analogous potentiality ascriptions.

However, such observations are consistent with potentialities being dispositions nevertheless. The ordinary-language connotation of disposition claims, that the manifestation has a high probability of occurring, is defeasible; some particular instantiations of dispositions are unlikely to manifest. Furthermore, it is a misnomer to talk of "the" disposition to so-and-so. Two different dispositions could have the same manifestation, but not be the same disposition. For example, being shy and being passive-aggressive can both manifest in anti-social behavior, yet they are different behavioral dispositions. So, there are some cases where the expressions "the potential to be *F*" and "the disposition to be *F*" pick out different properties, both of which are dispositions. Admittedly, this has a somewhat counter-intuitive implication that, for some property F, the potential to be F is a disposition that is not commonly called "the disposition to be F."

Though the imperfect interchangeability of dispositions-talk and potentiality-talk is suggestive, a better way to gauge whether potentialities are dispositions is to consider whether they bear the marks of dispositionality. Consider an embryo's potential for rationality: (1) It has a manifestation—being rational; (2) this manifestation will occur given certain, albeit very complicated to specify, circumstances of a favorable environment, nurturance, and so on; (3) an embryo can possess the potential to be rational without being rational; (4) a certain counterfactual is, other things being equal, true of the embryo (if a certain favorable environment and nurturance were to obtain, the embryo would become rational); and (5) it is not inappropriate to call the potential for rationality "the disposition to become rational." It is also worth noting that, like many dispositions, potentialities seem to have causal bases. An embryo's potential to be rational is not a brute, fundamental feature, but is presumably based on its genetic code and other biological factors, intrinsic as well as (possibly) extrinsic.

There is a slight complication with respect to the expression "the potential to be rational": It is ambiguous between the disposition to *engage* in rational behavior, and the disposition to *be capable of* rational behavior. On the second reading, "being rational" is itself a capability, that is, a disposition, its manifestation being, very roughly, rational behavior. You can say of someone, while he is sleeping, that he is a rational person, though clearly he is not exhibiting any rational behavior. On that second reading, the potential to be rational is what you might call a second-order disposition—a disposition to acquire a disposition. So, while both a fetus and a normal sleeping adult human can both be said to have the potential to be rational, I take it that the adult has the first-order disposition for rational behavior, whereas the fetus has the second-order disposition to acquire the disposition for rational behavior. The same could be said about the potentiality for agency, for one does not have to be currently exercising one's agency in order to be "an agent." Likewise, an oak tree is photosynthetic at night as well as during the day, which suggests that being photosynthetic is a matter of being disposed to photosynthesize in the right circumstances, and that an acorn's potential for being photosynthetic is a second-order disposition to acquire the disposition to photosynthesize.

So, a potentiality can be a disposition to acquire a disposition. What about its locus of manifestation? Given that the manifestation of *x*'s potential to be *F* is "*x* being *F*," it may seem as though the manifestation of *x*'s potentiality must occur where *x* is. When *x* manifests *x*'s potential to be rational, "being rational" happens where *x* is. This is not true of dispositions in general. A thing can be disposed to have an effect on something else: roses are disposed to smell sweet, provocative capes make bulls charge, and soporific lullabies put babies to sleep. In those cases, the locus of manifestation is not where the disposed object is.

However, the manifestation of potentialities can occur elsewhere as well. For example, when one has the potential to *do* something, such as score a goal, the effect that one has might not be where one is. Also, if someone has a potential to instantiate a disposition, the manifestation of that disposition may occur somewhere other than the location of the object that had the potential. For example, some people have the potential to be dangerous, funny, or annoying. When someone manifests being dangerous, funny, or annoying, it is often someone else that is hurt, laughing, or annoyed. One might argue that, while the manifestation of being funny is someone else laughing, the manifestation of "the *potential* to be funny" is "the person who had potential to be funny being funny" (and likewise for the other cases). So, the locus of manifestation is with the individual who had the potential. But, if the person does not count as being funny unless other people are laughing, then it is not clear that the locus of manifestation is with the person with the potential after all. Having the potential to instantiate a relational property is a similar sort of case. Consider the potential to be president of the United States. When that potentiality is actualized, it is the person who had the potential who now has the property of being the president of the United States. However, since having that property depends on complicated historical and social relations that go beyond the bounds of the individual, it is not clear that the locus of the manifestation is with the individual who had the potential. Rather than talk about the locus of manifestation being where the potentiated individual is, perhaps it is better to stick with the claim that the manifestation is a matter of the potentiated individual instantiating a certain property, where that property may be intrinsic, extrinsic, or relational.

As mentioned, potentialities, like dispositions, can be possessed without manifesting. But can they be possessed *while* manifesting? When a disposition manifests, the disposed object may or may not continue to instantiate the disposition. Sometimes, a thing loses a disposition when it manifests it, or even ceases to exist. The bomb is no longer explosive after it explodes. The match is no longer flammable once it has been lit. However, elastic bands are still elastic when stretched. Magnets are still magnetic even when they are manifesting their magnetism. What about potentialities? Does a person have the potential to be a person? Does a healthy person have the potential to breathe? Perhaps saying that *x* is potentially *F* is not equivalent to saying that it is possible *x* will be *F* in the future. There is no tension between saying that *x* is *F*, and that it is possible that *x* will be *F* in the future. But there does seem to be a tension between saying that x is F and x is potentially F. This suggests that when potentialities have been and continue to be actualized, it is often no longer appropriate to say that they are possessed. However, there are exceptions. Someone may have the potential to grow and the potential to learn, realize those potentialities, and yet still have the potential for further growth and learning. So, it is false to say that a potentiality is never both actualized and possessed. Sometimes, saying that an F is potentially F is misleading and inappropriate, but perhaps it is not false.

For all these reasons, I suggest that a potentiality is a type of disposition. Typically, potentialities are dispositions whose manifestation occurs where the disposed individual is, whose manifestation is a matter of the disposed individual acquiring a property, possibly another dispositional property, and/or becoming a member of a kind, and arguably potentialities often cease to be instantiated once they are manifest. However, manifestations of dispositions also involve things acquiring properties. And since there are potentialities whose manifestation does not happen where the potentiated individual is, or where a thing manifests a potential and still has it, potentialities do not seem to have any essential characteristics that distinguish them from dispositions. So perhaps potentialities just are dispositions.

Counterfactual Analysis of Potentiality

Masks, mimics, and finks were problematic for accounts of dispositions insofar as those accounts analyzed disposition ascriptions in terms of counterfactual conditionals. If these cases are also problems for an account of potentiality, that account must likewise analyze potentiality ascriptions in terms of counterfactuals. Such an account may look something like this:

(A) x has the potential to be F in circumstance C iff
(B) if x were in C, x would become F.

It would be too quick to dismiss this proposal based on the observation that an embryo has the potential to be rational, but if you put an embryo in a womb, it will not immediately become rational. The circumstances of manifestation of the potentiality for rationality are not merely being placed in a womb. To make the account more plausible, we can stipulate that circumstance C has a duration and is dynamic over the course of that duration, providing all that is necessary at each stage of x's development into an F.

Nevertheless, it would still be difficult, if not impossible, to specify in detail the circumstances of manifestation for the kinds of potentialities we are interested in. Recall the difficulty in specifying the conditions under which *fragility* manifests!

If the view is that something has a certain potential if and only if a certain counter-factual is true, then it is fair to expect to be told what that counterfactual statement is. But, in order to say what that counterfactual statement is, one would have to articulate the precise conditions which are sufficient for a thing to realize its potential. It would be inadvisable to make them too precise, lest you deny that potentiality to other things which may aptly be said to have it. Moreover, even if one were able to devise such a counterfactual, the analysis would still be stymied by masks, mimics, and finks, which suggests that a counterfactual analysis of potentiality is not going to be much help in dealing with problematic cases.

Surely, a thing's potential can be masked. An acorn could be placed in fertile soil, but if it were coated in hard plastic, the seed could not break through and grow. In that case, the seed might still have the potential to become an oak tree, but the associated counterfactual is false. The general problem is that, even if the specification of the circumstances of manifestation articulates all that must be present in order for the thing to realize its potential, the specification cannot rule out all of the possible factors which may interfere. To add to the analysis "and nothing interferes" would trivialize it. It would be a matter of explicating "x has the potential to be F" as "x will become F, unless it doesn't."

Interestingly, some of the most talked-about counterexamples to the moral relevance of potentiality appear to be variations on mimicking cases. Consider "super-kitten," a kitten that intuitively does not have the potential to be a person but is injected with a special serum that turns it into something with the characteristics of a person (Tooley 1972). A kitten receiving such extraordinary treatment is perhaps analogous to a wooden block being taken to Neptune, in the sense that, in both cases, unusual circumstances result in unusual behavior, and this challenges our application of concepts in normal circumstances. In effect, the kitten could exhibit the manifestation of the potentiality for personhood without having that potential at the outset. In that case, the potentiality ascription is false, but some associated counterfactual turns out to be true.

A potentiality could also be finkish. Consider again an acorn with the potential to become an oak tree. The circumstances of manifestation of that potentiality include dropping onto fertile soil. But suppose the gardener does not want any more oak trees in the yard, so he collects and crushes any acorn that drops. The circumstances that would normally result in an acorn manifesting its potential lead to its destruction. If the acorn has the potential to be an oak tree, that is a case in which the potentiality claim is true, but the associated counterfactual is false.

Something could finkishly lack a disposition as well. If some cloning or nano-technology could turn something nonhuman into a human fetus, and if that procedure is initiated only if that something is placed in a uterus, then that thing would, at the outset, lack the potential to be a human being. However, if it gets placed in the circumstances of manifestation, it would acquire that potential. Again, at the outset, the potentiality claim would be false, but the associated counterfactual would be true. I suppose the super-kitten could be recast as something that finkishly lacks the potential to be a person, if those who would provide the transformative agent would do so only on the condition that the kitten gets adopted by a family that intends to raise it as a human child, teaching it to speak and so on. It would be true of the kitten "if it is nurtured and educated, it will become a person," even though, at the outset, it lacks the potential to become a person.

It is not surprising that a counterfactual analysis of potentialities would be subject to the same difficulties as a counterfactual analysis of dispositions. What is perhaps of greater interest is the possibility that what are presented as counterexamples to the moral relevance of potentialities could be construed as counterexamples to a counterfactual understanding of potentialities. It seems to be open to the defender of the moral relevance of potentialities to deny that the thing in question has the relevant potentiality, even though a certain counterfactual is true of it. Just because a counterfactual is true of something does not mean that it has the relevant potentiality—it may be a mimic, or it may finkishly lack that potential. So, on what basis do we attribute potentialities to things? The defender of morally relevant potentialities may look to causal bases (Lewis 1997). One may argue that, in order for something to have the same potential as a human embryo, it must also have the causal basis for that potential. This would help explain why we say that something retains its potential even when the associated counterfactual is not true of it, as when that potential is masked or finked. In those cases, the thing in question still has the causal basis of that potential. It would also explain tendencies to deny the potentiality claim even when the counterfactual is true, if the thing in question lacks the causal basis for that potentiality.

Suppose you have two duplicate acorns, the first of which will sprout if you place it in fertile soil, and the second of which will be picked up by the gardener if you place it in fertile soil. Even though the counterfactual "if you place it in fertile soil, it will sprout" is not true of both acorns, you may be tempted to say that, because they are perfect duplicates, they have the same potentiality, regardless of their differing with respect to the truth value of the relevant counterfactual. If you do say that, perhaps you are thinking that since the acorns are intrinsic duplicates, they must have the same causal basis for the potential to sprout, and therefore they must both have the same potential to sprout. However, note that you would be assuming that perfect duplicates must have the same potentialities—that potentialities are intrinsic. But given the possibility of extrinsic dispositions, this assumption is open to doubt.

Extrinsic Potentialities

When determining whether a disposition or potentiality is extrinsic, it is important to distinguish "circumstances of manifestation" from "circumstances of possession." Recall that the circumstances of manifestation of a disposition are those factors that trigger a disposition to manifest. In the case of fragility, the circumstances of manifestation were, roughly, dropping or striking. However, the circumstances of possession are whatever makes it true that the thing in question has the disposition. And since a disposition can be possessed without being manifest (an unbroken glass can be fragile), then the circumstances of possession can obtain while the circumstances of manifestation do not. If the circumstances of manifestation do not obtain, a thing can still have a potentiality without actualizing it. But if the circumstances of possession do not obtain, the thing does not have the potentiality at all. Having extrinsic circumstances of manifestation does not make a disposition extrinsic, and does not make potentialities extrinsic either. A fragile glass typically needs a strike from something extrinsic to it in order to break, yet that does not make the fragility extrinsic. A perfect duplicate in any circumstance may still be equally fragile. Likewise, an embryo needs many external factors in order to manifest its potential to become rational. By parity of reasoning, that fact alone does not show that the embryo's potential is extrinsic.

In order for a fetus to be potentially rational or be disposed to become rational, there must be circumstances in which it would become rational. But in what sense is it the case that "there are" such circumstances? Since it is possible to possess this potential without manifesting it, it cannot be the case that these circumstances must actually obtain for the particular embryo to be potentially rational. However, saying that there are such circumstances, as long as such circumstances are logically or metaphysically possible, would allow too many things to count as potentially rational. Even given a metaphysically possible scenario in which rocks are turned into rational beings, we want to say embryos are potentially rational in the actual world while rocks are not. So, the circumstances which enable an embryo to become rational must be at least physically possible. We might want to place more restrictions on the range of possible circumstances and say that they must not only be possible in this world, but that circumstances of this kind are instantiated at some point in this world. Even further restrictions would be needed if, for example, one wants to say that an embryo is potentially rational while an ovum is not, since there is a commonly occurring physically possible causal process that leads from the ovum to a rational being.[2]

These decisions about which possible circumstances are going to count as circumstances of manifestation for a potentiality have implications for whether the potentiality is extrinsic or intrinsic. As with looking for examples of extrinsic dispositions, the strategy for finding cases of extrinsic potentialities is to consider perfect intrinsic duplicates and see if they could differ with respect to their potentialities. This fits well with the moral principle that we should treat like cases alike. Perhaps, if two individuals have the same potentiality, there is reason to treat them both alike. Consequently, an argument for the moral conclusion that it is permissible to treat two individuals differently might do well to challenge the assumption that they have the same potentiality, even if they are intrinsically alike.

So, consider an acorn with the potential for "treehood" and a perfect duplicate of that acorn in a different world, all by itself. If the duplicate acorn lacks the potential for treehood, then that potential is extrinsic. So, does the lonely duplicate acorn have the potential? If the metaphysical possibility of the circumstances of manifestation was sufficient, then the duplicate acorn must have the potentiality too, and the potentiality turns out to be intrinsic, for it is necessarily shared by perfect duplicates. If the circumstances of manifestation must be somewhere occurring in that world, then the lonely duplicate acorn lacks the potential, and the potentiality must be extrinsic. If the circumstances of manifestation must be physically possible, then the duplicate acorn can still lack the potential for treehood, if it is in a world where the laws of nature would not permit any circumstance which would enable it to develop into a tree. In that case, too, the potentiality would be extrinsic.

However, some philosophers think that the relevant sense in which dispositions are intrinsic is that they are "intrinsic, keeping the laws of nature fixed" (Lewis 1997). A more interesting and relevant case, at any rate, is whether duplicates in the same kinds of worlds or different parts of the same world could differ with respect to a potentiality. Perhaps, if F is an extrinsic property, and one can be disposed to have extrinsic properties, then the disposition to be F will be an extrinsic disposition. For example, since *being popular* is an extrinsic property, the disposition to be popular is an extrinsic disposition. In addition, if something's being F is determined by convention, then the disposition to be F could be an extrinsic disposition. For example, an entertainer might lose her disposition to be shocking in virtue of a change in her audience's sensibilities.

This source of extrinsicality seems even more plausible in the case of potentialities. For example, one can potentially be an uncle, famous, or *Time*'s "Person of the Year"—each of which is partly determined by extrinsic factors. I could lose my potential to become an aunt by all of my siblings dying childless. Recall that when x has the potentiality to be an F, then "F" refers to a class or a kind of which x can become a member. Furthermore, there are at least two ways to become a member of a class or kind. One way is to acquire the properties which are sufficient for membership in that kind. Another way is for the determinants of membership in that class to change. While such classes might not be considered "natural kinds," there are some classes the membership of which is socially determined or determined by convention. Some argue that even so-called natural kinds are determined by convention (Dupre 1981). Consider Eris, an astronomical body beyond Pluto discovered in 2003. At that time, Eris was potentially a planet. Then, in 2006 the criteria for membership in the class of planets were refined by the International Astronomical Union. Now Eris is not potentially a planet. I assume that Eris did not change intrinsically in any relevant way. So, it seems Eris's potentiality for "planethood" was extrinsic. In the case of human beings, an embryo might be potentially a citizen or a voter and could lose potentialities via changes in the political landscape in which she is located.

Sometimes, class membership is determined by the powers that be, by fiat, or any number of decisions procedures, about who or what to include in the class. For example, a beauty contestant is potentially Miss America 2012, but ceases to have that potentiality when she is not chosen to be one of the five finalists. Some social process decides who is included in the class, and if that process determines that one is no longer in contention, one can lose the potential without changing intrinsically. These types of extrinsic potentialities may seem to have little relevance to the types of potentialities the medical ethicist is interested in. But if being a person is more like being a member of a community rather than a biological kind, it is liable to having its membership determined by convention. If the extension of personhood is determined by convention, then the disposition to be a person could be an extrinsic potentiality. Something could gain or lose potential not by changing intrinsically, but by the powers that be determining a different standard of membership. For example, if members of a certain race were to be no longer considered persons, then their unborn children would no longer be considered potential persons (which may be an argument for not allowing arbitrary conventions to determine the category of personhood).

Perhaps there is another way for a potentiality to be extrinsic, keeping the standards of kind membership fixed, as well as the laws of nature. It would be helpful here to consider end of life cases, where one makes claims such as a coma victim is potentially conscious, or a terminal condition is potentially reversible. A patient might not be capable of recovering or becoming conscious, given current medical technology. However, it is possible that some future medical technology could reverse his condition. Do we want to say that the patient currently has the potential to recover? That could be cruelly misleading at best. Perhaps it would be more correct to say that they are not now potentially conscious, but if extrinsic factors were different, they would be. Then the patient's potential for recovery is an extrinsic potentiality. It is plausible that similar considerations apply if the necessary medical technologies exist but are not practically accessible, if they are very far away or prohibitively expensive, for example. Two patients with the same condition could have different potentialities due to the differing circumstances, and this entails that those potentialities are extrinsic.

Do similar considerations apply in beginning of life cases? We can consider cases of perfect duplicate embryos in different circumstances and consider whether they could have different potentialities. For instance, consider an embryo outside of a uterus and its perfect duplicate inside of a uterus. If there are no available means for implanting the embryo into a favorable environment, then by parity of reasoning with the end of life cases, we should say that the embryo lacks the potentialities enjoyed by its duplicate inside of a uterus. Therefore, the embryo's potentiality for rationality is an extrinsic potentiality. But how far can we push this idea that an embryo's potentiality can vary according to extrinsic circumstances? One thing to consider is what counts as "available means" for implanting an embryo. Surely, the medical technology must exist in this case, too. So, if we consider two duplicate frozen embryos, one in a fertility clinic with all the staff and equipment necessary for successful implantation, and the other in a remote location with no such amenities, perhaps we should say that those embryos have different potentialities. And if perfect duplicates can differ with respect to having a certain potentiality, then that potentiality is extrinsic.

However, another factor is necessary for successful implantation—people with the desire and resources to have the embryo implanted. If so, then the potentialities of frozen embryos depend on interests and resources of would-be fertility clinic patients. An egg selected for implantation would have different potentialities than one not selected. If we go that far, we should consider what to say about eggs conceived in other circumstances unfavorable to normal development, such as an ectopic pregnancy. Perhaps such an embryo would have less potential than a duplicate in more favorable circumstances. Another salient unfavorable circumstance for an embryo is to be in the uterus of a woman who does not want to be pregnant. It seems that there a sense in which an unwanted embryo has diminished potential as compared to its perfect duplicate with willing and able parents. If that is true, then that potentiality is extrinsic. But other extrinsic factors might be relevant to potentialities as well. If the availability of means to implant an embryo in a uterus were relevant to its potentialities, then the availability of means to remove an embryo from a uterus should be relevant as well. So, the potentiality of an unwanted embryo in the uterus of a woman with access to abortion services will be less than the potentiality of an embryo in the uterus without access to those services. In that light, debates about the morality of access to abortion would seem to be less about how to respond to the potentialities that embryos antecedently have, as they are about what potentialities we are required to ensure that embryos have.

As we saw when considering problems for counterfactual accounts of potentialities, these considerations about the nature of potentialities suggest different ways to frame disagreements about the moral relevance of potentialities. Rather than disagreeing about whether the potentiality of an unwanted embryo or terminally ill patient is morally relevant, parties to the debate could reconsider whether the embryo or patient actually has, or should have, the potentiality in question. If these potentialities are extrinsic, the fact that the individual is intrinsically like another individual who does have that potentiality is not decisive.

This conclusion seems to be in tension with the response to masks and finks in which attributions of potentialities were made in virtue of whether the thing in question had the appropriate causal basis of that potentiality, regardless of whether it was situated in circumstances in which that potentiality could be actualized. Typically, those who think that causal bases are essential to dispositions are thinking of those causal bases as intrinsic (Lewis 1997). However, an alternative position is that not only can dispositions be extrinsic, but the causal bases of dispositions can be extrinsic too (Nolan 2005). So, the mistake of those who claim that intrinsic duplicates have the same disposition is not that they are only focusing on the causal basis of that disposition, but rather that they are only focusing on *part* of the causal basis of the disposition, and not taking into account the properties extrinsic to the disposed individual that are part of the causal basis of its disposition. In other words, if an embryo's potentiality is extrinsic, then the causal basis of its potentiality does not merely consist of the intrinsic properties of the embryo but also includes properties of its environment.

Conclusion

It seems as though whether potentialities for consciousness, rationality, agency, and so on are intrinsic or extrinsic has potentially (no pun intended) significant moral consequences. If arguments against terminating care rely on individuals having such potentialities, and if these potentialities are extrinsic, then these arguments can be undermined in cases where individuals do not enjoy the extrinsic circumstances of possession of these potentialities. But *are* these potentialities extrinsic? I think there is a case to be made that they are. However, embryos and coma patients have many potentialities, some of them intrinsic, some of them extrinsic. In the case where an individual lacks an extrinsic potentiality because of current circumstances, it will often be true to say that they would have that potentiality if circumstances were different. In other words, even if one lacks the extrinsic potentiality in question, one still has a second-order potentiality, a potentiality to have that potentiality. That second-order potentiality might be intrinsic.[3] Now, which potentialities are morally relevant: the extrinsic potentiality for consciousness, rationality, and agency, or the intrinsic potentiality to acquire those potentialities, or both? I take it that is a moral question which is not settled by the forgoing metaphysical considerations.

I have tried to outline a number of options regarding the nature of potentialities for those who would like that notion to play some role in their theorizing in bioethics, or elsewhere. There still are a number of decisions to make about how to explicate the concept of potentiality that is most relevant for one's purposes. How should one flesh out the associated counterfactuals, regardless of whether they hope to reduce potentiality claims to counterfactual conditionals? How should one circumscribe the relevant possible circumstances of manifestation for a given potentiality? Are the circumstances necessary for the actualization of a given potentiality to be counted circumstances of possession or circumstances of manifestation? Is the kind of which something is potentially a member a natural kind or a class whose membership is determined by convention? My anticipation, and perhaps my worry, is that these questions do not have answers that can be determined independently from the conclusions about the moral relevance of potentiality that a given theorist aims to establish.[4]

NOTES

1. "Potential" also has many uses in physics and other sciences, though comparing how these may be related to the concept at issue would take us too far afield.

2. I am not suggesting that there are good reasons to make such a distinction. If you do, you would have to place further restrictions on what counts as circumstances of manifestation. For an example of the claim that an embryo is a potential person but an ovum is not, see Covey (1991).

3. Complicating matters further, if as discussed earlier rationality is dispositional, the intrinsic potential for acquiring rationality would in fact be third-order: It would be the potential to have the potentiality to have the disposition for rational behavior.

4. Many thanks to John Lizza for inspiration and helpful comments on multiple drafts. Also thanks to Joe Mendola, Harry Ide, and the audience at my presentation of this paper at the University of Nebraska, Department of Philosophy, Faculty-Grad Presentation Series, March 2, 2012.

REFERENCES

Armstrong, D. M. 1996. Dispositions as categorical states. In T. Crane (ed.), *Dispositions: A Debate*, 15–19. New York: Routledge.

Bird, A. 1998. Dispositions and antidotes. *Philosophical Quarterly* 48:227–34.

Choi, S. 2006. The simple vs. reformed conditional analysis of dispositions. *Synthese* 148:369–79.

Covey, E. 1991. Physical possibility and potentiality in ethics. *American Philosophical Quarterly* 28(3):237–44.

Dupre, J. 1981. Natural kinds and biological taxa. *Philosophical Review* 90(1):66–90.

Exploratorium. 1997. Your weight on other worlds. www.exploratorium.edu/ronh/weight/.

Goodman, Nelson. 1983. *Fact, Fiction, and Forecast*. 4th ed. Cambridge: Harvard University Press.

Gundersen, L. 2002. In defense of the conditional account of dispositions. *Synthese* 130:389–411.

Harre, R. 1970. Powers. *British Journal for the Philosophy of Science* 21:81–101.

Johnston, M. 1992. How to speak of the colors. *Philosophical Studies* 68(3):221–63.

Lewis, D. 1997. Finkish dispositions. *Philosophical Quarterly* 47(187):143–58.

Martin, C. B. 1994. Dispositions and conditionals. *Philosophical Quarterly* 44:1–8.

McKitrick, J. 2003. A case for extrinsic dispositions. *Australasian Journal of Philosophy* 81:155–74.

Molnar, G. 2003. *Powers: A Study in Metaphysics*. Oxford: Oxford University Press.

Mumford, S., and Anjum, R. L. 2011. *Getting Causes from Powers*. Oxford: Oxford University Press.

Nolan, D. 2005. *David Lewis*. Durham, NC: Acumen Publishing.

Noonan, J. 1970. An almost absolute value in history. In John Noonan (ed.), *The Morality of Abortion: Legal and Historical Perspectives*, 51–59. Cambridge: Harvard University Press.

Smith, A. D. 1977. Dispositional properties. *Mind* 86:439–45.

Tornaletti, S., and Pfeiffer, G. P. 1996. UV damage and repair mechanisms in mammalian cells. *Bioessays* 18:221–28.

Tooley, M. 1972. Abortion and infanticide. *Philosophy and Public Affairs* 2:37–65.

Vetter, B. 2010. Dispositions without the stimulus. Paper presented at the Dispositions Workshop, Center for the Study of Mind in Nature, Oslo, Norway, March 22–23.

CHAPTER THREE

The Paradoxes of Potentiality

JOEL FEINBERG

Having conceded that rights can belong to beings in virtue of their merely potential interests, we find ourselves on a slippery slope; for it may seem at first sight that anything at all can have potential interests, or much more generally, that anything at all can be potentially almost anything else at all! Dehydrated orange powder is potentially orange juice, since if we add water to it, it will be orange juice. More remotely, however, it is also potentially lemonade, since it will become lemonade if we add a large quantity of lemon juice, sugar, and water. It is also a potentially poisonous brew (add water and arsenic), a potential orange cake (add flour, etc., and bake), a potential orange-colored building block (add cement and harden), and so on, *ad infinitum*. Similarly a two-celled embryo, too small to be seen by the unaided eye, is a potential human being; and so is an unfertilized ovum; and so is even an "uncapacitated" spermatozoan. Add the proper nutrition to an implanted embryo (under certain other necessary conditions) and it becomes a fetus and then a child. Looked at another way, however, the implanted embryo has been combined (under the same conditions) with the nutritive elements, which themselves are converted into a growing fetus and child. Is it then just as proper to say that food is a "potential child" as that an embryo is a potential child? If so, then what isn't a "potential child"? (Organic elements in the air and soil are "potentially food," and hence potentially people!)

Clearly, some sort of line will have to be drawn between direct or proximate potentialities and indirect or remote ones; and however we draw this line, there will be borderline cases whose classification will seem uncertain or even arbitrary. Even though any X can become a Y provided only that it is combined with the necessary additional elements, a, b, c, d, and so forth, we cannot say of any given X that it is a "potential Y" unless certain further—rather strict—conditions are met. (Otherwise the concept of potentiality, being universally and promiscuously applicable, will have no utility.) A number of possible criteria of proximate potentiality suggest themselves. The first is the criterion of causal importance. Orange powder is not properly called a potential building block because of those elements needed to transform it into a building block, the cement (as opposed to any of the qualities of the orange powder) is the causally crucial one. Similarly, any pauper might (misleadingly) be called a "potential millionaire" in the sense that all that need be added to any man to transform him into a millionaire is a great amount of money. The absolutely crucial element in the change, of course, is no quality of the man himself but rather the million dollars "added" to him.

What is causally "important" depends upon our purposes and interests and is therefore to some degree a relativistic matter. If we seek a standard, in turn, of "importance," we may posit such a criterion, for example, as that of the ease or difficulty (to some persons or other) of providing those missing elements which, when combined with the thing at hand, convert it into something else. It does seem quite natural, for example, to say that the orange powder is potentially orange juice, and that is because the missing element is merely common tap water, a substance conveniently near at hand to everyone; whereas it is less plausible to characterize the powder as potential cake since a variety of further elements, and not just one, are required, and some of these are not conveniently near at hand to many. Moreover, the process of combining the missing elements into a cake is rather more complicated than mere "addition." It is less plausible still to call orange powder a potential curbstone for the same kind of reason. The criterion of ease or difficulty of the acquisition and combination of additional elements explains all these variations.

Still another criterion of proximate potentiality closely related to the others is that of degree of deviation required from "the normal course of events." Given the intentions of its producers, distributors, sellers, and consumers, dehydrated orange juice will, in the normal course of events, become orange juice. Similarly, a human embryo securely imbedded in the wall of its mother's uterus will in the normal course of events become a human child. That is to say that if no one deliberately intervenes to prevent it happening, it will, in the vast majority of cases, happen. On the other hand, an unfertilized ovum will not become an embryo unless someone intervenes deliberately to make it happen. Without such intervention in the "normal" course of events, an ovum is a mere bit of protoplasm of very brief life expectancy. If we lived in a world in which virtually every biologically capable human female became pregnant once a year throughout her entire fertile period of life, then we would regard fertilization as something that happens to every ovum in "the natural course of events." Perhaps we would regard every unfertilized ovum, in such a world, as a potential person even possessed of rights corresponding to its future interests. It would perhaps make conceptual if not moral sense in such a world to regard deliberate nonfertilization as a kind of homicide.

It is important to notice, in summary, that words like *important, easy,* and *normal* have sense only in relation to human experiences, purposes, and techniques. As the latter change, so will our notions of what is important, difficult, and usual, and so will the concept of potentiality, or our application of it. If our purposes, understanding, and techniques continue to change in indicated directions, we may even one day come to think of inanimate things as possessed of "potential interests." In any case, we can expect the concept of a right to shift its logical boundaries with changes in our practical experience.

CHAPTER FOUR

Physical Possibility
and Potentiality in Ethics

EDWARD COVEY

I. Problems of Possibility

In recent years, especially since Michael Tooley introduced us to his potential super-kittens,[1] there has been much discussion about the role of potentiality in ethics. This discussion has unfortunately tended to revolve around the issue of abortion, where it is easy to argue that potential personhood is not a sufficient ground for a right to life. However, there are strong reasons to be found in other contexts for at least a *prima facie* thesis that an individual's possibility of development can put us under obligations to that individual. For example, such a thesis might underlie the common judgment that human babies have a right to be educated and brought up into full-fledged moral personhood, *at least if they are allowed to remain alive.* That infants do have such a right might be deniable, but only at a fairly high cost to our well-considered ways of thinking about human rights and duties.[2] I shall not try here to prove that we must acknowledge potentiality as a moral ground in such contexts. Rather, I shall simply take as a motivation for this study the working hypothesis that some sort of potentiality thesis ought to be able to generate judgments in favor of a human right to develop. At the same time, it seems almost obvious that no principle of potentiality in ethics should lead us to conclude that every human reproductive cell has a right to develop into a person, or any of the similar absurdities that critics often claim such principles would entail.

Anyone who wants to defend potentiality as a ground for ethical rights and duties should be able to show that there can be a coherent and well-founded account of the metaphysics of possible becoming which would support that ethical position. My aim here is to explore the concept of possibility as it might be relevant to the ethical contexts of becoming and development, focusing especially on the question of whether a full acknowledgment of the metaphysics of possibility would tend to support or undermine ethical principles of potentiality.

"*X* is potentially a person," it will be generally agreed, is to be understood as, "it is possible that *X* become a person," where "possible" is taken in the sense of "physically possible" rather than "logically possible." Physical, or nomic, possibility is normally analyzed in terms of nomic regularities, or the laws of nature; an event or state of affairs is nomically possible just in case its coming about is in accordance with the laws of nature, given the initial state of affairs that actually obtains in the world. For example, it seems to be nomically possible that a human baby (with a normal brain) should think but nomically impossible that a cactus should think, because the laws of nature are such that cacti cannot develop brains, and only things with brains (or analogous structures) think.

A typical characterization of the concept of physical possibility comes from Nicholas Rescher:

> A consideration of the "laws of nature" is indispensable to any theory of possibility, because laws and dispositions establish a dividing line between the *genuinely* possible (that which is *really* possible) and the *merely* possible (the sphere of purely speculative possibility), serving to separate proximate from remote possibility as it were. This acorn might possibly develop into an oak tree (it might not, too, for it might be eaten by a squirrel). Here we have a real possibility. One might also contemplate the "possibility" that the acorn develop into a pear tree; but this is clearly no *real* possibility—it is a *purely hypothetical* possibility, and a very far-fetched one at that. In the former case, things run in their lawful channel, while the latter case clearly requires us to abrogate or modify the laws of nature. This important amplification of the distinction between *real*, physical or natural possibility, and *strictly hypothetical* (or "merely logical") possibility—the former of which calls for preserving not only logical and conceptual principles, but the laws of nature as well—is one of the fundamental ideas of our subject.[3]

There is, however, an additional distinction to be drawn, not just between nomic and merely logical possibility but this time between what can be called remote and proximate possibility within the nomic category. David Annis appeals to such a distinction in "Abortion and the Potentiality Principle,"[4] where he points out that physical possibility must be analyzed partly in terms of subjunctive conditionals, and that subjunctives are not transitive. This is used to block the *reductio* argument which says that if potential personhood entails rights to development or to life, then every human sperm and every human egg has such rights. It is true that a human egg has the potential to become a zygote; *if* it were to be penetrated by a sperm a zygote *would* come about. It is also true that a zygote is a potential person (at least according to the view discussed by Annis); if the zygote were to develop long enough it *would* become a person. From the two propositions, "if the *egg* were fertilized it would become a *zygote*," and "if the *zygote* were allowed to develop it would become a *person*," it does not follow that if the egg were fertilized that egg would become a person, and therefore it does not follow that the egg is a potential person in any relevant sense of "potential." Its possibility of becoming a person is remote in the sense that the end state in question is not directly accessible (as a real possibility) from the initial state.

Although the general guidelines for the application of this sort of argument prove to be quite problematic, it is significant for many cases of what might be generically characterized as potential personhood (and other sorts of potential); if the intransitivity argument is correct, this removes *part* of the case against potential personhood as a ground for moral significance. Cells that could be cloned surely are only *remotely* potential persons, as are all of the millions of nonhuman reproductive cells that might be genetically engineered to develop humanlike capacities, so it should not follow that all of these things have rights of development.

It will be appropriate at this point to clarify that this sort of argument, along with those that follow, is important for this project for two reasons. (1) As I have suggested already, in fairness to potentiality theories, it is necessary to see whether not just anything that could in some sense become something morally significant has the real possibility of doing so in a morally significant sense. (2) Potentiality is most often discussed as a sufficient condition for moral consideration, but the potential to develop in a certain way is always a trivially *necessary* condition for any right of *becoming*, at least for any such right to be in any way applicable. Therefore, it is essential to have a clear account of the limits of possible becoming, no matter what the grounds for such a right might be.

Surely the sort of distinction drawn by Annis is correct in essence, and there are clear-cut cases in which it is applicable. The guidelines for applying it in general, though, are, of course, far from clear. Suppose that someone were to say, "A ten-year-old child is potentially a teenager, a teenager is potentially an adult, so a ten-year-old is only remotely potentially an adult," or, "The car door could be opened, and if it were opened you could get inside, so it is only remotely possible for you to get into the car," for it is always possible in such cases to find a subjunctive conditional which from the original state of affairs would take the envisaged transition only part of the way.

In all cases of this sort, we are faced with statements of the following types: (1) "The F would become a G if condition C_1 were to obtain, and the G would become an H if C_2 were to obtain," and (2) "The F would become an H if C_1 and C_2 were to obtain." The problem is in determining in which sorts of cases (2) is true not simply as an expression of (1) (though 1 might still be true), and in which cases (2) is true only in the sense that it is equivalent to saying that (1) is true. The case of the ten-year-old's development and the case of entering the car seem clearly to be of the former type.

It might be suggested that our only guidelines for the distinction are to be found in the continuity or discontinuity of the process leading from the initial state to the envisaged possible end state, and in the similarity or dissimilarity of the individual in the initial state to the individual in the possible end state. Remoteness or nearness of nomic possibility (or *N*-possibility, as I shall call it hereafter for convenience) would then be to some extent a matter of degree, with grey or fuzzy areas between the clear extremes. For example, the reason that transitivity fails from egg or sperm to person is because between egg and zygote there is a radical transformation of kind and form and function. Between zygote and person there is also such an extreme transformation, so that while the first change is great, but still, as it were, accessible from the initial state, the end state is discontinuous and dissimilar enough with the initial state only to be accessible from the intermediate state. Surely this would also apply to many of the other sorts of things that might be hypothetically thought potential persons: individual body cells, nonhuman germ cells, perhaps Tooley's potential-person-kittens. With respect to the latter, it would be easy to tentatively concede that they are analogous to early stages of human development, and if there is a grey area between remote and proximate potentiality, both those kittens and human fetuses would seem to be in that grey area through some part of their development. If remoteness of potentiality is a concept of this sort, analogous to geographical remoteness, there is much room for dispute about just how much remoteness is necessary for true inaccessibility between possible transitions.

Some philosophers draw a similar distinction between (mere) potentiality and (actual) capacity.[5] An adult comatose patient has the *capacity* for personhood, which is currently unfulfilled, while a fetus or even an infant may be thought to have merely the *potential* for personhood. In essence, this is an application of the same general kind of reasoning that is involved in the distinction between remote and proximate potentiality but often with differing judgments about what is *proximate enough* to count as genuine *capacity* rather than mere potential. In the form that would judge that all who have not yet actually become full-fledged competent persons lack the true capacity for personhood (and therefore do not have a right to develop it), this is to be tentatively rejected, since it is inconsistent with my proposed working hypothesis that infants have a right to be raised to become genuine persons.

I am not persuaded that there are potentialities which are genuinely remote in this sense except in cases where a possible change would entail a loss of identity. In such cases, the potential end state would be metaphysically inaccessible *to the initial individual*. For example, a cow is "potentially" a collection of steaks and hamburgers, which, if eaten, will "become" a collection of human cells and excreted waste matter, but surely by the time this transformation has taken place the cow would no longer exist. I would argue that this is the case with the obvious examples of remote potential which I have mentioned. Transitivity fails between the egg's possibility of becoming a zygote and the zygote's becoming a person because by the time that the person has developed, the egg has been superseded (at some perhaps indeterminate stage) by a subsequent individual. Person and egg are not identical.

It might be thought that distinctions of the preceding sort between proximate and remote potentiality also rest on a genuine metaphysical failure of transitivity across iterated possibilities. That is, it seems that iterations of physical possibilities do not reduce to a single possibility, as do logical possibilities in the S4 and S5 systems, where it is a thesis that $\Diamond\Diamond p$ iff $\Diamond p$. For example, if Melissa has removed the carburetor from Stan's car, he cannot drive the car today. Although in a sense she could reinstall the carburetor today without violating any of the laws of nature, she will not reinstall it until tomorrow. From the fact that it is *possible* for the carburetor to be back on the car today, and that with the carburetor installed it is possible to drive the car, it does not follow that it is possible for Stan to drive his car today.

In practice, we are rarely concerned with finding out whether a hypothetical state of affairs is *simply* N-possible or N-impossible without a context. Certainly all judgments of N-possibility are to be made with reference to the actual world and actual states of affairs, and the question to be asked is: would it be in accordance with the laws of nature for the actual state of affairs to be superseded by the state whose possibility is in question? In regard to the as-yet-unactualized possible, its becoming actual depends in most cases on other conditions which do not yet obtain, and which, in fact, may be purely counterfactual. To say, for example, that an infant is a potential autonomous agent is to assume that all of the nurture and training that are necessary for that transition are genuinely possible. In contexts such as this, where the hypothetical end state is possible only through the obtaining of various other nonactual events and states, there are in principle two sorts of answers that could be given to every question regarding the possibility of the end state: (1) it is impossible because the necessary conditions for it are not actually met (i.e., it is possibly possible, but not possible), or (2) it is possible because the necessary (and jointly sufficient) conditions for it are possible. I want to argue, though, that this apparent dichotomy rests on an ambiguity in the concept of N-possibility.

Here I would like to introduce yet another distinction between notions of nomic possibility. While we are often concerned with the true accessibility of possibilities from the actual world, given both its laws and its existent individuals and states of affairs, this is not always the case. We also make conjectures about what might be nomically possible in a less restricted sense, but one that is still short of the lawlessness of logical possibility. I shall say, then, that:

1. A hypothetical event or state of affairs, s, is *absolutely N-impossible* iff. s would be inconsistent with the most basic physical laws of the actual world in all logically possible worlds in which those laws operate.

For example, it is absolutely N-impossible for any two possible masses to be near one another without being affected by gravity. It is not absolutely N-impossible that an acorn grow into a pear tree, for there are logically possible worlds in which the laws of nature remain as in the actual world, but in which people exploit those laws by developing advanced techniques of genetic alteration which reprogram acorns with pear genes.[6]

2. An event or state of affairs is actually N-impossible iff. the actually-obtaining state of affairs, s_1, is such that s_1's being superseded by s_2 would be inconsistent with the physical laws of the actual world.

This is the notion of "real" or "genuine" possibility described by Rescher. It is not clear at this time whether it is actually N-impossible for some acorn at some time to develop into a pear tree, since it is not clear whether our technology could progress to that extent, given the physical, financial, and human psychological resources that might be available. It *is* actually N-impossible for *this* acorn to become a pear tree if it begins to germinate today.

In the contexts with which I am concerned, the apparent failure of physical possibility iterations to generate actual possibilities resolves into the following two principles.

1. Where the "transition" from s_1 to s_2 is possible only given an intermediate condition s_3, and where s_3 is merely absolutely possible, but not actually possible, the (*absolute*) possibility of s_3's obtaining, together with the (*absolute*) possibility of s_2's obtaining if s_3 obtains, will not yield the (*actual*) possibility of s_2's obtaining, so it might seem as if the possibility of a possibility does not yield a possibility.

This sort of reasoning is applicable where our own decisions do not form part of the conditions having the role of s_3. For example, it may not be actually possible that a giant meteor will destroy the Earth tomorrow, even though it is possible that if one is near and heading in our way the Earth will be destroyed, and it is possible that a giant meteor is in such a relation to the Earth. However, given that there is no such meteor, it is impossible that the Earth will be destroyed by a giant meteor tomorrow. This, though, is because given the rest of the actual state of the world, it is only *absolutely* possible and not *actually* possible that such a meteor is heading our way.

2. Where human choice and rational agency is involved, it is never correct for a person or group to consider their own choices of possible actions as part of the

given background conditions which would imply that certain outcomes are physically impossible.

Part of what is meant by saying that we are free agents (or true *agents* at all) is that the dispositional states which may determine our actual choices never count as criteria of physical necessity in our calculations of what we can and cannot do. This is part of what distinguishes free agency from cases of *true compulsion*, in which real agency is absent, and in which the "choices" must simply be taken as natural conditions of the actual world.

Melissa, who has removed Stan's carburetor, might say, "It is impossible for him to drive his car today because I've decided to keep the carburetor off his engine until tomorrow, even though if I reinstall it today he will be able to drive the car, and I can (but I won't) reinstall it." This has the apparent form of a judgment that *possibly possibly p*, but *not possibly p*. In ordinary discourse this is fine, but the more precise way for Melissa to characterize the situation would be to say that he could, indeed, drive the car today but *will* not because she chooses a particular one of the possibilities open to her. Stan, though, may rightly judge that given her actual decision, he is *personally* powerless to bring about the desired result (though he may also not be—he might be able to achieve the result through persuasion or some mechanical work of his own).

In such cases the issue is not whether a particular outcome is possible given that some controllable possible condition is unactualized. Rather it is a matter of whether one is willing to actualize certain members of inconsistent sets of possibilities. There are sets of possibilities which are absolutely N-impossible where the individual members are absolutely N-possible. Every conjunction of an actual state of affairs with any actually N-impossible subsequent state constitutes an absolutely N-impossible set. There are also sets of possibilities whose members are jointly actually impossible but individually actually possible. For example, given the actual world, including the fact that I have somewhat limited financial resources, I cannot *both* spend \$5,000 gambling in Las Vegas next week *and* keep a reserve of savings in the bank, although both might be (individually) genuinely possible.

To return to the ethical issues involving potentiality, let us imagine that researchers have just discovered that chimpanzees actually have about the same brain capacity as humans (despite appearances and measurements—their brains make use of the available neural tissue differently than ours). It has also been discovered that they do not develop human types of reasoning and communication except with special techniques of training, which have been tested and found effective. With this training, they can develop linguistic skills like ours and be brought to the point at which they can participate in our culture just as we do.

Now it seems probable that many people would be averse to training them in this way, but it would not even be plausible to argue that while our own children are potential persons these apes are not. The decision to withhold training and eventual human treatment would have to be made on some other ground, as, for example, that it is too expensive, and would lessen our own welfare, or that they are of a foreign kind, e.g., "ugly animals." The point is, if the *potential for personhood* is the ground for a human right to become persons, there should be no reason to withhold it from those apes, for they would have the same potential, and in both cases some significant human effort is necessary for actualization of the potential.

Suppose now that the discovery is, instead, that chimpanzees, through a simple, cheap, minor surgical procedure become able to be trained as in the above example. Here one might want to give either of two additional arguments against doing this to them. It might be claimed that the potential to become persons is so *remote* as not to count in any significant way (as in the egg or sperm-to-person argument). This certainly seems rather poorly founded, for there is no sequence of drastic physical metamorphoses of any kind. One might then argue that the potential is remote in the other sense discussed, that is, that it involves a possible change which could only occur given a previous possible change, and that since the development of person-traits is only *possibly possible*, it does not follow that it is a genuine possibility. Where this is not simply a judgment of remoteness of potential, though, it really reflects a *choice* not to bring about the conditions necessary for the end state's obtaining. It is actually impossible that both the apes become persons *and* we do nothing to modify them so that they will be able to be educated, but it is, in the imagined case, physically possible for the apes to become persons, because the sequence of events leading to their personhood is genuinely physically possible.

Since the possibility of human personhood depends on possible human action there is no genuine difference in potential based on the need for slight modifications of the organism in addition to the education and nurture that are expected. Of course, we acknowledge this in the case of humans, for if a child were born with a brain defect which rendered it incapable of being educated but which could be easily remedied with a minor operation, we would not say, "He can't develop into a normal adult, so he doesn't have any right to be educated." Instead we would say that he could *easily* become a normal adult, and we would even say that he had been wronged if he were not given the surgery.

The fact that the analogous cases involving animals are not blocked from moral rights of personhood does not in itself show that potentiality is an illegitimate ground for a right to develop. It is not at all clear that we should want to find any relevant difference between the case of infants and the cases of other sorts of things that might be found to have a genuine potential for personhood, for the aversion which people might feel toward granting that there are similar rights in those cases might be completely accounted for in terms of species prejudice and fears of conflicts of interests between groups.

II. Teleological Potentiality

So far, I have been discussing potentiality in terms of a simple physical possibility of becoming. There is another, stronger sense of potentiality which is sometimes invoked by opponents of abortion. This is what can be best called *teleological potentiality*. According to some views of human development, a human being in any of the early stages of development is to be understood as essentially an uncompleted or unfulfilled human being, rather than as an entity whose identity and nature are determined by its present properties. Thus, its development expresses a future-oriented nature until it has fulfilled its *telos* and become a full-fledged human being or person. The details of the argumentation for such theories do not matter for my purposes, since I am not concerned here with whether or not such a theory is correct but only with the implications which it would have if it is correct. More specifically, I am concerned with determining whether or not a theory of teleological potentiality would yield a right to become a person independently of the sort of potentiality principles I have been discussing, and whether the implications of those principles would be affected by substituting a concept of teleological potentiality for the previously considered concept of mere physical possibility of becoming.

Before taking up these questions, let me draw another distinction. There are two forms that teleological potentiality theses can take, involving (1) a physical-program account of potentiality, and (2) a conceptual account. According to the first, an individual x has the teleological potential to be an F just in case x has an internally determined disposition to become an F, as in the case of a fetus's genetic determination to become an independently surviving human being. According to the second type of account, an x has the potential to become an F just in case X essentially falls under a concept, f, which is defined in terms of a completed process of development such that x must be considered an uncompleted stage of an F.

The appeal to physical teleology of an infant or fetus adds little to mere physical possibility appeals with regard to establishing a right to become a person if we assume that a workable potentiality theory must be able to generate the right of infants to grow into full-fledged moral persons. A fetus's disposition to develop is the disposition to grow into an infant. Beyond the point of birth, further development requires positive efforts on the part of others. Therefore, while in the case of the fetus's disposition to become a baby it might make sense to prescribe a *lack of intervention* in an independently continuing process, the nurture required for full personhood makes that further transition a question of whether or not to *act* so as to bring about development which is partly determined by physical dispositions and partly determined by human decisions. So we should say that the development of personhood is *possible*, contingent on our actions, bringing us back to the same problem as in the case of physical-possibility potentiality. Therefore, the appeal to genuine *person-hood* as the teleological fulfillment of infant or fetal development does not involve a physically determined disposition, and thus is either mistaken or expresses, instead, a thesis about conceptual teleology.

The concept of an infant or fetus as essentially a future *person* expresses a normative judgment that the infant or fetus should become a person, since, after all, it is up to *us* (rather than determined by nature) whether or not it does become a person. This dependence on human agency, in fact, is more than just a matter of whether we intervene in a natural state or process; it is *we* who supply the *telos* of personhood. So it is impossible to separate the teleological concept of personhood from the prescriptions of development which we supply, and these are obviously not independent of the moral issue of whether we ought to bring about this development.

The judgment that an infant is essentially the person whom it will become might well *express* a moral judgment that it ought to become a person, but it cannot thereby also form a *ground* for that judgment, on pain of circularity. So, while it might involve an important moral intuition and might be quite significant to the issue of development, a teleological potentiality principle seems not to give grounds for the right to become a person over and above any that might be claimed to be established by a mere physical-possibility thesis.

III. Conclusion

In my analysis of some crucial aspects of possible becoming, I have presupposed that there are at least significant *prima facie* reasons for thinking that some sorts of potential entail rights of development (and/or duties to cause development). In this essay, I have neither sought nor found any firm grounds for an ethical potentiality principle. If there are such grounds, they would be found outside the sort of metaphysical considerations that are addressed here. For example, if the very form of our best-founded judgments about persons' rights is such as to extend them to nonactual persons, those judgments must have the form of either a potentiality thesis or a kind-based principle (or some combination of these). This is because, first, if there were *no* restrictions on the classes of things that have a right to develop, such a right would always be automatically (and trivially) limited by the *possibility* of the development in question. In a theoretically boundless moral community of that type, then, the potential for ethically relevant development would always be sufficient for the right to develop. Second, if there *are* restrictions (other than impossible develop-ment) on the range of things that have a right to become persons, such restrictions obviously would have to be in terms of actual qualities of things that are included or excluded (as, e.g., their being human, or being sentient, etc.). It may be that species (or other such kinds) cannot be defended as grounds for preferred moral status, even as plausibly as certain sorts of potentiality.

If there *is* some *prima facie* reason to suppose that our moral reasoning must in-clude a potentiality thesis, it is important to prove whether such a thesis coheres with the rest of our best-considered moral judgments. I have tentatively accepted the argument that a certain sort of "remoteness" of potentiality may block some of the most counterintuitive implications that are sometimes claimed to follow from the thesis that certain potentials (e.g., personhood) are grounds for moral rights of development. This notion of remoteness involves relative inaccessibility through chains of unactualized possibilities on which further possibilities depend. I have noted that loss of identity (i.e., extinction and replacement) during a process of pos-sible change would be a true metaphysical ground for judgments of ethically inac-cessible remoteness of this sort. This, in itself, would block the *reductio* argument, which would extend rights of development to such absurd candidates as sperm and foods that could be eaten to "become" a person.

I have also explored what might look like a further metaphysical ground for inac-cessibility of remote potentiality and have not found any metaphysical basis for an ethical distinction between the (physically) possible and the (physically) possibly possible. However, in many cases the possibly possible could make for remoteness of obligation in another way. Where a chain of as-yet-unactualized means is necessary for a possible end, there will be questions as to how we should order the priorities of our planned efforts, and the ethically allowable ordering of priorities may often ne-gate a *prima facie* judgment that a certain potential ought to be actualized.

This sort of reasoning would provide at least one important ground for the judg-ment that remoteness of potentiality in this second sense would correlate with weakness of obligation or absence of obligation. The more complicated and difficult the process of actualizing potential and the more stages are involved in arriving at a morally significant possible end stage, the more our time and efforts and resources would have to be channeled away from the maximization of our own interests and even from the actualization of other potentials which are more directly accessible from the current state of affairs. Just as remoteness of actual relationships com-plicates the weighing and balancing and resolution of *prima facie* rights and duties, so remoteness of potential would do the same. This, though, is a very different rea-son for blocking remote rights of development than would be given by a true meta-physical argument for inaccessibility of remote potentiality.

NOTES

1. Michael Tooley, "Abortion and Infanticide," *Philosophy and Public Affairs*, vol. 2 (1972), pp. 37–65.

2. For an extended discussion of this topic, see my doctoral dissertation, *Becoming Persons: The Ethical Problems of Potentiality, Identity, and Kinds* (University of Arizona, 1989).

3. Nicholas Rescher, *A Theory of Possibility* (Pittsburgh, 1975), p. 144.

4. David B. Annis, "Abortion and the Potentiality Principle," *Southern Journal of Philosophy*, vol. 22 (1984), pp. 155–58.

5. Tooley, for example, defends such a position in his more recent *Abortion and Infanticide* (Oxford, 1983).

6. This is in addition to the usual concern with those logically possible worlds in which the actual individuals remain unchanged, but in which we consider what might come about with alternations in the actual laws of nature.

CHAPTER FIVE

Abortion

Listening to the Middle

EDWARD LANGERAK

Says one critic of the philosophical debate on abortion: "Philosophers are not listened to because they do not listen."[1] Though I believe the charge is too strong, my own review of the literature makes it uncomfortably understandable. If there is any public consensus on abortion, as reflected in legal systems as well as in public opinion surveys, it is the middle-of-the-road view that some abortions are not permissible but that others are, and that some of the permissible abortions are more difficult to justify than others. But many of the most widely cited philosophical writings on abortion argue that the only coherent positions tend toward the extremes: all or most abortions are put into the same moral boat with either murder or, more frequently, elective surgery. In fact, proponents of the extremes tend to respect one another as at least being self-consistent, while joining in swift rebuttal of those who want it both ways and ignominiously try to be moderates on either murder or mandatory motherhood.

This reaction against the middle derives from some basic beliefs of those on the extremes. On the liberal side are those who believe that fetuses, and perhaps even very young infants, lack some necessary condition (say, self-consciousness) of personhood.[2] This view is often combined with the further assertion that the social consequences of society's conferring on the fetus a claim to life are such that the conferral should not be made until birth or shortly thereafter. On the conservative side there are those who believe that from conception (or very shortly thereafter) the fetus has as strong (or almost as strong) a claim to life as does any person. This claim resides either in some property thought sufficient for personhood (say, genetic endowment) that the fetus has in itself, or in the immediate conferral of personhood on the fetus by God or society.

Of course, as Schopenhauer said, arguments are not like taxicabs that you can dismiss when they become inconvenient; and the two extremes are quick to point out the problematic implications of each other's positions. The liberals are accused of courting infanticide and the conservatives of trivializing the moral category of murder. Such implications would be more damaging to the extremes were it not that most moderate positions have an equally problematic flaw—that of arbitrary line-drawing. My reading of the abortion literature suggests that there are two widely shared beliefs that moderate positions seek to incorporate in their approaches to the abortion issue. The first belief is that something about the fetus itself, not merely the social consequences of abortion, makes abortions (or at least many abortions) morally problematic. The second belief is that late abortions are significantly more morally problematic than early abortions. Not only are these beliefs widely shared by moderates, but I find that liberals and conservatives, whose positions implicitly reject one or both of these beliefs, often feel uncomfortable in rejecting them.

In accounting for these two beliefs, most middle positions maintain variations of what I call the "stage" approach and what its critics call the "magic moment" approach. The assertion is that at some point in the development of the fetus, say at the point of acquiring some vital sign, of sentience, of quickening, or of viability, the fetus suddenly moves from having no claim to life to having as strong (or almost as strong) a claim as an adult human. While the "stage" approach is consistent with the two beliefs underlying the moderate position, its difficulty has always been to explain the tremendous moral weight put on some specific point in what really amounts to a continuum in development. Critics on both extremes argue that, no matter what stage is picked as the "magic moment," the whole approach is prima facie arbitrary.

The implications of the liberal and conservative positions, including their denial of one or both of the moderate beliefs, and the prima facie arbitrariness of the stage positions, motivate consideration of an alternative that both is coherent and listens to the middle by accounting for the two beliefs.

Without examining all the alternatives, I will argue that the potentiality principle is plausible and accounts for the first belief—that something about the fetus itself makes abortion morally problematic—but that, by itself, it cannot account for the second belief—that late abortions are significantly more problematic than early abortions. I will then argue that a conferred claims approach is plausible, consistent with the potentiality principle, and accounts for the second belief though it cannot account for the first.

I will suggest that combining the potentiality principle with a conferred claims approach provides moderates with a coherent framework for thinking through the central questions of the abortion debate: (1) When does an individual human being attain either an inherent claim to life or such properties that society ought to confer on it a claim to life? (2) When do a person's or a group of persons' claims to life, physical or mental health, freedom, privacy, and self-actualization override another human being's claim to life? (3) When should answers to the first two question be incorporated into the law of a pluralistic society?

The Potentiality Principle

I formulate the potentiality principle as follows: "If, in the normal course of its development, a being will acquire a person's claim to life, then by virtue of that fact it already has some claim to life." To understand this principle, one must distinguish among "actual person," "a capacity for personhood," "potential person," and "possible person." An *actual person* is a being that meets a sufficient condition (whatever that may be)[3] for personhood and thereby has as strong a claim to life as normal adult human beings. Roughly, a *capacity for personhood* is possessed by any being not currently exhibiting that capacity but who has proceeded in the course of its development to the point where it could currently exhibit it (for example, a temporarily unconscious person). A *potential person* is a being, not yet a person, that will become an actual person in the normal[4] course of its development (for example, a human fetus). A *possible person* is a being that could, under certain causally possible conditions, become an actual person (for example, a human sperm or egg).[5]

This technical set of distinctions is important because the potentiality principle asserts that potential persons, but not possible persons, have a claim to life. Some attacks on the principle confuse these categories.[6] Also, the principle is consistent with granting full personhood to those with a capacity for personhood, a fact ignored by those who collapse "capacity" and "potentiality" and argue, for example, that the category of "potential person" endangers sleeping persons. Moreover, the distinctions can help us avoid sloppy language, such as that of the Supreme Court in *Roe* v. *Wade*, when it asserted that at viability the state begins to have a compelling interest in "potential life." Clearly, a fetus is actually alive and is even an actual human being, genetically defined; its unique status is that, given most criteria of personhood, it is neither an actual person nor a merely possible person—it is a potential person.

Potentiality and Temporality

The potentiality principle asserts that a potential person has a claim to life, albeit one that may be weaker than the claim of an actual person. Many people find this assertion intuitively plausible but are unable to persuade those who challenge it. Here is my attempt to persuade.

It is clear that the unique status of the potential person has to do with its inherent "thrust" or predetermined tendency. A potential person is not simply a set of blueprints, it is an organism that itself will become the actual person toward which it is already developing. Controversial issues of personal identity arise here, but two points seem obvious. First, we cannot simply assume that its predetermined tendency already grants it the claims it will have in the future. To paraphrase H. Tristram Engelhardt, Jr., we must not lose the ability to distinguish between the claims of the future and those of the present,[7] or as S. I. Benn succinctly puts it, a potential president is not already commander-in-chief.[8] Second, those attracted to the potentiality principle do see some derivative relationship between the claims that a being will have in the normal course of its development and those that it has in the present.

I believe that the plausibility of the last point rests in perceiving humans as basically temporal beings. For actual persons this is true, first of all, from an internal point of view (a fact Heidegger uses for his entire ontology). Our self-consciousness so orients us to our past and our future that, in an important sense, we *are* our history and our projections as well as our present. A premedical student, for example, sees himself or herself as a future physician, not just as a science student. This temporal perception is also true from an external point of view, a point of view that extends to humans that are not yet persons. When we see a very young child, we see something of the adult it will, in the normal course of its development, become, as well as something of the baby that it once was. In this temporal perception lies, I believe, the respect we feel is due former persons (for example, respectful treatment of corpses) and, for that matter, former presidents. The respect we give former persons and presidents is not as great as that which we give actual ones, but that does not undermine the fact that some respect is due the former and that it is derivative from, indeed proportional to, the respect due to the latter.

Similarly, perceiving humans in a temporal context accounts for the respect many feel is due to humans by virtue of their potential. As an analogy, consider a potential president. Following my distinctions, such a person is not merely a possible president (something civics teachers used to say about every American child); he or she has already won the election but has not yet been inaugurated (on a somewhat arbitrarily selected date). The person is not yet commander-in-chief but, in the normal course, *will* (not *could*) be. Already that person receives some of the perquisites of the future office. The fact that the news media and others give the potential president more attention than the actual president, of course, may be the result of prudence, if not exploitation (the same derivation for much of the respect given actual presidents). But, at least in pre-Watergate times, some of the respect given actual presidents, and most of that given former presidents, derives from the high office that the person has or had, even when the person is not particularly deserving. Those who perceive a person in a temporal context and who, like myself, still respect an actual or former president by virtue of the office (apart from achievements in it), will derivatively have some respect toward a potential president by virtue of the office he or she will have.

Even those who deny that presidents ought to be respected simply by virtue of their office, should agree that some of the respect given persons derives from their "office" of personhood, apart from their achievements. In fact, traditionally the respect involving a claim to life derives from what persons are, rather than what they achieve or fail to achieve. If so, then perceiving humans in a temporal context should elicit some respect for former and potential persons, respect that is derivative from and proportional, though not identical, to the respect elicited by the actual persons they were or will become.

Temporality and Probability

Some may grant the strength of this argument as it applies to former persons, sensing that it accounts, for example, for our aversion to artificially keeping former persons "alive" in order to harvest their organs at a convenient time. However, whatever else we may say about former persons, they were certainly, at one time, actual persons. But the personhood of potential persons is still "outstanding" and there is no guarantee that it will be realized. The contingency of the "not yet" makes it asymmetrical with the "has been" even when we perceive humans in a temporal context.

This objection forces us to ask just what is the moral significance of the predetermined tendency of a potential person. Though the tendency does not guarantee personhood, it does distinguish the organism from possible persons by guaranteeing a dramatic shift in probabilities. This difference in probabilities is similar to that which distinguishes a potential president from a possible president. The potentiality principle asks us to respect a potential person by virtue not of what it *could* be, but of what it *will* be in the normal course of its development. Even those of us who refuse to mythologize the predetermined tendency in potential persons must agree that this tendency makes it highly likely that, without outside interference, they will become persons. Is this shift in probabilities of moral significance?

Consider the other end of the life-span. Those who believe that it is sometimes permissible to cease striving officiously to keep humans in an irreversible coma artificially alive must agree that the irreversibility of the coma is seldom, if ever, absolutely guaranteed. But we believe it is morally irresponsible to allow the rare "miraculous recovery" to prevent acting on the best medical prognosis, when it indicates no reasonable hope of recovery. To shut off a respirator when there is a 50 percent chance of recovery (or even a 5 percent chance, given our laudable bias toward erring in favor of personal life), is morally wrong, but not when the probability of recovery approaches (without reaching) zero. In an uncertain world, judgments of high probabilities are often the only kind we have. This makes dramatic shifts in probabilities morally significant.[9]

So I believe that the high probability of future personhood, inherent in a potential person, is of moral significance to those who perceive humans in a temporal context and that this makes plausible the assertion of the potentiality principle. I hope I have at least shifted the burden of proof onto those who deny that the high probability of a fetus's becoming a person with a strong claim to life already grants it some (proportional) claim to life and respect.

Conferred Claims

Although the potentiality principle, as defended, accounts for the first belief—that something about the fetus itself makes abortion morally problematic—it leaves open the question of just how strong a claim to life should be attributed to the fetus. There are extreme liberals on the abortion issue who may grant the fetus some claim to life but simply argue that the claims of an actual person—claims to freedom and mental health—always override the claim to life of a fetus. Among those who use the potentiality principle, there will be intramural debates on how strong a claim to life it implies. I cannot argue the case here, but I believe that the most plausible use of it is one that allows the use of IUDs and "morning after" pills (both of which probably act as abortifacients), as well as abortions during the first trimester for such reasons as the woman's being too young for motherhood.[10] But then the claim to life attributed to the very early fetus cannot be very strong. The incidence of early spontaneous abortion is estimated variously from 15 percent to over 50 percent,[11] and second-trimester fetuses have a somewhat higher natural death rate than postviable fetuses. In other words, the probability of an older fetus becoming an actual person is perhaps double the probability of a zygote becoming a person. While this shift in probability is noteworthy, and marks implantation as a point of some moral significance, it is not nearly as significant as the difference in moral seriousness moderates see between a very early abortion and a late one. Consequently, if the inherent claim to life of a potential person is derived from and proportional to the probability of its becoming an actual person, one cannot in good faith allow the claim to life of a zygote to be easily overridden and then assert that the inherent claim to life of an older fetus is so vastly stronger that it all but cannot be overridden. Therefore, although the potentiality principle can account for the belief that something about the fetus itself makes abortion morally problematic, it cannot by itself account for the belief that late abortions are significantly more morally problematic than very early abortions.

However, the conferred claims approach can account for the second belief, although it cannot account for the first. Assume that, whatever moral claim to life an older fetus may have by virtue of its potentiality, the claim may not be strong enough to override the claim of a pregnant woman for an abortion. At what point should society confer a stronger claim to life on the fetus? At what point should society treat it as if it were a person?

The conferral approach to the status of the fetus is not an unusual one,[12] though it is sometimes thought incompatible with an approach that asserts an inherent claim in the fetus itself. But an approach that *confers* claims rubs an approach that *recognizes* inherent claims only if the inherent claim to life is thought to be as serious as an actual person's claim to life. In this case it would be futile (rather than contradictory) to ask what claims society ought to confer on it. However, when the recognized inherent claim is weaker than a normal adult's claim to life, as can be the case with the potentiality principle, one can coherently ask whether society ought, in addition, to confer on the fetus a stronger claim to life.

The argument in favor of such a conferral basically appeals to the social consequences of abortions and infanticide. For example, infants are so similar to persons that allowing them to be killed would generate a moral climate that would endanger the claim to life of even young persons. And older fetuses are so similar to infants that allowing them to be killed without due moral or legal process would endanger infants. Of course, there must be a cutoff for this sort of argument. For example, most would agree that preventing the implantation of zygotes would have no discernible effect on our sympathetic capacities toward persons. At what point would abortions begin to have such effects, especially on medical personnel, that it is in society's interest to endow the fetus at that point with a stronger claim to life? This seems largely an empirical question and one not easily answered,[13] though I will suggest some guidelines below.

One difficulty with the conferral approach has always been that the relevant considerations are the interest and sympathies of actual persons, rather than moral claims inherent in the fetus itself. Indeed, the above argument is reminiscent of Kant's view that we ought not beat our dogs merely because beating our dogs might make us more inclined to beat people. Such arguments derive protection for some beings from the rather variable, even capricious, sympathies of other beings. Thus the conferral approach by itself does not account for the belief that something about the fetus itself makes abortion morally problematic, but this belief is accounted for by the potentiality approach.

Implantation, Quickening, Viability, and Birth

My combined approach escapes the problematic implications of the extremes but does it escape the flaw of arbitrary line-drawing that I attributed to those moderate positions that appeal to the stage or "magic moment" approach? Two related considerations show that it does. First, notice that the word "arbitrary" should not be used loosely. For example, there is a certain arbitrariness in making eighteen the age of majority rather than seventeen or nineteen. But the relevant criteria nonarbitrarily imply that, if a legally precise line must be drawn within the continuum of growth, the debate must focus on that time span rather than, say, the span between seven and nine.

Second, I submit that the two criteria I use—important shifts in probabilities and dangerous social consequences—nonarbitrarily suggest four spans (beyond that of conception) for moral and legal line-drawing in a potential person's continuum of growth. Although these criteria imply distinct spans for definite increments in the strength of the claim to life, at no stage does a potential person move from having no claim to having one as strong as an adult.

The first span, as we saw, is that of implantation, when the shift in probabilities of actual personhood signifies a somewhat stronger inherent claim to life, at least from the moral point of view. The recognition of this change is due apart from any consequentialist considerations about the difference between more or less unknowingly preventing implantation and knowingly detaching an implanted embryo. However, the remaining spans are suggested by consequentialist considerations about the psychological and social impact of abortions, considerations in favor of conferring an even stronger claim to life on the fetus.

The second span involves the traditional indicator of "quickening." When the fetus begins making perceptible spontaneous movements (around the beginning of the second trimester), its shape, its behavior, and even its beginning relationship with the mother and the rest of society (every father recalls when he first felt the fetus's movements) all suggest that abortions after this point will have personal and social consequences specifiably more serious than those of earlier abortions.

The third is that of viability, when a fetus is capable of living, with simple medical care, outside the womb (around the end of the second trimester). Recall the "infanticide" trials of physicians who, claiming they were inducing abortions, were charged with participating in premature births and murders. This controversy is only one indication that killing potential persons after viability has social consequences (apart from legal ones) even more serious than abortions soon after quickening.

Finally, consider that allowing infanticide is generally regarded as a *reductio* of those positions that allow it. The aversion to infanticide is shared even by most of those whose criteria for personhood imply that a newborn is still only a potential person and not an actual one. This suggests that most people agree that at birth the potential person attains properties and relationships so close to those of actual persons that the consequences of killing at this point are practically the same as killing young persons.

If these observations are true, they justify conferring on newborns a claim to life as strong as that of adult persons. They also suggest partial wisdom in the Supreme Court's decision allowing states to grant a rather strong claim to life to postviable fetuses, a claim overridden only by the claim to life or health (I would specify "physical health") of the mother. But the court decision, in effect, mandates the allowing of abortion on demand for all previable fetuses. If my observations about quickening are correct, we should also draw an earlier line, conferring a claim to life on the fetus at the beginning of the second trimester, a claim less strong than that conferred at viability, but one overridden only by such serious claims as that of the mother to mental or physical health.[14] Probably the moral line drawn at implantation should remain outside the legal realm.

I admit the difficulties in legally implementing such an approach, but I doubt that they are insurmountable or as deep as the moral and legal difficulties of alternative approaches. Therefore I believe I have presented a plausible approach to the abortion issue that is coherent, is not arbitrary, and listens well to the considered intuitions of those in the middle.[15]

NOTES

This essay was written during a fellowship at the National Humanities Institute, University of Chicago.

1. Roger Wertheimer, "Philosophy on Humanity," in *Abortion: Pro and Con*, ed. Robert L. Perkins (Cambridge: Schenkman Publishing), p. 127.

2. For brevity I use "fetus" in a generic sense to refer to unborn humans at any stage of development, including that of zygote, conceptus, and embryo. I assume the fetuses are human beings, genetically defined, and use "person" to refer to those human beings that have as strong a claim to life as a normal adult. I use "as strong a claim" rather than "same claim" because, if very young human beings are persons, their claim to life clearly involves the claim to be nurtured as well as the claim not to be killed, a feature that is not clearly true of a normal adult's claim to life. I use "claim" to life rather than "right" or "prima facie right"

because my argument entails that a fetus's (though not a person's) claim to life can be held with varying degrees of strength, and I agree with Joel Feinberg (*Social Philosophy* [Englewood Cliffs: Prentice Hall, 1973], pp. 64–7) that this is a feature of claims rather than rights. Though Feinberg may object to my use of his distinction, I agree with him that the "right" or "valid claim" in a given instance is the strongest of competing claims. For an account of the relationship between claims and rights that I believe is consistent with my argument, see Bertram Bandman's "Rights and Claims," in *Bioethics and Human Rights*, ed. Elsie L. Bandman and Bertram Bandman (Boston: Little Brown, 1978).

3. One advantage of the potentiality principle is that one need not specify the necessary or sufficient conditions for actual personhood. One need only note that, whatever they are, a potential person will acquire them in the normal course of its development. My own position is that self-consciousness is a necessary and perhaps a sufficient condition for personhood: "The fact that man can have the idea 'I' raises him infinitely above all the other beings living on earth. By this he is a *person*" (Immanuel Kant, *Anthropology from a Pragmatic Point of View*, trans. Mary J. Gregor [The Hague: Martinus Nijhoff, 1947], p. 9). See also H. Tristram Engelhart, Jr. ("The Ontology of Abortion," *Ethics*, 84/3 [April 1974], p. 230): "Only self-conscious subjects can value themselves, and, thus, be ends in themselves, and, consequently, themselves make claims against us." While Joel Feinberg seems to object to thinking of personhood as a property, he does appeal to the fact that persons are "equally centers of experience, foci of subjectivity" (*op. cit.*, p. 93).

4. Although using the phrase "in the normal course of its development" rather than "in the normal course of events" emphasizes the teleological ("nature's aim") rather than the statistical probability aspect of "normal development," my later argument about probability and claims assumes that even a teleological notion of normal has statistical implications: if the natural end of (a) is to become (A) then it is highly probable that, without interference, (a) will become (A). I believe I am referring to what some Thomists call "active, natural potentiality," though I deny potential personhood is as claim-laden as actual personhood.

5. The class of potential and possible persons must be distinguished from the class (membership unknown) of future persons, namely the class of future actual persons who do not now exist but will in fact exist in the future. One must be careful with analogies between our duties to potential persons and our duties to future persons (for such an analogy, see Werner S. Pluhar, "Abortion and Simple Consciousness," *Journal of Philosophy*, 74/3 [March 1977], p. 167). If there are future persons (as is so likely as to be certain), they will be actual persons whose quality of life will be affected by actions we now perform, while it is debatable whether killing potential persons affects the quality of their lives *as persons*.

6. A point I argue in reply to Michael Tooley's "Abortion and Infanticide," *Philosophy and Public Affairs* 2/4 (Summer 1973), pp. 410–16.

7. Engelhart, p. 223.

8. "Abortion, Infanticide, and Respect for Persons," *The Problem of Abortion*, ed. Joel Feinberg (Belmont: Wadsworth Publishing, 1973), p. 103.

9. In this I agree with John T. Noonan, "An Almost Absolute Value in History," in *The Morality of Abortion*, ed. John T. Noonan, Jr. (Cambridge: Harvard University Press, 1970), though he seems to argue wrongly that an abortion involves a high probability of killing a person. Instead, it kills a human that had a high probability of becoming a person.

10. Notice that if one uses the potentiality principle to attribute a very strong claim to life for the fetus, one has, in effect, denied the belief that late abortions are significantly more morally problematic than early abortions.

11. See Malcolm Potts, Peter Diggory, and John Peel, *Abortion* (Cambridge: Cambridge University Press, 1977), chap. 2. The highest estimate I have seen, at variance with most others, is 69 percent, by Harvard physiologist John D. Biggers (*Science*, 202 [October 13, 1978], p. 198).

12. See R.B. Brandt, "The Morality of Abortion" (The *Monist*, 56 [1972], pp. 504–26), for a quasi-Rawlsian development of this approach. See also Ronald M. Green, "Conferred Rights and the Fetus," *Journal of Religious Ethics*, 2/1 (1974), and Benn, *op. cit.*

13. See Magda Denes, *In Necessity and Sorrow: Life and Death in an Abortion Hospital* (New York: Penguin Books, 1977), for one description of the different social effects of abortions at different stages of pregnancy.

14. Notice that adding the conferred claims approach highly qualifies a possible implication of my defense of the potentiality principle, namely, the implication that it is somewhat easier to justify aborting fetuses with defects that lower their probability of attaining personhood. Any arguments for conferring a stronger claim to life on fetuses at a given point would apply to most defective fetuses as well.

15. Patricia Fauser, James Gustafson, Gary Iseminger, Daniel Lee, and Frederick Stoutland gave me very helpful comments on an earlier draft of this essay.

PART TWO

POTENTIALITY
AT THE BEGINNING OF LIFE

CHAPTER SIX

Persons with Potential

JASON T. EBERL

The moral status of human embryos and fetuses is one of the most vexing questions in bioethics, and various responses often stand or fall on the answer to the more foundational, and just as vociferously debated, question of the *ontological* status of such entities—whether they count as "persons," "potential persons," or merely "human biological material."[1] The *argument from potential*, as it is often termed, is typically formulated as follows: (1) Persons possess a high, perhaps infinite, degree of moral value; (2) persons thereby possess certain basic rights, including a right to life; (3) human embryos and fetuses[2] typically possess the potential to develop into persons; (4) having the potential to develop into a person suffices for something to possess the moral value of a person; (5) hence, embryos and fetuses also typically possess a high, perhaps infinite, degree of moral value and thereby the same basic rights. This conclusion is open to a standard counterargument that the rights possessed by an *actual* entity are not transferable to a *potential* forerunner. For example, when President Barack Obama was growing up in Hawaii, he did not possess the right, as a potential commander-in-chief, to order U.S. troops into Afghanistan (Feinberg 1986, 267; Benn 1984, 143).

Despite the merits or demerits of this and other counterarguments, the search is motivated for a stronger foundation to assert that embryos and fetuses have a moral status sufficiently equivalent to that of mature human persons to bear the same basic right to life. The most direct argumentative route is to establish that embryos and fetuses are not potential, but *actual* persons, and thus bypass the above counterargument.[3] Of course, embryos and fetuses do not yet engage in any of the activities typically understood to define the essence of personhood;[4] however, they arguably possess the *intrinsic potentiality* to develop themselves—with the assistance of a protective, nutritive environment (something upon which all organisms, including mature human persons, are dependent as well)—into beings who can immediately engage in the definitive activities of persons. The crucial premise here is the claim that possessing the intrinsic potentiality to develop oneself into a fully actualized person[5] suffices for an organism to be, both ontologically and morally, a person already (Gómez-Lobo 2004, 205; Schwarz 1998, 271). If this premise holds, an embryo or fetus is not a "potential person" but a "person with potential" (Finnis 2006, 18; Lee 2004, 262; Oderberg 1997, 263), specifically, the potential to develop oneself, while preserving one's numerical identity,[6] into an entity that actually thinks in a self-conscious rational fashion (Ford 1988, 85).

Concept of Potentiality[7]

Aristotle provides a well-developed definition of potentiality—later adopted and further elaborated upon by Thomas Aquinas—which is distinguished into two types: *active* and *passive*. Something has an active potentiality if it has within itself everything necessary, given its proper *design environment*, to actualize itself in the relevant manner.[8] The locus of a substance's set of active potentialities is its *substantial form*.[9] By contrast, something has a passive potentiality if it can be the subject of externally directed change such that it can become what it is not already (Perrett 2000, 192; Reichlin 1997, 13–17; Lee 1996, 24–26; Larmer 1995, 243–44).

Furthermore, active potentiality comes in two varieties. The first is what Robert Pasnau (2002, 115) refers to as a "capacity in hand" to perform an operation, which means that no further development or significant change is required for the potentiality to be actualized. For example, a person may have a capacity in hand to speak Spanish if, for example, she majored in it in college; but it may be the case at any one moment that she is not using this capacity and so it is not in actual operation, which it would be if she were speaking Spanish at that moment. The second is what Norman Kretzmann (1999, 39) refers to as a substance's "natural potentiality" to develop a capacity in hand to perform an operation. For example, before having learned Spanish and thus developed a capacity to do so, a person would have a natural potentiality to develop this capacity, as opposed to a dog or a plant that lacks such a natural potentiality. Any human person is born with an innate cognitive architecture that allows her to acquire a language, Spanish or otherwise (Chomsky 1968; Pinker 1994); other sentient animals apparently lack such cognitive architecture. Of course, actualizing a human person's natural potentiality for language acquisition requires external input—textbooks, teachers, exposure to native speakers, and so on—but the natural potentiality itself must be *active* if such input is to be effective. Although the actualization of this potentiality may alter a person from being a non-Spanish-speaker to being a Spanish-speaker, it does not alter her essential nature as a human person with a natural potentiality to acquire languages such as Spanish. Any natural substance has numerous natural potentialities as defined by its essence, some of which may be developed into capacities in hand while others are left undeveloped.[10]

Because a substance possesses its essential set of active potentialities by virtue of its substantial form, which also grounds a substance's persistent numerical identity (Stump 2003, 46), it follows that (a) something which has an active potentiality for self-conscious rational activity *already* possesses the essential nature definitive of personhood, and (b) something which lacks such a potentiality, even though it may have the passive potentiality to obtain it, does *not yet* possess the nature of personhood and thus must undergo a change in both specific and numerical identity if it is to become a person.[11]

Returning to the central argument, active potentiality refers to something's capacity to *be* in a certain way, as opposed to merely the possibility of its *becoming* something (Witt 1995, 264). For example, a sperm or ovum possesses the relevant active potentialities definitive of personhood only if it could come to actualize those potentialities while preserving its numerical identity. It remains the *same* substance identical with itself throughout its development from a germ cell to an actually self-conscious rational person. A change, however, from a germ cell to a person does not appear to be an identity-preserving transformation: a sperm loses its substantial identity when it fuses with an ovum, and vice versa, to form a new substance—an embryo (DiSilvestro 2006, 149; Perrett 2000, 189; Hershenov 1999, 265; Reichlin 1997, 4; Burke 1996, 497–500; Lee 1996, 26–28; Covey 1991, 239; van Inwagen 1990, 151–52; Buckle 1988, 233–38; Ford 1988, 84–55, 109–10; Stone 1987, 816–18).

Michael Lockwood (1988, 197) thus errs, in discussing the ontological status of an embryo produced through in vitro fertilization, when he claims that, "to the extent that a fertilized human ovum in vitro has an active potential for developing into a human person, so do the contents of the petri dish prior to fertilization."[12] Lockwood neglects to take into account the lack of *numerical* identity between a sperm and ovum in a petri dish prior to fertilization and the zygote produced once they conjoin.[13] Therefore, the only sense in which a germ cell may plausibly be called a "potential person" is in the weak sense that it provides the *makings* of a person.[14]

Embryonic/Fetal Personhood

With the Aristotelian concept of potentiality in mind, I follow Aquinas in contending that *all that is required for something to be a person is for it to have <u>at least an active potentiality</u> to perform self-conscious rational operations.* The actual performance of such operations is accidental to a person's existence.[15] A developing embryo or fetus possesses an active potentiality for self-conscious rational thought, although it cannot yet actually think in such a manner.[16] By contrast, sperm and ova do not have such an active potentiality:

> [Things] are always in potentiality to actuality when they can be reduced to actuality by their proper active principle with nothing external hindering them. However, seed is not yet such. For it must be by many changes that an animal comes from it. But when by its proper active principle, namely, something actually existing, it can already become such, it is then already in potentiality. (Aquinas 1950, bk. IX, lect. 6, sec. 1837; my translation)

A sperm or ovum is best understood as having a passive potentiality to become a person. Each must undergo a change brought about by an extrinsic principle: sperm must be changed through union with an ovum and vice versa, which transforms them into a substance with active potentialities for the definitive operations of personhood. Once this substantial change occurs, a person exists even if she is not actually exercising all of her definitive operations.

The change required for something to actualize an active potentiality is brought about by its "proper active principle." An active principle is required because a potentiality can be actualized only by something that is already in a state of actuality. Something can be moved from a state of potentiality to a state of actuality only by some active principle that is either internal or external to it. A sufficient condition for something's having an active potentiality is if it can actualize the potentiality by some active principle *internal*—that is, "proper"—to it. Furthermore, for a natural living organism, its ordered natural development, the principle of which is active and internal to it, is sufficient for it to *be* that toward which it is developing. As Aristotle concludes in *De generatione animalium:*

> When we are dealing with definite and ordered products of nature, we must not say each *is* of a certain quality because it *becomes* so, rather that they *become* so and so because they *are* so and so, for the process of becoming attends upon being and is for the sake of being, not *vice versa*. (Aristotle 1984a, bk. v, ch. 1, 778b2-6.)

Consider a key difference between a natural living organism and an *artifact*, namely, the location of their respective "formal causes."[17] When a builder is building a house, the formal cause of the house is the idea the builder has in her mind of how the house should appear, that is, what structure it is to have once completed. Perhaps this idea has been materially instantiated in a blueprint. Once the house is completed to the builder's satisfaction, in accord with the mental or printed blueprint, the formal cause is now located in the house itself. The matter, having been assembled in the proper fashion, has taken on the form of the house that had previously been found only in the blueprint. The form of the house is not present in the matter composing it until the building process is complete.

For a living organism, however, there is no analogue to the builder in whose mind the formal cause of the organism is located—putting aside the possibility that God acts as such a builder. Rather, the formal cause must be located in the organism itself as it is developing toward its final appearance and structure: "The living thing is dynamic, and it has within itself the source of what it will become" (Lee 1996, 25; see also Wade 1975, 242; Oderberg 1997, 287–89; Reichlin 1997, 12). A living organism's blueprint is internal to it in a way that a house's blueprint is not, since the latter has an *external* efficient cause that brings it from being potentially a house to being actually a house. A living organism, which has an *internal* efficient cause of its development, must be guided in its development by the formal cause already instantiated in it as it moves from being, for example, a person with the potential for rational thought to a person who actually thinks rationally after having developed the requisite organic structure. A person's substantial form is thus present in the matter composing her from the moment her development begins. Once conception occurs,[18] an embryo has a complete human genome and other cytoplasmic factors that are sufficient—given a supportive environment—for it to develop a functioning cerebral cortex supportive of self-conscious rational thought. From this fact, one can infer that an embryo, well before it forms a functioning cerebral cortex, possesses an active potentiality for self-conscious rational thought insofar as it has a natural potentiality to develop a capacity in hand to engage in such operations.

Objections to the Argument from Potential Concerning Embryos and Fetuses
Moral Symmetry and Potential Feline Persons

Michael Tooley presents one of the earliest and most powerful challenges to the argument from potential. He begins by drawing two sets of distinctions: between "immediately exercisable capacities" and "blocked or suppressed capacities"; and between "capacities" in general and "potentialities." Both categories of capacities correspond to Pasnau's concept of a "capacity in hand." Tooley's "potentialities" include both Kretzmann's "natural potentiality," as a form of active potentiality, as well as passive potentiality insofar as both forms of potentiality require an entity to undergo change "involving more than the mere elimination of factors blocking the exercise of a capacity," regardless of whether such change is wrought by an external agent or by means of "factors within the entity itself" (Tooley 1983, 150).[19] He then argues that an entity does not possess the ontological or moral status of a person by virtue of its capacities—and *a fortiori* its potentialities, whether active or passive (1983, 151–57).

The central premise of Tooley's argument is the "basic moral symmetry principle":

Let C be any type of causal process where there is some type of occurrence, E, such that processes of type C would possess no intrinsic moral significance were it not for the fact that they result in occurrences of type E.

Then:

The characteristic of being an act of intervening in a process of type C that prevents the occurrence of an outcome of type E makes an action intrinsically wrong to precisely the same degree as does the characteristic of being an act of ensuring that a causal process of type C, which it was in one's power to initiate, does not get initiated. (Tooley 1983, 186)

Relevant to the issue at hand, Tooley concludes: "Therefore it is intrinsically wrong to destroy something possessing an unexercised capacity for rational awareness only if it is equally wrong intentionally to refrain from producing something with the capacity for rational awareness" (1983, 156). This conclusion applies *a fortiori* to any type of active potentiality relevant to the properties definitive of personhood, implying a *reductio* that if intrinsic moral value accrues to entities that possess such an active potentiality, then the same degree of moral value accrues to entities that possess even a mere passive potentiality to be changed by an external agent into an actually self-conscious rational person. Thus, not only would the use of contraceptives—whether abortifacient or barrier—be morally wrong, but so would any act of refraining from procreative activity that may result in conception; and not only would contraception or refraining from procreative activity be morally wrong, but they would be *just as* wrong as aborting a developing embryo or fetus or killing an actually self-conscious rational person.

Tooley (1983, 191–93) bolsters his *reductio* by devising an illustrative thought experiment in which a drug is developed that, when injected into a kitten, would allow it to develop a brain capable of self-conscious rational thought. Injecting the kitten thus bestows upon it an intrinsic active potentiality for self-conscious rational thought no different from a human embryo or fetus. *Per* my view, even before the kitten has actually developed a functioning cerebrum capable of self-conscious rational thought, it would be intrinsically morally wrong either to kill the injected kitten or to inject it with an antidote that stops or reverses its neural development.[20] *Per* the moral symmetry principle, however, it would be equally morally wrong to kill a kitten that has not been injected with the available drug, as well as to refrain from injecting a kitten with the drug.

Tooley's argument rests on the moral symmetry principle, which in turn rests on "our ordinary moral intuitions" and his defense of those intuitions, along with the principle itself, against a slew of arguments to the effect that *positive interference* with a causal process, *C,* leading to an intrinsically valuable occurrence, *E,* is morally distinct from *refraining* to initiate *C* (Tooley 1983, 186–90, 205–41). I offer two critical points concerning his argument. First, it seems evident that the moral-symmetry principle is not a sound *general* principle but is applicable only to certain types of cases and is likely so for reasons other than the principle itself. The principle's intuitive appeal thus stems from its formulaic *description* of how such types of cases are morally evaluated, based on other criteria, and not because the principle fundamentally drives the normative evaluation of such cases.

For example, the moral symmetry principle appears to describe accurately a case in which the use of life-sustaining medical treatment, such as a ventilator, is required for a patient to survive. In this case, it seems that interfering with the ventilator's operation would be morally equivalent to not utilizing the ventilator in the first place—both result in the patient's death. Furthermore, there is a general consensus among bioethicists that there is no moral distinction, *ceteris paribus*, between withholding and withdrawing life-sustaining medical treatment if there are sound moral reasons not to utilize such treatment, for instance, the patient has explicitly stated in an advance directive that she would not want to live in a state of total dependence upon such machinery, or the medical team has deemed that the use of a ventilator would be futile in maintaining the patient's life beyond a few hours or days with no hope of recovery, or it has been rationally concluded that use of a ventilator would not be in the patient's best interest insofar as it would produce more pain and discomfort to the patient than benefit (Beauchamp and Childress 2009, 155–58). Once again, there appears to be moral equivalency between interrupting a causal process—discontinuing use of a ventilator—that has value only insofar as it would sustain a patient's life, and not initiating that process in the first place. This moral equivalency, however, is not an intrinsic element of the moral evaluation of the situation at hand; rather, it is out of respect for the patient's autonomy, or due to a judgment of practical ineffectiveness, or in reference to what would objectively be in the patient's best interests, that the decision either to withhold or withdraw the ventilator is morally justified.

Consider a different case, in which a patient is being sustained by a ventilator, such that without it the patient would die, but the patient has not expressed an autonomous wish to have the ventilator removed, continued use of the ventilator is not futile to sustaining the patient's life, and the benefits provided by its continued use are not outweighed by whatever pain or discomfort it may cause. This is akin to the first iteration of the ventilator case above. But now an emergency situation arises in which two other patients require temporary use of the ventilator—assume it is the only one on hand—or they will suffer severe pulmonary damage and may even die; however, by the time each of the latter patients could be weaned from the ventilator, the first patient will have expired. In this case, unless one adopts a strict utilitarian moral framework,[21] it is arguable that the first patient has a justified *claim* to continued use of the ventilator and it would thus be unjust to remove him from the ventilator against his will in order to help the other two patients. Hence, in this case, interrupting a causal process, *C,* that sustains the life of one patient would be morally worse than refraining to initiate the same causal process in order to sustain the lives of two other patients.

One might contend that this last example complicates the issue unfairly since the case involves multiple persons: one from whom we would be removing the ventilator, and the others to whom we would not be applying it. So here is another example in which there is only a single indirect object of one's action.[22] Imagine that a benefactor, *S,* sets up a trust fund for a temporarily comatose individual, *C,* so that *C* will have financial support to help cover her living expenses and hospital bills once she recovers from her coma. If, before *C* wakes up, *S* removes money from the trust fund or completely empties it, then it seems that *S* has *harmed C* insofar as *C* will now be financially worse off than she was before *S* removed the money from the trust fund—in fact, the fund having been designated *ab initio* for *C, S* may in fact be culpable of having "stolen" from *C.* However, *S* is perfectly free to have elected not to set up the trust fund for *C* in the first place. Thus, while *S* arguably is obliged not to remove money from the trust fund once it is established—interrupting the process by which *C* will have money available to her once she awakens from her coma—*S* is under no obligation to establish the trust fund for *C.*

Tooley's moral symmetry principle thus provides a proper mode of analysis for certain types of cases, but not others. Furthermore, when the principle does apply, the symmetry is due to some more foundational moral principle or value; the symmetry principle itself does not function *normatively* to help one arrive at the proper moral evaluation, as Tooley intends it to do.

If my contention regarding the restricted applicability of the moral symmetry principle holds, then I may justifiably assert my second point—namely, that the *reductio* does not follow in Tooley's "kitten" thought experiment. *My* intuition—reasonably assumed to be shared by others—is that there is a moral distinction between killing an already injected kitten or administering a counteragent and refraining from injecting a kitten in the first place, regardless of whether or not the latter kitten is killed.[23] The moral symmetry principle does not accurately describe my intuition about this case and does not provide any normative reasons to challenge this intuition. The same goes for the type of case under debate for which the thought experiment is an analogue: there is a moral distinction between interfering with a human embryo or fetus's development into an actually self-conscious rational person and refraining from procreative activity.

Tooley's thought experiment putatively counters what he terms the "biologically restricted" or "modified" potentiality principle, which limits the applicability of the argument from potential to already existing biological organisms. Tooley (1983, 178–79; 1998, 223–25) argues that this principle implies what he terms the "unrestricted" or "generalized" potentiality principle, which applies also to any "entity or system of entities" that may give rise to a person. The latter principle would entail that, if the argument from potential holds, it would be morally impermissible to turn off a machine that, once turned on, would carry a large number of sperm via a conveyor belt to an ovum inside an artificial womb where, if fertilization takes place, gestation would follow with the birth of an infant nine months later—no further human intervention being required.

Tooley neglects to take into account the *identity criterion* utilized above to distinguish how the active/passive potentiality distinction is applied in different cases. There is no reasonable warrant to extend the moral regard that putatively applies to *actually existing entities* to *systems* that may produce such entities. Tooley is conflating a potential person—or person with potential, in my view—with a *possible* person (Pahel 1987, 98). Sperm and ovum may each possibly help give rise to a person if fertilization occurs because the system that brings them together proceeds uninterrupted, but an embryo or fetus is already a person under development with no further system—other than a supportive nutritive environment—being required to allow its intrinsic potentiality to be eventually actualized.

Tooley attempts to provide reasonable warrant for extending moral regard to systems that may produce a person. He devises a "thought experiment" in which a woman may undergo a "two-step abortion": first, her womb is irradiated so that the embryo becomes a frog embryo; second, the frog embryo is aborted. Tooley claims that an anti-abortionist would not accept this two-step process as justifiable and thereby would accept the above generalization to the moral equivalence of "systems" by means of which a person may come into existence or, in the thought experiment, to be killed. Tooley's thought experiment takes the two-step process, or system, as the *object* of moral evaluation by the anti-abortionist. But, as Tooley notes, aborting a frog embryo is not generally considered morally objectionable; hence, the proper object of the anti-abortionist's negative moral evaluation must be the *irradiation* of the human embryo that destroys its active potentiality for self-conscious rational thought. In other words, destroying a human embryo's active potentiality for self-conscious rational thought actually constitutes an act of abortion, regardless of whether it is brought about through irradiation, genetic manipulation, or physical disaggregation; whatever is done with the frog embryo that results is a completely separate issue that merits its own moral evaluation. Hence, an anti-abortionist need not accept the *generalized* version of the potentiality principle and the absurd consequences that seem to follow.[24]

In Vitro versus In Utero Embryos[25]

R. Alta Charo (2001) raises the question of whether the potentiality of an embryo or fetus *in utero* differs in relevant respects from that of an embryo *in vitro*, which must be implanted in a supportive uterine environment if its development is to continue beyond the first week of cell division:

> A fertilized egg or early embryo in a petri dish most certainly has an intrinsic tendency to continue growing and dividing. Without the provision of an artificial culture medium, however, it will never grow and divide more than about 1 week. If the provision of such a medium is considered a form of external assistance akin to that at issue in passive potentiality, then the fertilized egg is a potential week-old embryo, not a potential baby. (Charo 2001, 86)[26]

Contra Charo, the discretionary provision of a uterus or artificial culture medium is not "a form of external assistance akin to that at issue in passive potentiality." Though obviously a form of external assistance, what the agent provides is merely a supportive environment for an embryo to exercise its own developmental potential.[27] Uterine implantation or placement into a culture medium does not alter the intrinsic nature of an embryo itself or bestow upon it more inherent potentialities than it already possesses (Gómez-Lobo 2005, 106–7). Responding to the claim that an *in vitro* embryo is merely a "possible" person that could become a person only through the deliberate decision of an external agent to implant it, Reichlin (1997) contends,

> To speak of the potentiality of a being implies affirming something about the *nature* of that being, something about the kind of being it actually is: the biological facts about it cannot be but *a posteriori* confirmations and empirical expressions of an underlying ontological structure. This structure is completely independent of other people's choices: these can prevent an embryo from realizing its inherent potential, but they cannot prevent it from having such potential, that is, they cannot prevent it from being what it is. (Reichlin 1997, 11–12)[28]

John Lizza notes, by reference to a classic analogy utilized in the potentiality debate, that "an acorn . . . eaten by a pig would still have the potential to develop into an oak tree, since we could intervene, remove the acorn, and transplant it into a more conducive environment. We might have good reasons for choosing not to remove the acorn. However, the acorn still has the potential for becoming an oak tree" (Lizza 2005, 49).[29]

The form of external assistance a uterus provides is analogous to an astronaut's spacesuit or an underwater explorer's submarine. Each provides what the person needs to exercise her vital metabolic functions; the lack of such support does not entail that she lacks the relevant potentialities for those functions. If an astronaut's spacesuit malfunctions and stops supplying oxygen, her vital metabolic functions will cease shortly thereafter. If, however, a fellow astronaut fixes her suit in a timely fashion and restores the flow of oxygen, her vital metabolic functions will resume. This indicates that the astronaut's active potentiality for such functions remained despite the temporary loss of the requisite supportive environment.[30] Another relevant example is the incubator most prematurely born infants require to continue their postnatal development. Although such infants cannot survive without the incubator's assistance, their dependence on it does not entail that their potentiality for full development is merely passive and not self-directed.

Thus, the requirement of external assistance to further one's development does not entail that one's potential for such development is merely passive. There is a relevant difference between *mere* external assistance and external *directive* assistance. The former aids a substance to become fully what it already *is* due to its essential nature; the latter directs a substance to change into something it is not yet in such a fashion that its numerical and specific identity is altered through the change. For example, mature human persons require external assistance—namely, a supportive biosphere—in order to exercise their active potentialities relative to living, sensing, and thinking—that is, in order to exist fully as living rational animals; but the biosphere does not alter the essential nature of mature human persons as such. The activity of an *in vitro* fertilization technician, however, in bringing sperm and ovum into union to produce an embryo, is *directive* insofar as the technician is bringing something into existence—an embryo—that had not previously existed and, in the process, causing the individual sperm and ovum to go out of existence through the fertilization process.

I conclude that an *in vitro* embryo's potentiality for development into an actually self-conscious rational person does not preclude its existence as a person already. This is because the potentiality at issue is an active potentiality that is part of the embryo's intrinsic nature:

> An embryo is, by definition and by its nature, potentially a fully developed human person; its potential for maturation is a characteristic it *actually* has, and from the start. The fact that embryos have been created outside their natural

environment—which is to say, outside the woman's body—and are therefore limited in their ability to realize their natural capacities, does not affect either the potential or the moral status of the beings themselves. A bird forced to live in a cage its entire life may never learn to fly. But this does not mean it is less of a bird, or that it lacks the immanent potentiality to fly on feathered wings. It means only that a caged bird—like an in vitro human embryo—has been deprived of its proper environment. (President's Council on Bioethics [PCB] 2002, 156)

This argument may be criticized, however, for proving too much. Charo and others argue that since a person can be cloned from a somatic cell, any such cell that currently constitutes my body is potentially another person (Charo 2001, 86–87; Savulescu 2001, 220; PCB 2002, 148–49; McHugh 2004, 210; Hanson 2006). But this argument fails to apply properly the active/passive potentiality distinction. Many changes, requiring the *directive* activity of an external agent, must accrue to a somatic cell before it can, in the relevant sense, have the potentiality to become a person. First of all, a somatic cell requires extensive reorganization of its internal structure—namely, removal of its nucleus, which is then implanted in an enucleated ovum. Furthermore, as Gómez-Lobo (2004, 203) notes,

the nucleus of a somatic cell, by itself, does not have the potentiality to become an embryo. It is only after the DNA has been reprogrammed thanks to the cytoplasm of an ovum that the crucial potentiality arises. A significant change involving two separate factors has to take place. In other words, we should not confuse the potentiality that an element of a somatic cell has by itself with the potentiality of the cell that has been generated by [cloning]. It is only the latter that can develop into the sort of adult we all agree deserves respect. (Gómez-Lobo 2004, 203)[31]

The primary reason a somatic cell fails to have an active potentiality to develop into a fully actualized person is that the *identity criterion* is violated insofar as the cell must be disaggregated, through enucleation, and only a part of it—the nucleus—be implanted in another already extant cell—the ovum. This entails a *substantial change* in specific and numerical identity for both the somatic cell and the ovum (Guenin 2008, 24–25; Eberl 2006, 81–82; DiSilvestro 2006, 149–50; Hershenov 1999, 265). Michael Burke (1996) affirms this conclusion by contending that a somatic cell cannot be considered to be of the same *natural kind* as an embryo insofar as the latter, but not the former, is an animal—an organism:

An ordinary (undoctored, uncultured) body cell is not an animal. But since animals are *essentially* animals, *non*animals are essentially *non*animals. This means that an ordinary body cell could not survive changes that would make it, if it survived, an animal. So there is no identity across time between an ordinary body cell and any animal that develops from it. Therefore, an ordinary body cell has no strong *potential* to become an animal and, *a fortiori*, none to become a *rational* animal. (Burke 1996, 504–5)[32]

Burke further contends,

> In general, it is reasonable to say that in order for an entity to be an embryonic animal, the entity must be able, given a favorable environment (of the sort natural to the species in question), *but without prior reorganization*, to undergo embryo-logical development, that is, to commence or continue developing into a mature animal [emphasis mine]. (Burke 1996, 509)

Additionally, to countenance the possibility that a somatic cell has the same potentiality as an embryo to become a fully actualized human person is to presume that it is *already* a human person. This presumption is implausible because a somatic cell that is *part* of a human person cannot itself be such an entity (Burke 1996, 510).[33] All parts of a person's body are proper parts of her and not substances in their own right, unless they become separated from the body.[34] Since a somatic cell is not a substance in itself, but only part of a substance, it cannot be a person; nor does it have an active potentiality for further self-directed development into a fully actualized person. As Robert George and Christopher Tollefsen conclude, "Somatic cells that may be used in cloning are not analogous to embryos but to gametes":

> Functionally, they are parts of other human beings. They are not distinct, complete, self-integrating organisms. They are not members of the species *Homo sapiens*. But human embryos, by whatever method they are generated, are. (George and Tollefsen 2008, 187)[35]

A cloned embryo is not a proper part of a person—particularly since it is produced *in vitro*—and thus nothing precludes it from being a person with an active potentiality for further development as such. To compare a cloned embryo's potentiality to that of a somatic cell is illegitimate insofar as there are metaphysical reasons why a somatic cell, unlike a cloned embryo, lacks an active potentiality to develop into a fully actualized person (Lee and George 2008, 129–30).

Potentiality and Moral Value

There are various strategies to establish the inherent moral value of an embryo or fetus by virtue of its active potentiality to develop a capacity in hand for self-conscious rational thought (e.g., Williams 2008; DiSilvestro 2005; Poplawski and Gillett 1991). In keeping with the Thomistic viewpoint I have elucidated here, I will adopt a broadly construed *natural-law* ethic, which recognizes the intrinsic value of various types of beings by reference to their essential capacities and, by extension, the active potentiality to develop such capacities in hand. As Jim Stone concludes,

> Nature, good, and identity are intimately related. An animal's nature determines a developmental path which guarantees identity, a path that produces the animal's adult stage. In human animals, that stage involves the attainment of conscious goods, which are produced by the nature as it actualizes itself along an identity-preserving path that evolved because it produces those goods. Nature, good, and identity each determine the other, each is an aspect of the other; they are bound in unity. What the fetus *is* finally, is something that makes *itself* self-aware; that good is the fetus's good—this is its nature. Anything benefits from the good which it is its nature to make for itself. I submit that we have a prima facie duty to all creatures not to deprive them of the conscious goods which it is their nature to realize. (Stone 1987, 821)[36]

It is worth noting that Stone's conclusion does not depend on whether an embryo or fetus is a person; nevertheless, if an embryo or fetus has the ontological status of a person, it is certainly arguable that it should be regarded as having the moral status of a person as well.

The moral conclusion, however, does not immediately follow from the ontological conclusion. According to Brown (2008, 602), an active potentiality for self-conscious rational thought becomes relevant only when it is present by virtue of a functioning human brain. This is based on the contention that psychological properties are necessary for someone to possess *interests* that ground the rights they should be recognized to possess (DeGrazia 2008, 305–6). Tooley (1983, 151) also denies that fully actualized persons possess the moral rights they do by virtue of their ontological constitution, but rather by virtue of certain psychological states that allow them to have *desires*, the fulfillment of which rights are designed to protect. Jeff McMahan (2002, 307), in contrast, allows that a late-term fetus, which is not yet actually self-conscious and rational, but has developed a cerebrum capable of at least some degree of consciousness and further development into a self-conscious rational person, may be understood as possessing an interest—albeit a weak "time-relative" interest—in its own further development into a person.[37] Unfortunately, I cannot delve into a more extensive discussion here of the moral relevance of an entity's possessing an active potentiality to develop itself into an actually self-conscious rational person, except to contend that *at minimum* such an entity merits consideration as the object of a *prima facie* moral obligation not to kill it or deprive it of the goods that it may reasonably be expected to come to possess absent external interference with its natural, self-directed development. As Don Marquis (1989) argues, the same principle that grounds the wrongness of killing an adult human being—namely, loss of an objectively valuable future—renders abortion impermissible since an embryo or fetus also possesses an objectively valuable future insofar as it is numerically identical to an adult human person who will actually have such experiences. There may also be a positive prima facie moral obligation to assist such an entity's development by providing it with a supportive environment and removing any impediments to the actualization of its active potentialities.[38] Whether the negative moral obligation rises to the level of grounding an *inviolable right* or should be weighed against other competing moral values merits a separate discussion.[39]

NOTES

1. Another way this issue is often couched is in terms of whether embryos and fetuses count as "human beings" or "potential human beings." In this essay, I address the issue in terms of *personhood* rather than *humanity* insofar as the former concept unambiguously refers to a being with a high degree of–if not an inviolable–moral status with attendant basic rights, such as the right to life. The latter concept, in contrast, is debated as to whether it inherently refers to a being that merits a different level of moral regard than other species of living, sentient animals; consider, for example, Peter Singer's (1975) famous charge of "speciesism." Eschewing a debate here of the relative merits of Singer's argument, I will accept for the sake of discussion that being "human" does not automatically confer an inviolable right to life, although it would if it is the case that all human beings are persons. For a counterpoint concerning the ontological and moral status of a "non-person human being," see Brown 2008.

2. From here on, the modifier "human" will be understood.

3. This argument differs also from the argument based on *probability* found in Noonan (1970).

4. There is no settled list of which activities–or, more generally speaking, properties–are definitive of personhood. The earliest philosophical definition of personhood comes from Boethius (1918, sec. 3), who defines a person as an "individual substance of a rational nature." John Locke (1975, bk. II, ch. 27, sec. 9) offers an alternative definition of a person as "a thinking intelligent Being, that has reason and reflection, and can consider itself as itself, the same thinking thing in different times and places." Contemporary philosophers have perpetuated the thesis that a person is any being that exhibits *a capacity for self-conscious rational thought*, augmented perhaps by other capacities, such as using language to communicate, having nonmomentary self-interests, and possessing moral agency or autonomy (e.g., Singer 1992, 84; Warren 1973, 55; Tooley 1983, 146; Baker 2005). These various ways of defining personhood are not inherently contrary to each other, since they all include the criterion of either *rationality* or *self-consciousness*, such that any being who possesses the capacity for both would undoubtedly qualify as a person. Thomas Aquinas (1996, prop. 15), for example, implicitly augments the Boethian definition to include self-consciousness when he refers to the human intellect having the capacity to "turn upon" and "know itself."

5. By "fully actualized person," I do not intend to refer to a *perfect* person—one who has no unactualized potentialities; certainly no person, other than God as defined in classical theism, fits that criterion. Rather, I mean an individual who has actualized the definitive potentialities associated with self-conscious rational thought such that she unquestionably counts as a person.

6. The qualification that an embryo or fetus preserves its *numerical identity* as it develops is crucial insofar as I understand personhood to be a *substance sortal*, meaning that an entity is a person *essentially* and thus cannot become or cease to be a person without becoming a numerically distinct entity. The contrary view is that personhood is a *phase sortal*, referring to a mode of existence that an entity can begin or cease while remaining the numerically same entity, like being a father or a professor (Olson 1997, 30). For elucidation of the distinction between substance and phase sortals, see Wiggins 1980.

7. This section and the following include material derived from Eberl 2008 and 2005.

8. I derive the concept of a "design environment" from Alvin Plantinga's (1993, ch. 2) concept of something fulfilling its *proper function*, according to its *design plan*, in an *appropriate environment*. This concept coheres with Aristotelian-Thomistic ontology insofar as the way in which Aristotle defines a substance's essential nature makes reference to how the substance is *teleologically* oriented to actualize its definitive set of proper potentialities in an environment which is suited for the actualization of such potentialities.

9. The term *substantial form* refers to the essential configuration of a material substance that includes the set of properties that define the substance's essential nature as individuated by the form inhering in a particular quantity of designated matter, such that a change of substantial form would entail a change in numerical identity and perhaps also a change in its species membership. In contrast, an accidental form, such as "being red," defines a way in which a thing may or may not be without altering its essential nature or changing its numerical identity. The concept of substantial form includes both the *universal* set of essential properties that are shared by all individual members of the same natural kind, and the *individuated* set of properties that inhere in a particular material substance. Once individuated, a particular substance's substantial form grounds its persistent diachronic identity. Typically, the substantial form of a human person informs a material body that is suitable for actualizing the soul's definitive potentialities for life, sentience, and self-conscious rational thought. However, it may suffice for a human person to persist if his or her soul informs a material body, such as a cerebrum, that suffices only for the last category of potentiality to be realized insofar as the potentiality for self-conscious rational thought marks the "specific difference" between human persons and all other sentient animals. For further discussion of the individuation of the substantial form of human persons and the persistent identity of a person by virtue of the individual's substantial form, see Eberl 2004, 347–59. For further discussion of cerebrum-transplant thought experiments through the lens of the same ontological viewpoint adopted in this paper, see Hershenov 2008.

10. For further elucidation of this distinction in types of active potentiality, sometimes construed as "proximate" vs. "remote" active potentiality, see Lee and George 2008, 136–38; Lee 1996, 28n33; Gómez-Lobo 2005, 109; Schwarz 1998, 265–66; Reichlin 1997, 15; Joyce 1978, 99–100; Wade 1975, 249.

11. By "specific and numerical identity," I mean that something not only ceases to be the same *individual* but also the same *kind* of thing. For example, something changes from being a nonperson to being a person.

12. See also Warren 1997, 206–7; Bigelow and Pargetter 1988, 177. Lockwood's assertion would stand if one held mereological composition to be "unrestricted." In the present context, I stipulate a restricted notion of composition premised on the Aristotelian view that certain natural ontological kinds, such as "animal," cannot exist as "scattered objects." For discussion of the ontological status of embryos and fetuses given unrestricted mereological composition, see Hudson 2001, 151–58.

13. Jeff McMahan (2002, 304–5) also draws an explicit distinction between "identity-preserving" and "nonidentity" potential, applying the latter to the case of a sperm or ovum. McMahan further denies identity-preserving potential to an embryo or early-term fetus that has yet to develop a cerebrum capable of at least some degree of consciousness. This conclusion, however, depends upon his ontological account of human persons as "embodied minds," which fundamentally differs from the Aristotelian-Thomistic account of human nature I advocate here; see Eberl 2004. Space does not permit me to provide a detailed comparative analysis of these two ontological views.

14. For a similar argument based on the concept of "sortal essentialism," see Burke 1996.

15. See Aquinas 1948, 1a, q. 118, a. 1 *ad* 4; Aquinas 1984, a. 13; Kretzmann 1999, 379n27.

16. See Lee 2004, 252–53.

17. Aristotle defines four causes of any being. The *material cause* is the matter that composes it, that out of which it is produced. The *formal cause* is the substantial or accidental form that defines it as the type of thing it is. The *efficient cause* is the agent or activity that instantiates the form in the matter, that which produces the thing. The *final cause* is the end or purpose for which the thing is produced. See Aristotle 1984b, bk. II, ch. 3, 194b24–195a3.

18. Clarifications are in order regarding the term *conception*. First, in reference to the typical process of *fertilization*, there is some debate concerning when in this 24-hour-long process the beginning of an embryo's existence, in the form of the monocellular zygote, should be pinpointed. Ronald Hamel and Michael Panicola (2004, 238) assert that syngamy–when the 23 maternal chromosomes line up with the 23 paternal chromosomes—would be the best candidate insofar as that is when the zygote first exists as a single totipotent cell with a diploid human genome. This view is challenged by Maureen Condic (2009). For further elucidation of the fertilization process relative to the question of when a human person begins to exist, see George and Tollefsen (2008, 36–42). Second, there are at least three alternative ways through which an embryo may be brought into existence that do not involve the fusion of sperm and ovum: parthenogenesis, monozygotic twinning, and cloning through somatic cell nuclear transfer. I will thus adopt a conceptually expansive definition of "conception," following Oderberg (1997, 293): "Conception is that event, typically involving the union of sperm and egg, which consists in a change in the intrinsic nature of a cell or group of cells, where that change confers on the cell (or its descendants in the case of division) the intrinsic potential to develop, given the right extrinsic factors, into a mature human being." *Parthenotes* are embryos produced through induced mitosis of an unfertilized ovum with concomitant doubling of its 23 chromosomes–by injecting the nucleus of another ovum

with its own set of 23 chromosomes–to produce a diploid genome without any contribution from the male gamete. For claims and arguments that at least certain types of parthenotes should count as persons due to their intrinsic developmental potential, see Huarte and Suarez 2004.

19. In addition to distinguishing active from passive potentiality, Tooley (1983, 167) adds the in-between concept of "latent" potentiality, in which an entity possesses all the positive causal factors needed for it to acquire some property, but there is some internal inhibitor that blocks the action of such factors.

20. My conclusion regarding this thought experiment differs from Kenneth Pahel (1987, 103–5), who contends that a kitten does not bear the same *natural right* to develop into a person as a human fetus does due to its being of a distinct natural kind whose intrinsic *telos* is to develop into a mature cat, not a mature person. Rather, I concur with Katherin Rogers (1992, 250–51), who contends that an injected kitten has become a distinct entity altogether from the kitten before the injection, although they share some characteristics in common: The essential nature of felines precludes possessing or developing an active potentiality for self-conscious rational thought. Of course, there is *material continuity* between the kitten before and after the injection, as well as continuity of various subrational cognitive and vegetative processes. Nevertheless, coming to possess an active potentiality for self-conscious rational thought results in an *ontological* change from the kind "non-rational animal" to the kind "rational animal/person" (Eberl and Ballard 2009).

21. Note that I neither advocate nor disallow the applicability of utilitarian considerations to this type of case but merely put them to the side, as there are many bioethicists who explicitly eschew such considerations.

22. I owe this example to David Hershenov (pers. comm.).

23. I agree with Elizabeth Harman (2003, 188–89) that interference with the injected kitten could justifiably occur until the serum has "sufficiently interacted" with the kitten's own cells and tissues.

24. I agree with Tooley (1983, 180), however, that the *biologically* restricted version of the potentiality principle may be too restrictive insofar as not only nonhuman (such as Tooley's kitten) but also nonbiological entities (such as artificially intelligent androids) may be created that possess an active potentiality for self-conscious rational thought. For an analogous discussion concerning animal-human chimeric embryos, see Eberl and Ballard 2009. Such nonhuman or nonbiological entities still qualify, though, as *individual substances* of a classic Aristotelian sort and thereby are understood to be informed by the relevant substantial form. *Systems* do not qualify as such.

25. This subsection is derived from Eberl and Brown 2011.

26. See also Mahowald 2004, 210; Singer and Dawson 1990, 87.

27. It is the case that epigenetic factors from the mother can differentially influence genetic expression as the embryo develops; however, such factors do not affect the embryo's possession of the genes, which may be subject to expression in various ways. I thank Al Howsepian (pers. comm.) for raising this point to me.

28. Reichlin is responding to Tauer (1985, 264). It is worth noting in this context that, given that the intentions of external agents are irrelevant to a being's intrinsic potentiality, there is no distinction in potentiality between embryos created solely for research purposes (e.g., to derive human embryonic stem cells) and those created initially for reproductive

purposes that were never utilized and are thus considered "spare" (Agar 2007, 204; Devolder 2005, 180).

29. Lizza (2005, 49) goes on to assert, though, that the acorn's potentiality in this case is "remote," unlike the more "proximate" potentiality of an acorn planted in the earth.

30. Could one counter that the astronaut's dependence on her fellow astronaut's assistance in restoring her supportive environment implies that her potentiality for being alive is merely *passive*? No, because the assistance provided does nothing to alter or replace the astronaut's organic structure by which she is able to breathe in and circulate oxygen once it is made available to her again.

31. See also Brown 2008, 616n6; Rogers 1992, 250.

32. It is important to note that Burke's argument against a somatic cell having the same potentiality as an embryo rests on conceiving the embryo as an "animal," not necessarily as a *human* animal or person. Thus (*pace* Oderberg 1997, 263) Burke does not beg the question at hand of the embryo's ontological and moral status.

33. As Russell DiSilvestro (2006, 150–51) notes, there is a relevant distinction between the term *human* functioning in the "stuff sense" and in the "count sense." The former applies to the proper parts of a human person, including each of her somatic cells, while the latter refers to the person herself. This same conclusion would apply, *contra* Brown (2007, 607–8), to the totipotent cells composing an embryo in its earliest stages of development (Oderberg 1997, 280).

34. A somatic cell that has been separated from a person's body is not a proper part of her as it is no longer informed by her substantial form; it has its own substantial form. Such a cell, though, could not be considered to have the same potentiality as a cloned embryo either, because it is not *totipotential*. External intervention is required to enucleate the cell and implant its nucleus into an enucleated ovum in order for a person to be produced from it. As noted above, this process alters the cell's specific and numerical identity. Therefore, there are no grounds for asserting that a somatic cell that has been separated from its body and may be enucleated for the purpose of generating a cloned person has in itself an active potentiality to become a fully actualized person.

35. See also Oderberg 1997, 292.

36. Stone does not explicitly label his moral conclusion as falling under "natural-law" theory, but I find it to be at least commensurate with such an ethic as described in Eberl 2006, 9–16. Roy Perrett (2000, 192–93) criticizes this argumentative strategy by stating that natural-law theorists have failed to deliver the goods, so to speak, with respect to the question of why we ought not to interfere with a being's natural development. Space does not permit me to mount a full-fledged defense of natural-law theory, but I call attention to a few key formulations and defenses of classical natural-law theory to cast doubt on Perrett's global negative assessment: Finnis 1980; Lisska 1996.

37. For a critical response, see Liao 2007.

38. Such a positive obligation arguably includes "rescuing" frozen embryos created through *in vitro* fertilization, and no longer needed by their genetic parents, by means of prenatal *adoption* (Brown and Eberl 2007).

39. I wish to thank Brandon Brown, Michael Burke, Russell DiSilvestro, Michael Gorman, David Hershenov, Al Howsepian, Christopher Kaczor, John Lizza, and Christopher Tollefsen for helpful comments on an earlier draft of this essay.

REFERENCES

Agar, N. 2007. Embryonic potential and stem cells. *Bioethics* 21:198–207.

Aquinas, T. 1948. *Summa theologiae.* English Dominican Fathers (trans.). New York: Benziger.

———. 1950. *In duodecim libros metaphysicorum Aristotelis expositio.* R. Cathala and R. Spiazzi (eds.). Turin: Marietti.

———. 1984. *Quaestio disputata de anima.* J. Robb (trans.). Milwaukee: Marquette University Press.

———. 1996. *Commentary on the Book of Causes.* V. A. Guagliardo, C. R. Hess, and R. C. Taylor (trans.). Washington, DC: Catholic University of America Press.

Aristotle. 1984a. *De generatione animalium.* In J. Barnes (ed.), *The Complete Works of Aristotle.* Princeton, NJ: Princeton University Press.

———. 1984b. *Physics.* In J. Barnes (ed.), *The Complete Works of Aristotle.* Princeton, NJ: Princeton University Press.

Baker, L. R. 2005. When does a person begin? *Social Philosophy and Policy* 22:25–48.

Beauchamp, T. L., and Childress, J. F. 2009. *Principles of Biomedical Ethics.* 6th ed. New York: Oxford University Press.

Benn, S. 1984. Abortion, infanticide, and respect for persons. In J. Feinberg (ed.), *The Problem of Abortion*, 135–44. 2nd ed. Belmont, CA: Wadsworth.

Bigelow, J., and Pargetter, R. 1988. Morality, potential persons and abortion. *American Philosophical Quarterly* 25:173–81.

Boethius. 1918. Contra eutychen et nestorium. In H. F. Stewart, E. K. Rand, and S. J. Tester (trans.), *Tractates and the Consolation of Philosophy*, 72–129. Cambridge: Harvard University Press.

Brown, B. P. 2008. *Ergon* and the embryo. MA thesis, Indiana University–Purdue University, Indianapolis.

———, and Eberl, J. T. 2007. Ethical considerations in defense of embryo adoption. In S. Brakman and D. F. Weaver (eds.), *The Ethics of Embryo Adoption and the Catholic Tradition*, 103–18. Dordrecht: Springer.

Buckle, S. 1988. Arguing from potential. *Bioethics* 2:227–53.

Burke, M. B. 1996. Sortal essentialism and the potentiality principle. *Review of Metaphysics* 49:491–514.

Charo, R. A. 2001. Every cell is sacred: Logical consequences of the argument from potential in the age of cloning. In P. Lauritzen (ed.), *Cloning and the Future of Human Embryo Research*, 82–89. New York: Oxford University Press.

Chomsky, N. 1968. *Language and Mind.* New York: Harcourt, Brace & World.

Condic, M. 2009. When does human life begin? A scientific perspective. *National Catholic Bioethics Quarterly* 9:141–43.

Covey, E. 1991. Physical possibility and potentiality in ethics. *American Philosophical Quarterly* 28:237–44.

DeGrazia, D. 2008. Must we have full moral status throughout our existence? A reply to Alfonso Gómez-Lobo. *Kennedy Institute of Ethics Journal* 17:297–310.

Devolder, K. 2005. Human embryonic stem cell research: Why the discarded-created-distinction cannot be based on the potentiality argument. *Bioethics* 19:167–86.

DiSilvestro, R. 2005. Human embryos in the original position? *Journal of Medicine and Philosophy* 30:285–304.

———. 2006. Not every cell is sacred: A reply to Charo. *Bioethics* 20:146–57.

Eberl, J. T. 2004. Aquinas on the nature of human beings. *Review of Metaphysics* 58:333–65.

———. 2005. Aquinas's account of human embryogenesis and recent interpretations. *Journal of Medicine and Philosophy* 30:379–94.

———. 2006. *Thomistic Principles and Bioethics.* New York: Routledge.

———. 2008. Potentiality, possibility, and the irreversibility of death. *Review of Metaphysics* 62:61–77.

———, and Ballard, R. A. 2009. Metaphysical and ethical perspectives on creating animal-human chimeras. *Journal of Medicine and Philosophy* 34:470–86.

———, and Brown, B. P. 2011. Brain life and the argument from potential: Affirming the ontological status of human embryos and fetuses. In S. Napier (ed.), *Persons, Moral Worth, and Embryos,* 43–65. Dordrecht: Springer.

Feinberg, J. 1986. Abortion. In T. Regan (ed.), *Matters of Life and Death: New Introductory Essays in Moral Philosophy,* 256–93. 2nd ed. New York: Random House.

Finnis, J. 1980. *Natural Law and Natural Rights.* Oxford: Clarendon Press.

———. 2006. Abortion and health care ethics. In H. Kuhse and P. Singer (eds.), *Bioethics: An Anthology,* 17–24. 2nd ed. Oxford: Blackwell.

Ford, N. M. 1988. *When Did I Begin? Conception of the Human Individual in History, Philosophy and Science.* New York: Cambridge University Press.

George, R. P., and Tollefsen, C. 2008. *Embryo: A Defense of Human Life.* New York: Doubleday.

Gómez-Lobo, A. 2004. Does respect for embryos entail respect for gametes? *Theoretical Medicine and Bioethics* 25:199–208.

———. 2005. On potentiality and respect for embryos: A reply to Mary Mahowald. *Theoretical Medicine and Bioethics* 26:105–10.

Guenin, L. M. 2008. *The Morality of Embryo Use.* New York: Cambridge University Press.

Hamel, R., and Panicola, M. R. 2004. Emergency contraception revisited: A response to Eugene Diamond. *National Catholic Bioethics Quarterly* 4:236–39.

Hanson, S. S. 2006. More on respect for embryos and potentiality: Does respect for embryos entail respect for *in vitro* embryos? *Theoretical Medicine and Bioethics* 27:215–26.

Harman, E. 2003. The potentiality problem. *Philosophical Studies* 114:173–98.

Hershenov, D. B. 1999. The problem of potentiality. *Public Affairs Quarterly* 13:255–71.

———. 2008. A hylomorphic account of thought experiments concerning personal identity. *American Catholic Philosophical Quarterly* 82:481–502.

Huarte, J., and Suarez, A. 2004. On the status of parthenotes: Defining the developmental potential of a human embryo. *National Catholic Bioethics Quarterly* 4:755–70.

Hudson, H. 2001. *A Materialist Metaphysics of the Human Person.* Ithaca, NY: Cornell University Press.

Joyce, R. E. 1978. Personhood and the conception event. *The New Scholasticism* 52:97–109.

Kretzmann, N. 1999. *The Metaphysics of Creation: Aquinas's Natural Theology in Summa contra Gentiles,* vol. 2. Oxford: Clarendon Press.

Larmer, R. 1995. Abortion, personhood and the potential for consciousness. *Journal of Applied Philosophy* 12:241–51.

Lee, P. 1996. *Abortion and Unborn Human Life*. Washington, DC: Catholic University of America Press.

———. 2004. The pro-life argument from substantial identity: A defence. *Bioethics* 18:249–63.

———, and George, R. P. 2008. *Body-Self Dualism in Contemporary Ethics and Politics*. New York: Cambridge University Press.

Liao, S. M. 2007. Time-relative interests and abortion. *Journal of Medicine and Philosophy* 4:242–56.

Lisska, A. 1996. *Aquinas's Natural Law Theory: An Analytic Reconstruction*. Oxford: Clarendon Press.

Lizza, J. P. 2005. Potentiality, irreversibility, and death. *Journal of Medicine and Philosophy* 30:45–64.

Locke, J. 1975. *An Essay Concerning Human Understanding*. P. H. Nidditch (ed.). New York: Oxford University Press.

Lockwood, M. 1988. Warnock versus Powell (and Harradine): When does potentiality count? *Bioethics* 2:187–213.

Mahowald, M. B. 2004. Respect for embryos and the potentiality argument. *Theoretical Medicine and Bioethics* 25:209–14.

Marquis, D. 1989. Why abortion is immoral. *Journal of Philosophy* 86:183–202.

McHugh, P. R. 2004. Zygote and "clonote": The ethical use of embryonic stem cells. *New England Journal of Medicine* 351:209–11.

McMahan, J. 2002. *The Ethics of Killing: Problems at the Margins of Life*. New York: Oxford University Press.

Noonan, Jr., J. T., 1970. An almost absolute value in history. In Noonan, Jr., J. T. (ed.), *The Morality of Abortion: Legal and Historical Perspectives*, 51–59. Cambridge: Harvard University Press.

Oderberg, D. S. 1997. Modal properties, moral status, and identity. *Philosophy and Public Affairs* 26:259–76.

Olson, E. T. 1997. *The Human Animal: Personal Identity without Psychology*. New York: Oxford University Press.

Pahel, K. 1987. Michael Tooley on abortion and potentiality. *Southern Journal of Philosophy* 25:89–107.

Pasnau, R. 2002. *Thomas Aquinas on Human Nature*. New York: Cambridge University Press.

Perrett, R. W. 2000. Taking life and the argument from potentiality. *Midwest Studies in Philosophy* 24:186–97.

Pinker, S. 1994. *The Language Instinct*. New York: Harper Collins.

Plantinga, A. 1993. *Warrant and Proper Function*. New York: Oxford University Press.

Poplawski, N., and Gillett, G. 1991. Ethics and embryos. *Journal of Medical Ethics* 17:62–99.

President's Council on Bioethics. 2002. *Human Cloning and Human Dignity: An Ethical Inquiry*. www.bioethics.georgetown.edu/pcbe/reports/cloningreport.

Reichlin, M. 1997. The argument from potential: A reappraisal. *Bioethics* 11:1–23.

Rogers, K. A. 1992. Personhood, potentiality, and the temporarily comatose patient. *Public Affairs Quarterly* 6:245–54.

Savulescu, J. 2001. Should we clone human beings? Cloning as a source of tissue transplantation. In M. Ruse and A. Sheppard (eds.), *Cloning: Responsible Science or Technomadness?* Amherst, NY: Prometheus Books.

Schwarz, S. 1998. Personhood begins at conception. In L. P. Pojman and F. J. Beckwith (eds.), *The Abortion Controversy 25 Years after* Roe v. Wade*: A Reader*, 257–73. Belmont, CA: Wadsworth.

Singer, P. 1975. *Animal Liberation*. New York: Random House.

———. 1992. Embryo experimentation and the moral status of the embryo. In E. Matthews and M. Menlowe (eds.), *Philosophy and Health Care*, 81–91. Brookfield, VT: Avebury Publishing.

———, and Dawson, K. 1990. IVF technology and the argument from potential. In P. Singer, H. Kuhse, S. Buckle, K. Dawson, and P. Kasimba (eds.), *Embryo Experimentation: Ethical, Legal and Social Issues*, 76–89. New York: Cambridge University Press.

Stone, J. 1987. Why potentiality matters. *Canadian Journal of Philosophy* 17:815–30.

Stump, E. 2003. *Aquinas*. New York: Routledge.

Tauer, C. A. 1985. Personhood and human embryos and fetuses. *Journal of Medicine and Philosophy* 10:253–66.

Tooley, M. 1983. *Abortion and Infanticide*. New York: Oxford University Press.

———. 1998. In defense of abortion and infanticide. In L. P. Pojman and F. J. Beckwith (eds.), *The Abortion Controversy 25 Years after* Roe v. Wade*: A Reader*. Belmont, CA: Wadsworth.

van Inwagen, P. 1990. *Material Beings*. Ithaca, NY: Cornell University Press.

Wade, F. C. 1975. Potentiality in the abortion discussion. *Review of Metaphysics* 29:239–55.

Warren, M. A. 1973. On the moral and legal status of abortion. *Monist* 57:43–61.

———. 1997. *Moral Status: Obligations to Persons and Other Living Things*. New York: Oxford University Press.

Wiggins, D. 1980. *Sameness and Substance*. Cambridge: Harvard University Press.

Williams, R. 2008. Abortion, potential, and value. *Utilitas* 20:169–86.

Witt, C. 1995. Powers and possibilities: Aristotle vs. the Megarians. *Proceedings of the Boston Area Colloquium in Ancient Philosophy* 11:249–66.

CHAPTER SEVEN

The Moral Status of Stem Cells

AGATA SAGAN AND PETER SINGER

1. Introduction

Most ethical objections to the use of stem cells are directed at the use of human embryonic stem cells—in particular, at the destruction of human embryos in order to obtain these cells. In an attempt to deflect these objections, some have proposed ways of obtaining cells that have the properties of embryonic stem cells but do not involve destroying embryos. One of these techniques involves taking a single cell from an embryo and using it to generate an embryonic stem cell line, while the embryo can continue to develop unaffected by the removal of the cell (Lanza et al. 2006). Another technique is to take cells from an embryo that we know will cease to develop soon—and so is in a kind of dying state anyway (Landry and Zucker 2004). A third proposal is to create defective embryos—for example, ones that cannot form a placenta and so would never develop into adults—and take cells from them (Hurlbut 2004). A fourth is to induce parthenogenesis, so that an egg begins to develop without any sperm and cells can be removed (Huang et al. 2003). A fifth proposal is to reverse the potency of more mature cells so that they revert to the same state as embryonic stem cells (Melton et al. 2005).

These proposals have been criticized. Some question whether the effort put into developing these alternative methods is worthwhile and raise questions about how much use they are likely to be (National Institutes of Health NIH Stem Cell Task Force 2005; Coalition for the Advancement of Medical Research Dedicated to Advancing Stem Cell Research, n.d.). Leaving aside for now the issue of whether those methods really avoid the destruction of embryos, we want to ask a different question: Is the destruction of embryos really the key ethical issue concerning the use of human embryonic stem cells?

Embryonic stem cells are mainly derived from the inner cell mass of the embryo, from which the later stages of a human being develop. (The remainder of the embryo contributes to the development of the placenta.) This inner cell mass can, if moved to another trophoblast, develop into an adult. Do these cells perhaps have some moral status themselves, independently of the status of the embryo of which they once formed a part? This last question is not usually asked, because embryonic stem cells are equated with other cells that have no special moral status (American Association for Advancement of Science and Institute for Civil Society 1999, 11–12). Nevertheless, there are some who have put forward such views, among them Julian Savulescu and Ronald Bailey, and opponents of the use of embryonic stem cells have responded to them (Savulescu 1999; Bailey 2001a, 2001b; Lee and George 2001a, 2001b). We will try to go further into this issue. To set the stage for that discussion, we need to give closer attention to the nature of embryos and to the question of what human entities can develop into a mature human being. Once we have done this, we will consider to what moral status these human entities are entitled.

2. The Beginnings of Human Life
2.1. The Definition of the Embryo

The standard sense of the term *embryo,* in reference to mammals, is usually understood to refer to the entity resulting from the fertilization of the egg by the sperm, creating the zygote, until around the time organs begin to form. Once the organs begin to form, the developing entity is usually referred to as a *fetus* until it is born, although sometimes the term *embryo* is retained and *fetus* is understood merely as the name of a particular stage of development of the embryo. For a time, it was common to refer to the embryo prior to implantation as a *pre-implantation embryo,* or, for short, *preembryo.* The latter term never gained general acceptance, however, perhaps because opponents of embryo experimentation thought of it as a specious attempt to deny that an embryo exists from the moment of fertilization.

The term *embryo* is used in relation not only to mammals but also to other animals or even plants and can be used metaphorically to describe any initial stage of a development. Such uses are questionable. More significant, for our purpose, is the opposite phenomenon that the absence of a potential to develop does not negate the fact that an entity is an embryo. Although the very concept of something being an embryo suggests that it has the capacity to or is likely to develop into some more mature stage or adult form, in practice the term is also applied to entities that— perhaps because of some defect or because they have developed in the fallopian tube rather than in the uterus—have no possibility of developing to maturity. It seems that the term is used to refer to any member of the class of entities that would, when normal and in appropriate circumstances, develop to the mature stage. Until recently, it has been only in extreme cases, when the entity is severely abnormal—for example, when it is a chaotic mass of cells resembling a teratoma—that there has been any uncertainty about whether to call it an embryo. Now, however, the question "What is an embryo?" has been raised anew in the context of manipulations on entities that resemble embryos (Austriaco 2005).

2.2. Do We All Begin at Fertilization?

Most of us think that we can trace our existence back to fertilization, but this is not entirely accurate. Some humans, approximately 1 percent, are one of a pair of identical twins or higher multiples, and this figure is even higher if we include cases in which the other siblings die, perhaps undetected, during pregnancy. It is plausible to maintain that these humans begin to exist only when the embryo splits into two or more embryos. Any other view leads to paradoxes about how two distinct individuals can be said to have begun to exist at a time when there was only one individual. It has been suggested that in the case of an embryo that splits into twins there were two individuals present at the beginning. This may be defensible if the split is due to some factor internal to the embryo, but surely it is not if the split is caused by some external, perhaps entirely unpredictable, event.

In addition to these humans who are one of identical twins or higher multiples, there are others—the exact percentage is unknown—who come into existence as a result of the reverse process, that is, the fusing of two or more embryos into a single embryo. Then too we should say that the human individual came into existence not at fertilization but only after the fusing occurred. Otherwise we would have to specify which one of the two or more embryos the human being was, and why that one survived fusing and the other, or others, did not. The parallel here to the suggestion that in the case of an embryo splitting there were always two individuals would have to be the suggestion that in the case of embryos fusing there was always only one individual, located in two places. That is implausible, and it becomes untenable if the fusing is a result of a cause external to the embryos.

The difficulty of identifying the individual or individuals at this early stage becomes even more acute if we consider splitting an embryo, then fusing the split parts with parts of other embryos, then splitting them again, and fusing them again, and so on.

2.3. Might We Begin Life as Something Other Than an Embryo?

To the best of our present knowledge, a single egg will not develop into a mature human being. It will quite quickly cease to develop. Eggs, like sperm, have only half the number of chromosomes required for normal development. Even if the number of chromosomes is doubled, however, some of the genes will not be properly expressed unless the chromosomes come from specifically an egg or a sperm. In mice, it has been shown to be possible to produce a mature individual by joining two immature and appropriately altered eggs (Kono et al. 2004). This has renewed speculation about the possibility of parthenogenesis, but questions have been raised about the results achieved with mice eggs. The same problem of gene expression prevents sperm from developing, and in addition sperm lacks cytoplasm, which is indispensable for growth.

What about other possibilities, some of which we mentioned above when referring to possibilities that can occur in nature? A single cell can be the beginning of a new being. We can, for example, take a two-cell embryo and isolate the two cells. Each cell will develop into a complete individual. Only cells from the early stage of embryo development have this ability; as the embryo develops, the cells lose it. Around the morula stage, they also become more compact and harder to separate, but groups of cells may retain the ability to develop into a new being (Willadsen 1979). If we cut the blastocyst (a later stage of the embryo before implantation) into two halves, each half may develop, if it contains enough of both the inner cell mass and the trophoblast (Ozil 1993).

We do not know exactly how far into the process of development this is possible. But experiments that have been conducted for many years show that if we take a cell, or even just the nucleus of a cell, from a much later embryo and transfer it to an egg from which the nucleus has been removed, this entity is capable of developing into a mature being (Willadsen 1986). As Ian Wilmut famously showed with Dolly—the world's first cloned sheep—and as many subsequent experiments have confirmed, this can even be done if the cell is taken from an adult (Wilmut et al. 1997; Colman 1999). For ethical and legal reasons, experiments of these kinds using human cells have not been continued beyond the point of implantation, but there is no reason to think that our species would be significantly different from other mammals in this respect (Stojkovic 2005).

2.4. What Is Crucial for Development into a Being with Uncontested Moral Standing?

What, then, is crucial for the entity to be able to develop into a being that has uncontested moral standing? It seems that there must be a nucleus, with the genes needed for development, and probably some cytoplasm. (The cytoplasmic components contain resources in addition to those in the nucleus.) Everything else that is required seems to be the environment in which life develops. With adults, there is usually no problem in deciding what is an entity and what is its environment— human beings and the air they breathe, for example, are clearly distinct. But during the earliest stages of human life, the distinction is less clear. How, for example, does one draw the distinction in the case of the nucleus that is placed in an enucleated egg? One possible test for these circumstances—although it does not necessarily hold in other situations—is to ask whether we could change something without changing the identity of the being so dramatically that it would no longer be the same being. (We stress "dramatically" because modifying a gene responsible for a disease like muscular dystrophy, for example, is a change in the entity but would not be seen as changing the identity of the being, any more than losing a limb later in life would be seen as changing one's identity.)

If we transfer the nucleus to a different egg with different cytoplasm, does that affect the identity of the being who eventually develops? Some differences would be apparent, but we do not think they are identity-changing differences, any more than they would be if an embryo were transferred to a different woman's womb or a child were adopted at birth and reared in a different family.

At the moment we have no reliable adequate substitute for an egg's cytoplasm except perhaps the cytoplasm of blastomeres from early embryos. (Perhaps whole polyploid embryos could also be regarded as a substitute, because although their cells have nuclei, those nuclei will mostly be eliminated during the development of the embryos [Nagy et al. 1993].)[1] One day, however, we may be able to develop a cell in a fluid or some other structure or even just by triggering appropriate genes in the nucleus (Takahashi and Yamanaka 2006; Silva et al. 2006). If this becomes possible, it will be more readily apparent that the cytoplasm is the environment in which new life develops, rather than part of its identity.

3. Stem Cells
3.1. Where Do Stem Cells Fit among the Possible Origins of a New Individual?

It is clear that even a single embryonic stem cell can, by the transfer of its nucleus into an enucleated egg, be the beginning of a new human life (Wakayama 1999). Indeed, other stem cells (with the possible exception of germ stem cells) can also be the beginning of a new human life, but it seems that embryonic stem cells, because they are not so differentiated, are better suited for cloning than any other cells. We are not claiming that all cells have the potential to become mature humans, because there are significant differences between cells. We can do nuclear transfer with a nucleus from a terminally differentiated cell like an olfactory neuron or lymphocyte, but it is much less efficient than when we use embryonic stem cells (Jaenisch et al. 2004; Hochedlinger and Jaenisch 2002). We can't do it at all with red blood cells, for example, because they don't have a nucleus. There may also be other kinds of cells whose ability to give rise to a more mature human being we do not know about.

If something can develop into a new human being, should we think of it as having the moral status of an embryo? If what is important is that an entity can become an adult human being, then should not that entity have the same status as an embryo that can develop into a mature human being?

One of us has argued elsewhere that, despite its potential, the normal human embryo lacks the moral status that would give it a right to life or require us to protect it from destruction (Singer 1993, chap. 6). Here, however, we are not arguing on the basis of that position.[2] Rather, our point is that those who do think that the embryo is precious because of its potential to become a mature human being seem to be required to regard an embryonic stem cell as precious for the very same reason. One could imagine differences in the value accorded to the stem cell and the embryo, just as there could be differences between the embryo and the newborn infant, but it would seem that if the human embryo has moral standing and is entitled to protection in virtue of what it can become, then the same must be true of human embryonic stem cells. We can even imagine provisionally evaluating other kinds of cells on the basis of their ability to support development to maturity, with adult stem cells ranked below embryonic stem cells but above somatic cells, unless further experiments show otherwise (Yang and Cheng et al. 2006).

3.2. Implications of Granting Stem Cells Moral Status

If a new life is precious and entitled to protection, it seems that a minimal implication of this is that we should, if other things are equal, protect the new life from destruction and do our best to enable it to develop. What, then, would the inclusion of stem cells in the circle of precious entities require from us?

The most obvious implication is that we would not be permitted to use stem cells, no matter whether they originated from newly destroyed embryos or from stem cell lines that have been in existence for many years, or were obtained by some other method not involving the destruction of embryos at all. We would not even be permitted to use stem cells derived from adults, children, fetuses, or umbilical-cord blood. All these entities can develop into adult human beings. But that is not all. Should we allow all embryonic stem cells to grow into adults? If we accept that such entities are precious, then we would have to take the same view of all the cells of the embryo. Should we then split the early embryo and, when the resulting embryos have grown, split them again? This process cannot be repeated indefinitely, but when it can no longer be done, we could still, by means of nuclear transfer, use the cells of the embryo to allow as many of them as possible to develop into adults (Stice 1993; Wakayama 2000). Should we also try to locate all other cells in our body that have the potential to develop into more mature human beings, take as many as possible, and enable them to do so? There are billions of such cells, and new cells are created in our bodies all the time. Hence the number of possible new human beings who could be created from just one human, while not literally infinite, is so vast that it is difficult to name it without mathematical shortcuts. Multiplying it by the 6.5 billion people now in existence makes this number even larger.

No society on earth, no matter how strongly it says it supports the protection of human life, does any of this. We do not even consider ourselves obliged to split the early embryo, which is an easy and reliable way of allowing its cells to develop into human beings. Nor do we support research that will facilitate future attempts to allow all of these entities to realize their potential. We don't seriously entertain the notion of striving to actualize the potential of every entity that could become an adult human being. But even if we would come to the conclusion, in the light of what we've been discussing here, that our neglect of these entities is wrong, we would simply be unable to actualize the potential of more than a tiny fraction of the already existing entities that could develop into adults.

Some may say that we should not interfere to save the lives of the potential beings in an embryo, because we would then be killing the embryo, and it is prohibited to kill one innocent being in order to save others.[3] We could, however, take some cells from an embryo without destroying it. Or we could take a very large number of cells from an adult without causing any harm. (It is an interesting question, by the way, how many cells we could take before we end up destroying the adult.) We may not consider ourselves justified in killing one innocent human being to save others, but we do justify taking some risks, even substantial ones, with human lives, if a human life will otherwise certainly be lost. (For example, we may drive an ambulance much faster than we would normally consider safe.) Obviously, on the view we are considering here, when we contemplate taking cells from an embryo in order to allow them to develop, if we decide not to do this, a human life will otherwise be lost, in just the same sense that if we fail to protect a human embryo and it ceases to exist, a human life will be lost.

Others may oppose any interference at all on the grounds that, as physicians sometimes say, we should "let nature take its course." But this view implies an end to medicine as a whole, for all medicine is an interference in nature. We would need to be told why we should carry out, at considerable expense, some life-saving medical procedures—for example, saving extremely premature infants—whereas there is no obligation to perform others, such as saving the lives of cells that can become mature human beings. Again, if having the potential to become a mature human being is what entitles the embryo to have its life protected, many other cells are also entitled to have their lives protected.

Of course, in practice—at least at the moment—it would be costly to allow all these entities to realize their potential. Cloning from adult cells, especially, is a demanding procedure and even in animals is not yet entirely safe. There may also be objections to the loss of genetic diversity that could result from extensive cloning from a small number of people in a particular area. The existence of so many identical beings may cause psychosocial problems as well, a sufficiently important reason against that form of cloning. As for embryo cloning, whether by embryo splitting or by nuclear transfer using a nucleus from an embryonic cell, only embryos created in vitro could be considered for this procedure; few women are likely to consent to the removal of an embryo from their uterus so that it can be split and each of its cells can live. We already have hundreds of thousands of frozen embryos in reproductive clinics, so it would be possible to split them without encountering the problem of removing embryos from the uterus. But the very fact that we already have so many frozen embryos, and don't really know what to do with them, gives the idea of creating more of them a ludicrous air. Nevertheless, for those who think that the embryo is precious and entitled to protection because of its potential to develop into a mature human being, the issue remains.

We are aware that many opponents of killing embryos are also opposed to in vitro fertilization, or to the creation of surplus embryos. Once the embryos exist, however, if they are precious and must be protected, it should not matter how they were created. Others will think that cloning is against God's law and hence forbidden (Congregation for the Doctrine of Faith 1987, part 1, sec. 6), but that will not move those who do not share that particular religious belief. In any case, a prohibition on cloning does not exclude other things we could do to enable entities to develop into more mature human beings, including taking cells from embryos that are lost during the natural course of development. It has been estimated that 30 percent of embryos created by sexual intercourse spontaneously miscarry (Wilcox et al. 1988). It is not inconceivable that research could enable us to retrieve these embryos and enable them, or their constituent cells, to live and develop into mature human beings. Yet those who regard embryos as precious do not suggest that such research is a high priority.

4. Objections
4.1. Was Dolly Ever a Somatic Cell?

In a recent essay, Patrick Lee and Robert George (2006a) have responded to claims that are in some respects similar to those that we have made above. It is worth quoting the key passage of their argument, both in order to show why it fails to rebut the claims it addresses, and also why the claims we have made are significantly different. Lee and George write:

> [I]t is simply false to say that a somatic cell has the potential to become a mature whole human being. In the cloning process, the somatic cell (or its nucleus), which is part of a larger organism, ceases to be, and its constituents enter into the make-up of a new and distinct organism, a new member of the species that is cloned (e.g., sheep, mouse, or human, if that should occur). By contrast, when the embryo grows, it continues to be, and simply matures. You and I once were human embryos, just as you and I once were adolescents, children, toddlers, infants, and fetuses. But a cloned animal organism, such as Dolly the sheep, never was a somatic cell, and so too a cloned human being would not come to be until the cloning process was successfully completed. Thus, a human embryo does, but a somatic cell does not, have the potentiality—in the sense of active disposition and intrinsic power—to grow (indeed, to *self-develop*) toward the mature stage of a human being.

There are several problems with this argument as a response to what we have said here. The passage is directed to cloning from somatic cells and thus does not address some of the possibilities that we have mentioned, such as nuclear transfer using nuclei from embryonic cells and other methods of creating new individuals that blur the significance, for present purposes, of the boundary between somatic cells and other cells. If we split a two-cell embryo into its two constituent cells, each of them would have been the original cell that existed before the split. In any case, even if we consider somatic cells, it isn't clear to us, as we have tried to show, that we are justified in asserting that Dolly "never was a somatic cell" (Lee and George 2006a). There are different modes of reproduction, and they require different judgments about what was, or was not, something else. Suppose a friend admires my potted pelargonium. I break off a short piece of stalk, with a leaf or two on it, and put it into some potting mix. Nine months later, on my friend's birthday, I present her with a flourishing, blooming pelargonium that has grown from the cutting I took. Was this plant ever the stalk with its leaf or two? We think it was. But is that so different from saying that Dolly was once the somatic cell? Of course, the somatic cell needed an enucleated egg for it to develop, but the stalk needed potting mix and regular watering, and some cuttings are more likely to develop if dipped in a hormone to stimulate root growth. With plants, we have no difficulty in seeing that they have different ways of reproducing, including sexual reproduction through seeds and asexual reproduction through taking cuttings. That we do more when we clone a mammal does not mean that we are adding something that was not there before. There is no inherent reason why the same two different modes of reproduction cannot exist in humans as well, and if they ever do, we may well come to see the child as having once been the somatic cell from which he or she grew, just as we now see the pelargonium as having once been the stalk.

To the objection that the new plant didn't exist until we cut off the piece of stalk, we can respond that it is not so clear whether separation is necessary for being a distinct individual—think of conjoined twins, for example. We should also be aware that an adult body is continuously releasing thousands of cells (for example, during sneezing), so insistence on physical separation as a criterion for the existence of a distinct individual may not avoid the problem of protecting the many potential lives constituted by all these cells.

4.2. What Kind of Potentiality Matters?

There is, however, a more fundamental problem with the basic argument that Lee and George (2006a) present, even as applied to somatic cells. They appeal to a special sense of potentiality—parsed as "active disposition and intrinsic power"—to distinguish the embryo from the somatic cell. But they need to show not just that this is a possible way of understanding the concept of potentiality but also that it is the morally relevant way of understanding it. Should the answer to the question "Is it wrong to destroy an entity that has the potential to become a more mature human?" depend on whether or not the potential is that of "an active disposition and intrinsic power" or is a potential that only becomes active after scientists take some crucial steps?

Before we address this question, we should note that in the specific case of the embryos that would be destroyed to obtain stem cells, the distinction Lee and George (2006a) are seeking to make is more difficult to draw than they appear to realize. The embryos used by scientists to obtain stem cells are mainly surplus embryos produced during in vitro fertilization. There are hundreds of thousands of them, as we have said. Very few of them will have a chance to develop into mature human beings. For this to happen, there must be a woman willing to accept into her body an embryo that is not genetically related to her or to her partner. Scientists must then carefully thaw the embryo and transfer it to the woman's uterus. The "intrinsic power" of the embryo in these circumstances is impotent—in other words, there is no such power—without modern medical technology, and it can only "self-develop" with assistance from that technology. There is therefore not such a sharp distinction as one might at first think between the "intrinsic power" of the frozen embryo and that of the stem cell. Lee and George might respond that the existence of frozen embryos outside the womb has created this unusual situation, and that we should not use it to assess the intrinsic power of embryos in a more natural situation. But as we have already noted, there is nothing unnatural about embryos failing to implant and being flushed out of the uterus, and once we know that this happens, and have the ability to preserve such embryos, we face an ethical decision about whether we have an ethical obligation to do so.

Opponents of embryo research have encouraged women to "adopt" unwanted frozen embryos and carry them to term. They gave this initiative the name "Operation Snowflake," recalling President George W. Bush's remark in his speech rejecting federal funding for research on stem cell lines that were not already in existence: "Like a snowflake, each of these embryos is unique, with the unique genetic potential of an individual human being" (Bush 2001). In May 2005, and again in July 2006 when he vetoed a bill that would have funded research on stem cell lines derived from surplus embryos, President Bush posed for photos holding babies born as a result of Operation Snowflake (Bush 2005, 2006). The appeal of the photo opportunity—and of Operation Snowflake itself—is, of course, the idea that these babies would not have existed if the embryos from which they developed had been destroyed. But that would also be true if the babies had developed not from embryos that resulted directly from the union of an egg and a sperm but from embryos that were created by removing cells from an embryo. We can even imagine an "Operation Xerox Snowflake" that seeks to rescue not just each cryopreserved embryo but also at least a few cells from each embryo, so that still more of these babies can be born.

4.3. Is the Embryo, But Not the Stem Cell, a Distinct Individual with a Rational Nature?

Notwithstanding their argument that the potential of the embryo is different from the potential of the somatic cell, ultimately Lee and George assert that the embryo has a right to life not because it is a potential human being but because "*as a matter of basic biological fact* human embryos are *actual* human beings in the earliest stages of their natural development" (2006a). To support this claim, they seek to draw a line between what is and what is not a human being in a way that does not imply that every cell that could become a human being is also an actual human being. Hence the discussion of potentiality that we considered in the previous section. We shall now examine their defense of the claim that embryos are actual human beings, to see whether their position is defensible and whether it can avoid the implication that stem cells are also actual human beings.

4.3.1. WHAT ENTITIES HAVE A RATIONAL NATURE?

The final two paragraphs of Lee and George's essay give the crucial steps in their argument:

> Some entities have intrinsic value and basic rights and other entities do not. Such a *radical* moral difference logically must be based on a *radical* ontological difference (that is, a radical difference among those entities themselves). And so the basis for that moral difference (a difference in the way they should be treated) must be the natures of those entities, not their accidental characteristics which involve merely quantitative differences, or differences in degree. (By "accidental" qualities, we mean those attributes that do not help to define the nature of an entity. In humans, age, size, stage of development, state of health, and so forth are accidental qualities.) The immediately exercisable capacity to reason and make free choices is only the development of the underlying basic, natural capacity for reasoning and free choice, and there are various degrees of that development along a continuum. But one either is or is not a distinct subject with a rational nature (the traditional definition of "person"). So, Singer is correct to say that the right to life must be based on what is true of the entity now, not just what is true of its future. But it is true of the human embryo now that he or she is a distinct individual with a rational nature, even though it will take him or her several years fully to actualise his or her basic, natural capacities so they are immediately exercisable.
>
> Our conclusion: Every human being, irrespective of age, size, condition of dependency, or stage of development—or the means by which he or she is produced—is intrinsically valuable as a subject of rights and deserves full moral respect. (2006a)

An obvious question to ask about this passage is whether the notion of "development" is sufficiently distinct from the notion of "potentiality" to bear the weight here placed upon it. Given that we all agree that the human embryo in its present form cannot reason, has never been able to reason, and will not be able to reason for a long time, or possibly will never be able to reason, is it more accurate to say that the human embryo "is a distinct individual with a rational nature" or to say that the human embryo "is a distinct individual with the potential to become a rational being"? In our view, the former description is misleading. The embryo does not have "a rational nature" (2006a). What it has is the genetic coding that may, under favorable circumstances, lead it to develop into a being with a rational nature.

As we have seen, Lee and George reject the idea that a somatic cell—in contrast to an embryo—could be "a distinct individual with a rational nature." But if having the genetic coding to develop, under favorable circumstances, into a being with a rational nature is crucial to the wrongness of killing, then our earlier account of the different entities that can become a human embryo shows that some unusual entities have this property. Lee and George's position implies that these entities are actual human beings with a right to life and in need of medical intervention to save their lives. We doubt that Lee and George would want to take this view.

Perhaps Lee and George would respond that the entities we have referred to as capable of developing into a mature human being do not have the "active disposition" or "intrinsic power" to "self-develop" into such beings and, hence, are not now beings with a rational nature. But suppose we have an embryo that, because of a genetic defect, will not develop into a mature human being. Would Lee and George say that for this reason it is not "a distinct individual with a rational nature"? If so, they would be opening a path to destroying such embryos, in order to create stem cells lines from them. Indeed, it would seem to follow that they would have to accept the legitimacy of doing this, even if we also had the means to remedy the genetic defect and make the embryo completely normal, for it would still be the case that the embryo's power to develop was not "intrinsic" to it, and it was unable to "self-develop." Again, we doubt that they would want to take this view. But it seems that they must take either this view or the one sketched in the previous paragraph. They must therefore either agree that we have an obligation to preserve the lives of all entities with the potential to develop into mature humans, or accept the destruction of embryos with remediable defects.

4.3.2. FROM THE FACTUAL CLAIM TO THE MORAL CLAIM

So far, we have explored the implications of Lee and George's position on human embryos but have not asked whether it is soundly based. If it were, we might have to accept it, even if it leads to some surprising consequences regarding some cells that we do not normally think of as having a right to life. But even if we were to accept Lee and George's ontological claim, that would bring us no nearer to the moral conclusion they set forth in the final paragraph of their essay, that the embryo "is intrinsically valuable as a subject of rights and deserves full moral respect (2006a)." For if we define "rational nature" as they define it, we can still resist the claim that having a *rational nature*—in the sense in which they are using the term—suffices for being a subject of rights, or being intrinsically valuable, or deserving of moral respect. Rather, it would seem that the morally relevant characteristic on which such claims of value should be based is "the immediately exercisable capacity to reason and make free choices."

Why do we say this? Consider the grounds on which we may hold that gratuitously killing a being "like us" is an especially grave wrong—that is, a wrong that far exceeds any wrong we may commit in gratuitously killing a dog or a pig. (We will not here discuss the claim that it is simply membership of the species *Homo sapiens* that makes it worse to kill the human being. One of us has argued elsewhere against this view [Singer 1993, 2001], and Lee and George, to their credit, do not defend it.) We might say that to kill a being like us is an especially grave wrong because it involves the violation of the autonomous will of the being who is killed. Or we might say that it is an especially grave wrong because it thwarts the hopes and desires that beings like us have for the future and, typically, renders vain much of what they have been doing—studying, training, saving their money, preparing to have children, and so on—in the expectation that they will have a future. But it is not a being's "rational nature" in the Lee and George sense that gives rise to a violation of autonomy or the thwarting of hopes and desires for the future. Rather, it is the immediately exercisable—or at least, to take account of cases of temporary unconsciousness, previously exercised—capacity to reason that is required for killing to have these effects. This strongly suggests that these aspects of a person's existence are more relevant to the wrongness of killing than whether the being is of such a nature that it will eventually be able to exercise a capacity to reason.

When Lee and George assert that a radical moral difference between entities that have intrinsic value and basic rights and entities that lack such value and rights must be based on "the natures of those entities, not their accidental characteristics" (2006a) they beg several questions. They seem to assume a sharp dichotomy between, on the one hand, beings that have intrinsic value and basic rights and, on the other hand, beings that lack such value and rights. Such a dichotomy may be convenient for law and public standards of ethics, but we should not assume that it exists in nature. We may grant that rocks have no intrinsic value or basic rights, and that beings capable of exercising a capacity to reason do have both intrinsic value and basic rights, but there are many intermediate cases. The gradual development of the embryo, fetus, and child suggests one ground for the existence of intermediate cases, but even for those who think that the human embryo is already a being with a rational nature, our knowledge of human evolution makes it implausible to believe that there was a sudden leap—in a single generation?—from beings with no intrinsic value or basic rights to beings with the intrinsic value and basic rights that normal mature human beings have now. Evolution is a gradual process that takes place over millennia, and there must have been intermediate cases between our nonrational ancestors and our rational ones.

The growth in the creation of chimeras and hybrids will raise further doubts about the idea of a dichotomy, rather than a continuum, between beings with a rational nature and beings without such a nature. Actual and possible chimeras and hybrids include, for example, a sheep with one human gene, a complete human nucleus inside an enucleated rabbit egg, and a chimpanzee-human hybrid (Schnieke et al. 1997; Chen et al. 2003; Wikipedia no date). We have no trouble in classifying sheep with one human gene, but what about a human nucleus in an enucleated rabbit egg? Even if it could not develop into a mature human being, is it not comparable to a human embryo with a defect that will prevent it from ever actually having the capacity to reason? If a human embryo is, from the beginning, a being with a rational nature, and for that reason has the rights and intrinsic worth due to all human beings, is that status to be negated by the fact that it has a disability, even one so severe that it will never develop into a mature being? If not, why should we not say the same about the human nucleus in the rabbit egg? What, finally, about a chimpanzee-human hybrid who could, in the view of some scientists, even grow to adulthood?

More significantly, the question of whether a given characteristic defines the nature of an entity or is accidental to it cannot be used as an argument that seeks to answer the question, What kind of beings have intrinsic value and rights? *First* we must decide what kind of being has intrinsic value and rights, and only then can we say what characteristics define its nature and what are accidental to it. We must not here say, "We already know that all and only human beings have intrinsic value and rights, so the answer is that you must be a human being." That assumes the conclusion that Lee and George need to establish. There may be better answers. We might, for instance, answer that it is conscious beings who have intrinsic value and rights. Or we could say that it is self-aware beings, or beings with an exercisable or previously exercised capacity to reason, who have this special moral status. If we give such answers, then "the nature of the entities" that gives them intrinsic value and basic rights just *is* their consciousness or self-awareness or exercisable or previously exercised capacity to reason, and these things are not "accidental" to that nature—they are its defining characteristics. Being human, on the other hand, or having a particular genetic code then becomes accidental, since conscious and self-aware beings do not have to be human or have any specific genetic code. Lee and George simply assume that we must be looking for the kind of "nature" that persists through all stages of a being's biological life, and they label some features as "accidental" from this perspective (2006a). Why they make this assumption is a matter of speculation, but it may be because they began their quest already committed to the conclusion that all members of the species *Homo sapiens* have intrinsic value and basic rights.

5. Conclusion

Once we understand the full range of biological possibilities of producing new human beings, we have a new perspective on the beginning of life. These biological possibilities raise particular difficulties for the claim that the embryo should be protected because it has the potential to become a more mature human being. To cling to this view, we would have to take seriously all its far-reaching implications and make choices over a vast number of potential human lives.

How would we make such choices? One possible answer is that, in a world with more than a billion people living below the World Bank's poverty line, and millions of people dying every year from poverty-related causes, any prima facie obligation we might have to facilitate the development of additional human beings is overwhelmed by the fact that they would compete for scarce resources with those who already exist and would add to existing pressures on the natural environment. If, however, we believe that we should protect at least some of those entities with the potential to become mature human beings, how are we to decide which ones to protect? If we have an abundance of normally developing cells and enough prospective parents who meet all the normal requirements of providing a good home for their children, what other criteria should we use? Some people will not be comfortable with making such choices, on a large scale, especially when the choices will be between identical cells from the same embryo or adult, and we have to decide which among them will live and which will not. But not choosing is a kind of choice too, because it means that the cell will never develop as it could. Not choosing means that a possible human being will not exist.

These implications amount to something very close to a reductio ad absurdum of the claim that human embryos must not be destroyed because of their potential. It is, if not strictly a logical absurdity, at least a position that no one could seriously set out to put into practice.

Finally, we have considered and rejected one argument for the view that the human embryo is not merely potentially but actually a being of intrinsic value with basic rights. There may be other arguments for this position that we have not considered, but it is a position that is not going to be easy to defend.

The most obvious way to avoid the difficulties we have considered is to turn to the alternative view that at the beginning of life human entities lack the requirements for moral status. They lack not only those attributes that are linked to personhood, like self-awareness, but also more basic things, like sentience or the capacity to feel pain. Therefore unless there is some other reason to keep them alive—for example, the wishes of their parents—we may use them as we please. There are many, among them even some arguing from a theological perspective, who believe that even if embryos have some moral status, we would still be justified in using them for research purposes if that research could advance our knowledge in a way that would lead to cures for diseases that afflict millions (Hudson, Scott, and Faden 2005, 15; Peters 2001; Peters and Bennett 2001). We do not need to consider this claim. The more plausible view, in our judgment, is that human entities at the beginning of life do not have moral status, and hence the use of them for research purposes is justifiable. Moreover, because this research could lead to cures for diseases that are now fatal, it might even be obligatory.

ACKNOWLEDGMENTS

We thank Lori Gruen and Laura Graber for their work on this essay. We also thank Elizabeth Harman, who was the commentator at a seminar at the Princeton University Center for Human Values at which the essay was discussed, and others who participated on that occasion or who were kind enough to read and give us comments on a draft of it, as well as others who saw the essay under other circumstances.

NOTES

1. For a distinct argument based on these experiments, see, for example, Silver 2006a, 141–43. For discussion, see Lee and George 2006b, Silver 2006b, and Lee and George 2006c.

2. Indeed, this position is not entirely shared by Agata Sagan, who sees more significance in the continuity of human development from earlier stages.

3. On the debate about the distinction between killing and letting die, see Steinbock and Norcross 1994; Kuhse 1987, chaps. 2–4.

REFERENCES

American Association for Advancement of Science and Institute for Civil Society. 1999. *Stem Cell Research and Application: Monitoring the Frontiers of Biomedical Research*, www.aaas .org/spp/sfrl/projects/stem/report.pdf (last accessed 12 December 2006).

Austriaco, Nicanor Pier Giorgio. 2005. "Are Teratomas Embryos or Non-embryos? A Criterion for Oocyte-Assisted Reprogramming." *National Catholic Bioethics Quarterly* 5, no. 4 (Winter): 697–706.

Bailey, Ronald. 2001a. "Are Stem Cells Babies? Only if Every Other Human Cell Is, Too." *Reason Online* (11 July), reason.com/rb/rb071101.shtml (last accessed 12 December 2006).

———. 2001b. "My Critics Are Wrong: Why Using Human Embryonic Stem Cells for Medical Research Is Moral." *National Review Online* (25 July), www.nationalreview.com /comment/comment-baileyprint072501.html (last accessed 12 December 2006).

Bush, George W. 2001. "President Discusses Stem Cell Research." White House news release (9 August), www.whitehouse.gov/news/releases/2001/08/20010809-2.html (last accessed 12 December 2006).

———. 2005. "President Discusses Embryo Adoption and Ethical Stem Cell Research." White House news release (24 May), www.whitehouse.gov/news/releases/2005/05 /20050524-12.html (last accessed 12 December 2006).

————. 2006. "President Discusses Stem Cell Research Policy." White House news release (19 July), www.whitehouse.gov/news/releases/2006/07/20060719-3.html (last accessed 12 December 2006).

Chen Ying, Zhi Xu He, Ailian Liu, Kai Wang, Wen Wei Mao, Jian Xin Chu, Yong Lu, Zheng Fu Fang, Ying Tang Shi, Qing Zhang Yang, Da Yuan Chen, Min Kang Wang, Jin Song Li, Shao Liang Huang, Xiang Yin Kong, Yao Zhou Shi, Zhi Qiang Wang, Jia Hui Xia, Zhi Gao Long, Zhi Gang Xue, Wen Xiang Ding, and Hui Zhen Sheng. 2003. "Embryonic Stem Cells Generated by Nuclear Transfer of Human Somatic Nuclei into Rabbit Oocytes." *Cell Research* 13, no. 4:251–63.

Coalition for the Advancement of Medical Research Dedicated to Advancing Stem Cell Research. No date. "Alternative Methods of Producing Stem Cells: No Substitute for Embryonic Stem Cell Research," www.stemcellfunding.org/resources/Why_Alternatives_Summary.htm (last accessed 12 December 2006).

Colman, Alan. 1999. "Review of *Somatic Cell Nuclear Transfer in Mammals: Progress and Applications.*" *Cloning* 1, no. 4:185–200.

Congregation for the Doctrine of Faith. 1987. *Instruction for Respect for Human Life*. Vatican City: Vatican Polyglot Press.

Hochedlinger, K., and R. Jaenisch. 2002. "Generation of Monoclonal Mice by Nuclear Transfer from Mature B and T Donor Cells." *Nature* 415, no. 6875:1035–38.

Huang, Steve C., et al. 2003. (Helen Lin, JingQi Lei, David Wininger, Minh-Thanh Nguyen, Ruchi Khanna, Chris Hartmann, Wen-Liang Yan, and Steve C. Huang). "Multilineage Potential of Homozygous Stem Cells Derived from Metaphase II Oocytes." *Stem Cells* 21, no. 2:152–61.

Hudson, Kathy L., Joan Scott, and Ruth Faden. 2005. *Values in Conflict: Public Attitudes on Embryonic Stem Cell Research*. Washington, D.C.: Genetics and Public Policy Center, Phoebe R. Berman Bioethics Institute, John Hopkins University, www.dnapolicy.org/images/reportpdfs/2005ValuesInConflict.pdf (last accessed 12 December 2006).

Hurlbut, William B. 2004. "Altered Nuclear Transfer as a Morally Acceptable Means for the Procurement of Human Embryonic Stem Cells." Commissioned working paper discussed at the President's Council on Bioethics at the meeting in December 2004, www.bioethics.gov/background/hurlbut.html (last accessed 12 December 2006).

Jaenisch, R., et al. (Kevin Eggan, Kristin Baldwin, Michael Tackett, Joseph Osborne, Joseph Gogos, Andrew Chess, Richard Axel, and Rudolf Jaenisch). 2004. "Mice Cloned from Olfactory Sensory Neurons." *Nature* 428, no. 6978:44–49.

Kono Tomohiro, Yayoi Obata, Quiong Wu, Katsutoshi Niwa, Yukiko Ono, Yuji Yamamoto, Eun Sung Park, Jeong-Sun Seo, and Hidehiko Ogawa. 2004. "Birth of Parthenogenetic Mice That Can Develop to Adulthood." *Nature* 428, no. 6985:860–64.

Kuhse, Helga. 1987. *The Sanctity-of-Life Doctrine in Medicine: A Critique*. Oxford: Clarendon Press.

Landry, Donald W., and Howard A. Zucker. 2004. "Embryonic Death and the Creation of Human Embryonic Cells." *Journal of Clinical Investigation* 114, no. 9:1184–86.

Lanza, Robert, et al. (Irina Klimanskaya, Young Chung, Sandy Becker, Shi-Jiang Lu, and Robert Lanza). 2006. "Human Embryonic Stem Cell Lines Derived from Single Blastomeres." *Nature* 444, no. 7118:481–85.

Lee, Patrick, and Robert George. 2001a. "Reason, Science and Stem Cells: Why Killing Embryonic Human Beings Is Wrong." *National Review Online* (20 July), www.national review.com/comment/comment-georgeprint072001.html (last accessed 12 December 2006).

———. 2001b. "The Stubborn Facts of Science: Human Embryos Are Human Beings." *National Review Online* (30 July), www.nationalreview.com/comment/comment -georgeprint073001.html (last accessed 12 December 2006).

———. 2006a. "Human-Embryo Liberation: A Reply to Peter Singer." *National Review Online* (25 January), www.nationalreview.com/comment/lee_george200601250829.asp (last accessed 12 December 2006).

———. 2006b. "Fundamentalists? We? Bad Science, Worse Philosophy, and McCarthyite Tactics in the Human-Embyro Debate." *National Review Online* (3 October), article. nationalreview.com/?q=OTNiYWM2ZjJiYWVIN2IyMzFjOWYwMDZmMTc4MzU2 MGU (last accessed 12 December 2006).

———. 2006c. "Silver Lining: A Reply to Lee Silver." *National Review Online* (19 October), http://article.nationalreview.com/?q=MjNmZmYyN2NhNjFkYWRhNmExMDA2Yzhi MDY5YzMyYTI = (last accessed 12 December 2006).

Melton, Douglas A., et al. (Chad A. Cowan, Jocelyn Atienza, Douglas A. Melton, and Kevin Eggan). 2005. "Nuclear Reprogramming of Somatic Cells after Fusion with Human Embryonic Stem Cells." *Science* 309, no. 5739:1369–73.

Nagy, A., J. Rossant, R. Nagy, W. Abramow-Newerly, and J. C. Roder. 1993. "Derivation of Completely Cell Culture–Derived Mice from Early-Passage Embryonic Stem Cells." *Proceedings of the National Academy of Sciences of the USA* 90, no. 18:8424–28.

NIH Stem Cell Task Force. 2005. "Alternative Methods of Obtaining Embryonic Stem Cells." Presented by James F. Battey, Subcommittee on Labor, Health and Human Ser- vices, Education, and Related Agencies, Committee on Appropriations, U.S. Senate (12 July), stemcells.nih.gov/policy/statements/20050712battey.asp (last accessed 12 Decem- ber 2006).

Ozil, J. P. 1983. "Production of Identical Twins by Bisection of Blastocysts in the Cow." *Jour- nal of Reproduction and Fertility* 69, no. 22:463–68.

Peters, Ted. 2001. "The Stem Cell Controversy." *Dialog: A Journal of Theology* 40, no. 4 (Winter): 290–293.

———, and Gaymon Bennett. 2001. "Theological Support of Stem Cell Research." *Scientist* 15, no. 17 (3 September): 4.

Savulescu, Julian. 1999. "Should We Clone Human Beings?" *Journal of Medical Ethics* 25, no. 2:87–98.

Schnieke, Angelika, E. Alexander, J. Kind, William A. Ritchie, Karen Mycock, Angela R. Scott, Marjorie Ritchie, Ian Wilmut, Alan Colman, and Keith H. S. Campbell. 1997. "Human Factor IX Transgenic Sheep Produced by Transfer of Nuclei from Transfected Fetal Fibroblasts." *Science* 278, no. 5346:2130–33.

Silva José, Ian Chambers, Steven Pollard, and Austin Smith. 2006. "Nanog Promotes Trans- fer of Pluripoteney after Cell Fusion." *Nature* 441, no. 7096:997–1001.

Silver, Lee M. 2006a. *Challenging Nature: The Clash of Science and Spirituality at the New Frontiers of Life.* New York: Ecco.

———. 2006b. "Human Issues." *National Review Online* (19 October), article.nationalre view.com/?q=Mjg2Y2RkNDM1MzlkMGMyMjl3NjhkYmE0ZTRjOTgyZDE (last accessed 12 December 2006).

Singer, Peter. 1993. *Practical Ethics.* 2nd edition. Cambridge: Cambridge University Press.

———. 2001. *Animal Liberation.* 2nd edition. New York: Ecco.

Steinbock, Bonnie, and Alastair Norcross (editors). 1994. *Killing and Letting Die.* 2nd edition. New York: Fordham University Press.

Stice, S. L., and C. L. Keefer. 1993. "Multiple Generational Bovine Embryo Cloning." *Biology of Reproduction* 48, no. 4:715–19.

Stojkovic, M., P. Stojkovic, C. Leary, V. J. Hall, L. Armstrong, M. Herbert, M. Nesbitt, M. Lako, and A. Murdoch. 2005. "Derivation of a Human Blastocyst after Heterologous Nuclear Transfer to Donated Oocytes." *Reproductive BioMedicine* 11, no. 2:226–31.

Takahashi, Kazutoshi, and Shinya Yamanaka. 2006. "Induction of Pluripotent Stem Cells from Mouse Embryonic and Adult Fibroblast Cultures by Defined Factors." *Cell* 126, no. 4:663–76.

Wakayama, Teruhiko, Ivan Rodriguez, Anthony C. F. Perry, Ryuzo Yanagimachi, and Peter Mombaerts. 1999. "Mice Cloned from Embryonic Stem Cells." *Proceedings of the National Academy of Sciences of the USA* 96, no. 26:14984–89.

———, Yoichi Shinkai, Kellie L. K. Tamashiro, Hiroyuki Niida, D. Caroline Blanchard, Robert J. Blanchard, Atsuo Ogura, Kentaro Tanemura, Makoto Tachibana, Anthony C. F. Perry, Diana F. Colgan, Peter Mombaerts, and Ryuzo Yanagimachi. 2000. "Cloning of Mice to Six Generations." *Nature* 407, no. 6802:318–19.

Wikipedia. No date. S.v. "Humanzee," en.wikipedia.org/wiki/Humanzee (last accessed 12 December 2006).

Wilcox, A. J., C. R. Weinberg, J. F. O'Connor, D. D. Baird, J. P. Schlatterer, R. E. Canfield, E. G. Armstrong, and B. C. Nisula. 1988. "Incidence of Early Loss of Pregnancy." *New England Journal of Medicine* 319, no. 4:189–94.

Willadsen, S. M. 1979. "A Method for Cultured Micromanipulated Sheep Embryos and Its Use to Produce Monozygotic Twins." *Nature* 277, no. 5694:298–300.

———. 1986. "Nuclear Transplantation in Sheep Embryos." *Nature* 320, no. 6057:63–65.

Wilmut, I., A. E. Schnieke, J. McWhir, A. J. Kind, and K. H. S. Campbell. 1997. "Viable Offspring Derived from Fetal and Adult Mammalian Cells." *Nature* 385, no. 6619:810–13.

Yang, X., Tao Cheng, et al. (Li-Ying Sung, Shaorong Gao, Hongmei Shen, Hui Yu, Yifang Song, Sadie L. Smith, Ching-Chien Chang, Kimiko Inoue, Lynn Kuo, Jin Lian, Ao Li, X. Cindy Tian, David P. Tuck, Sherman M. Weissman, Xiangzhong Yang, and Tao Cheng). 2006. "Differentiated Cells Are More Efficient Than Adult Stem Cells for Cloning by Somatic Cell Nuclear Transfer." *Nature Genetics* 38, no. 11:1323–28.

CHAPTER EIGHT

Potential

JEFF MCMAHAN

This essay is a reprint of chapter 4, section 6, 302–29, of Jeff McMahan, *The Ethics of Killing* (New York: Oxford University Press, 2002). Numbering of subheads and references in the text to earlier chapters and sections are from this 2002 work.

6.1. Potential and Identity

It is frequently claimed that, even though abortion is not *murder,* because it does not involve the killing of a *person,* it is nevertheless seriously objectionable because it thwarts the fetus's potential. The focus is often on the fetus's potential to become a person. It is, for example, often claimed that abortion is wrong because the fetus is a potential person and it is seriously wrong to kill potential persons, even if it is not quite murder. In this section I will seek to understand exactly what sort of potential the fetus has and what its moral significance is.

The claim that the fetus is a potential person, or has the potential to become a person, is ambiguous. There are at least three ways in which it might be interpreted. I will try to elucidate these three interpretations by noting what each asserts about the relation between me and the fetus from which I developed.

First, the claim might mean that the fetus from which I developed was not me but had the potential to become me. One might make this claim if one believed that we are essentially persons—that is, that we cannot exist except as persons.

Second, the claim that the fetus is a potential person is perhaps more commonly understood to mean that, although I once existed as a fetus, I was not then a person and, consequently, my moral status was different from what it is now. Understood in this way, the claim presupposes that we are *not* essentially persons. On this view, "person" is a phase sortal—that is, a predicate that may apply to us only during a certain phase, or certain phases, of our existence.

Third, the claim is sometimes interpreted to mean that the fetus in its *present* state is an uncompleted person, a person in the process of becoming, a being whose essential nature is to evolve into a full-fledged person. The person is understood to be somehow latently or even occultly present in the potential person. This is thought to explain why whatever is morally due to a person is also due to a potential person.

Whether the claim that the fetus is a potential person—however that claim is interpreted—can ground a forceful objection to abortion depends, in part, on what is meant by "person." Let us assume for the sake of argument that "being a person" is shorthand for the possession of properties that are the basis of a high moral status—so that, for example, persons come within the scope of the morality of respect, or possess rights such as the right to life. I will continue to use "person" to refer to any being with a comparatively highly developed set of psychological capacities. But this is compatible with the assumption that personhood is a basis of high moral status, for it is plausible to suppose that the possession of the relevant psychological capacities is a sufficient basis for commanding respect or possessing rights. [1]

The claim that the fetus is a potential person has to be examined in relation to the distinction that I have drawn between the early fetus and the developed fetus. If the Embodied Mind Account of Identity is correct, the developed fetus—but not the early fetus—is identical with (that is, is the same individual as) the person into whom it might develop. Thus the first interpretation of the claim that the fetus is a potential person can apply only to the early fetus, while the second interpretation can apply only to the developed fetus. (The third interpretation, which is rather more obscure, might be thought to apply to either. I will return to it later.) It will therefore be helpful to consider separately the potential of the early fetus and that of the developed fetus.

Consider first the claim that the early fetus has the potential to become a person. This must mean that, while the early fetus is not the same individual as the person, it can nevertheless become or develop into that person. As I indicated in section 1 of this chapter, I believe that this claim is false when understood in a way that would make it clearly morally significant, and true only when understood in a way that seems largely morally insignificant. To see why this is so, we need to distinguish between two understandings of the notion of potential.[2]

There is a sense in which X has the potential to become Y only if X and Y would be identical—that is, only if X and Y would be one and the same individual entity. Or, rather, since what an individual has the potential to become is normally a thing of a certain *sort,* perhaps we should say that X has the potential to become a Y in this first sense only if X will continue to exist as a Y. It is in this sense that Prince Charles has the potential to become the king of England, since he would continue to exist as king. If he realizes his potential to become the king, he and the king will be one and the same individual. I will call this kind of potential *identity-preserving potential.* (Notice that if X has the identity-preserving potential to become a Y, it seems that

"Y" must be a phase sortal. X cannot become an entity of a different substantial kind and continue to exist.)

Identity-preserving potential contrasts with what I will call *non-identity potential*. Non-identity potential may take a variety of forms, which are unified by two features: first, when X has the non-identity potential to become Y (or a Y), Y will not, when it exists, be identical with X (or Y will not just be a phase in the history of X); but, second, we nevertheless employ the idiom of "becoming" in describing the transition from X to Y. In the commonest case, when X has the non-identity potential to become Y, X gives rise to, or causally contributes to the production of Y when its constituent matter is transformed in such a way that, while X itself ceases to exist, a new and different individual, Y, is formed out of that same matter. We say, for example, that the sperm and egg together have the potential to become a zygote. This is a paradigm of non-identity potential, for when the sperm and egg fuse, they both cease to exist but the zygote is created out of the matter of which they were composed. Or, to take another example, consider the possibility of running my wooden desk through a wood chipper, which grinds wood into sawdust. We have no hesitation in saying that my desk would become a pile of sawdust and therefore that it is now potentially a pile of sawdust or has the potential to become a pile of sawdust. But this is a deviant form of *becoming,* since it would involve the ceasing to exist of the desk. The desk's constituent matter would continue to exist and would take a new form, but the desk itself would no longer exist. Thus the desk's potential to become a pile of sawdust is non-identity potential.

Not all forms of non-identity potential conform to this paradigm. In some instances in which X has the non-identity potential to become Y, X does not cease to exist when it is causally involved in the production of Y but coexists with Y without being identical to it. An example is the potential a lump of bronze has to become a statue. When the lump of bronze is shaped in a certain way, we say that it becomes a statue. But the common view is that the statue is a new and distinct individual entity: it is not identical with or the same thing as the lump of bronze. Thus the lump of bronze continues to exist when the statue begins to exist; they coexist, both sharing the same constituent matter.

(Some might challenge this example on the ground that the lump of bronze in fact has the identity-preserving potential to become a statue, since the statue is really not a distinct substance but is only a phase in the history of the lump of bronze, in the same way that a child is not distinct from the person but simply *is* that person during a certain phase of his or her life. But, to show that the lump of bronze and the statue are distinct substances, Derek Parfit has suggested that we imagine that the statue is hollowed out, with all the bronze removed from the interior collected in a single lump, leaving the surface material unaffected.[3] The bronze that has been extracted would be the original lump of bronze—since a lump of bronze can continue to exist if it loses only a tiny proportion of its constituent matter. But suppose the lump was then destroyed, by being turned into coins. The statue would nevertheless continue to exist, although it would now be hollow—or alternatively, it might be filled back in with a cheaper iron ore. That the statue could continue to exist after the lump of bronze had ceased to exist shows that they are distinct substances.)

Of the two types of potential, it is normally only identity-preserving potential that is capable of grounding an interest in its own realization. That is, it is normally only if X's potential to become Y is identity-preserving that X can have an interest in becoming Y, or that it can be good for X to become Y. In the commonest case, if X has the non-identity potential to become Y, the realization of the potential involves the ceasing to exist of X. And it is seldom in an individual's interest to cease to exist—though of course there are comparatively rare cases when it is. Thus a person whose life has ceased to be worth living may have an interest in the realization of his non-identity potential to become a corpse. In the case of non-identity potential whose realization does not involve the ceasing to exist of the original entity, it is in principle possible that X could have an interest in "becoming" Y because the existence of Y would somehow benefit X even though Y would be a different individual from X. But I cannot think of any instances in which this would be true.

Return now to the issue of fetal potential. Let us first consider the early fetus, then the developed fetus. Having distinguished between identity-preserving and non-identity potential, we can now see why the early fetus cannot have an interest in becoming a person. Most previous discussions have assumed that the potential of the early fetus to become a person is identity-preserving. But if, as I have argued, we are not identical with our organisms, this assumption is false. The early fetus is simply the human organism in its early stages. It therefore has the identity-preserving potential to become a mature or adult human organism. But the adult human organism will not be the same individual as the adult person or self. Therefore the early fetus does not have the identity-preserving potential to become a person. It has only the non-identity potential to become a person. Its non-identity potential is of the second sort described above: that is, as it matures, the fetal organism causally gives rise to the existence of the individual who will become a person but it does not thereby cease to exist. Rather, it continues to exist as a mature organism that coexists with the person.

Because the early fetus has only the non-identity potential to become a person, it lacks an interest in the realization of that potential. It could have an interest in becoming a person if it would actually *be* that person, but that is what we must deny if we accept that we are not identical with our organisms. Assuming that the early fetus has only the non-identity potential to become a person, the only way it could have an interest in the realization of that potential would be if the later existence of the person would somehow benefit the organism. But, as I noted earlier, a mere organism lacks the capacity for consciousness (or has it only derivatively) and therefore is not the kind of entity that can be benefited in the morally relevant sense.

It is, of course, strange that we describe the organism's giving rise to the existence of the person as its *becoming* that person. But the same sense of "becoming"— that is, one that does not presuppose the continued existence of the entity that becomes something else—also appears in other contexts: for example, when it is said that the sperm and the egg become a zygote. The basis for this locution is probably the persistence, in the same region of space, of the constituent matter of the original entity, as if the thing that does the becoming were the matter itself rather than the entity it composed.

I have argued that the early fetus cannot have an interest in the realization of its potential to become a person, for that potential is not identity-preserving. Yet those who believe that even the early fetus has significant potential could argue that there are ways in which potential can be morally significant other than by an individual's having an interest in the realization of its potential. We should distinguish three ways in which potential might be morally significant:

1. X's potential to become a Y might be morally significant because it would be good for X, or in X's interest or time-relative interest, to become a Y.
2. X's potential to become a person might be morally significant because it would be good or valuable, either for others or impersonally (though not for X), for there to be a Y, or more Ys than there already are.
3. X's potential to become a person might be morally significant because it would give X an enhanced moral status.

I will discuss the third of these in the following section. For reasons that I will give there, this way in which potential may be valuable is not relevant to the case of the early fetus. But the second of these ways in which potential might be valuable may well apply to the early fetus. For the early fetus has the non-identity potential to develop into (that is, to give rise to the existence of) a person. To the extent that it is good or desirable that new people should exist with lives worth living, the early fetus's potential is instrumentally important. In order for the early fetus's potential to be important in this way, it is not necessary that the early fetus should benefit from its realization; hence it does not matter that the early fetus's potential to become a person is not identity-preserving. For, on this view, the value lies in the *outcome,* not in the effect on the early fetus itself.

There are, however, two points that should be noted. First, the moral significance of the early fetus's potential lies wholly in the value of what it is a potential
for—that is, the existence of the person. If there is a reason to respect the early
fetus's potential, it has nothing to do with any alleged interests, good, or status of
the early fetus itself. It has to do instead with the desirability of a person's coming
into existence with a life worth living. Second, any healthy pair of sperm and egg
has the same non-identity potential that the early fetus has to become a person.
Thus, making allowances for differences in the probability that their potentials will
be realized, whatever reason there is to promote the early fetus's potential is equally
a reason to ensure that the potential of the sperm and egg is also realized. So if the
early fetus's potential counts against an abortion, the potential of the sperm and egg
counts equally in favor of conception and against contraception.

The claim that a sperm and egg together have the potential to become a person
is quite commonly advanced as a reductio ad absurdum argument against appeals to
fetal potential. The contention is that if one objects to abortion on the ground that
the fetus is a potential person, one must oppose contraception as well, since that,
too, actively thwarts the potential that the sperm and egg have to become a person.
While this argument has force, its scope is narrowly restricted. It is a plausible response to anti-abortion arguments that appeal to the fetus's potential when the only
relevant potential the fetus has is non-identity potential. For that is the sort of potential that the sperm and egg have. The argument is therefore quite forceful in ex-
posing the limited moral significance of the early fetus's non-identity potential to
become a person. But it has no force against the claim that late abortion is wrong
because it frustrates the potential of the developed fetus to become a person. For the
developed fetus's potential to become a person is identity-preserving, and is therefore completely different in kind from the potential of the sperm and egg.

Because the developed fetus's potential to become a person is identity-preserving,
the developed fetus itself can have an interest in its realization. Its potential, in other
words, may be morally significant in the first of the three ways I distinguished. The
claim that it is wrong to thwart the developed fetus's potential to become a person
might be based on the assumption that it is wrong to frustrate its *interest* in becoming a person. And to say that it has an interest in becoming a person is just to say
that it would be better for it to be a person, either because its acquisition of the attributes constitutive of personhood would enable it to have a much higher level of
well-being, or because in becoming a person it would become a higher form of
being, or both.

I accept that the developed fetus has an interest in becoming a person and that
the strength of this interest is commensurate with the extent to which it would be

worse for the fetus never to become a person. I have argued, however, that the morality of a late abortion is not determined by the effect that abortion has on the developed fetus's interests—that is, by the extent to which abortion makes the fetus's life as a whole worse than it would otherwise have been. Rather than focusing on what would be better or worse for the fetus (where the value of its life as a whole is concerned), we should weigh the reasons that favor an abortion against the effect that an abortion would have on the fetus's *time-relative interests*—that is, on what there is most reason to care about *for its own sake now*. It might, of course, be held that the moral significance of the developed fetus's identity-preserving potential to become a person just is that it has a present time-relative interest in becoming a person. That time-relative interest, however, is subsumed within its time-relative interest in continuing to live. Thus this claim about the developed fetus's potential adds nothing to the objection to late abortion that is implied by the Time-Relative Interest Account of the wrongness of killing.

Before concluding this section, we should briefly consider the idea that a human fetus has the potential to become a person in the third of the three senses distinguished at the beginning of the section. I have included this third interpretation of the notion that a fetus is a potential person because I have found it gestured at in the literature; but it is not clear that it is really a distinct interpretation. Although those who appeal to this notion of potential often say such things as that the fetus is an uncompleted person or that it somehow contains the person in inchoate form within itself, what is normally meant seems to be only that the fetus is an entity whose essential nature is to unfold itself into a person. And this, I take it, is just a dramatic way of emphasizing that the fetus's potential is suitably internal or intrinsic—that is, that it is *not* that the fetus becomes a person by having the elements of personhood added from without; rather, they develop from within. Understood in this way, the third interpretation is equivalent to the claim that the fetus has the identity-preserving potential to become a person; thus it is true of the developed fetus but false of the early fetus. There is, however, a way in which the third interpretation could be a distinctive claim. It might claim that the fetus (or, more specifically, the developed fetus) is a potential person because it is a *partially existing* person, a person in the making or in the process of coming into existence. This, as I suggested in section 2 of this chapter, is an interesting and intuitively appealing claim. But it does not, as I also argued earlier, offer a strong argument against abortion. Its implications for abortion seem instead to coincide closely with those of the Time-Relative Interest Account of the morality of killing.

In summary, then, the early fetus's potential to become a person is not identity-preserving but is only non-identity potential. It therefore has no interest, and no time-relative interest, in becoming a person. If it would be good if another person were to come into existence, the early fetus's non-identity potential could have instrumental value. But that could not ground a strong objection to early abortion, because the potential of any pair of sperm and egg would have a similar non-identity potential and thus a similar instrumental value. The developed fetus, by contrast, does have the identity-preserving potential to become a person, and thus has an interest in its realization. But we should not be guided by the developed fetus's interests. Rather, we should be guided by a respect for its time-relative interests, and its time-relative interest in realizing its potential to become a person is weak for the same reason that its time-relative interest in continuing to live is weak.

6.2. Potential as a Basis for Moral Status

We have yet to consider the idea that potential may be a source of moral status. It is sometimes claimed that, because the fetus has the potential to become a person, it therefore already has the moral status, or perhaps the rights, that persons have. This, surely, is excessively crude. The possession of the potential, whether identity-preserving or otherwise, to become a Y does not normally give one the rights of a Y. A tennis player, for example, may have the potential to be a Wimbledon champion, but he does not have a right to the trophy unless he realizes this potential. And Prince Charles's potential to become the king of England does not give him the rights of a king.[4]

Even if this crude view is certainly false as a general claim, there may be special instances in which X's having the identity-preserving potential to become a Y confers on it a special moral status—perhaps not exactly the status of a Y but something approximating it. It might be, for example, that an individual that has the identity-preserving potential to become a person thereby also has a high moral status, one that entails certain moral protections. People often have something like this in mind when they claim that abortion is wrong because the fetus is a potential person.

The idea that the potential to become a person confers a special moral status is plausible, if at all, only if the potential is identity-preserving. (It makes little sense to suppose that X's potential to become a Y confers a special status on X now if X will never actually *be* a Y, and especially if the transition to Y involves X's ceasing to exist. In these conditions, if X had a high moral status, that might be a reason to *prevent* the realization of its potential, thereby preventing its ceasing to exist.) In the following discussion, therefore, I will use the term "potential person" to refer only to individuals that have the identity-preserving potential to become a person. I have argued that, among fetuses, only developed fetuses are potential persons. Hence the subsequent discussion will apply only to developed fetuses. For convenience, however, in the remainder of this section I will drop the cumbersome term "developed fetus" and refer simply to "the fetus." Those who believe, on whatever basis, that the early fetus also has the identity-preserving potential to become a person may take my references to fetuses to apply to whatever it is they believe has the relevant identity-preserving potential: the fetal organism, the fetal soul, or whatever, at any point in its career as a fetus.

Our question, then, is whether the fetus's identity-preserving potential to become a person confers on it a special moral status that constrains the permissibility of abortion. Of particular importance for our inquiry is the more specific question whether the fetus's potential to become a person brings it within the sphere of the morality of respect—or, as I will say, whether its potential is a basis for respect. For if its being a potential person makes it worthy of respect, killing it must be as seriously wrong as killing an innocent person, if other things are equal. Aborting it may therefore be seriously wrong even if its time-relative interest in continuing to live is comparatively weak (just as it would be seriously wrong to kill a very elderly person without her consent, even if her time-relative interest in continuing to live was weak because there was little prospect of further good in her life). For if the fetus's potential makes it worthy of respect, the morality of abortion is not governed by the Time-Relative Interest Account of the morality of killing, as I have suggested, but by the morality of respect.

Recall that the property or properties that are the basis of respect must be intrinsic rather than relational. These properties must be what morally differentiates us from animals, making us worthy of respect in a way that animals are not. I have suggested that the most plausible candidates are certain psychological capacities, arguably those capacities that are constitutive of personhood: primarily self-consciousness, but perhaps minimal rationality and autonomy, as well. Fetuses lack these capacities, but they differ from animals in having the potential to develop these capacities—that is, to become persons. Perhaps, then, the basis of the worth that commands respect is the possession of the relevant psychological capacities *or* the potential to develop those capacities. The main aim of this section is to determine whether the fetus's potential can plausibly be regarded as a basis for respect—though for the most part I will refer more generally to the possibility that its potential is a basis for moral status.

What exactly do we mean when we say that the fetus has the potential to become a person? What is it about the fetus now that is the ground for our ascribing that potential to it? If its potential is to be a basis for moral status, and if the basis for status must be a property or set of properties that are intrinsic, there must be something intrinsic about the fetus now that justifies the claim that it is a potential person.

We can approach this question by considering the following three cases:

The Normal Fetus. This is a developed fetus that is in every way normal and healthy.

The Fetus with a Chemical Deficit. This is a fetus whose brain is developing normally—in that it will have a typical array of cortical neurons and synapses—except that it is deficient in a certain chemical (perhaps a neurotransmitter) that is important for the proper functioning of the cerebral cortex. In the absence of this chemical, its brain will never function above the level of a chimpanzee's brain. Without this chemical, the fetus will never be a person.

The Fetus with Cerebral Deficits. This is a fetus whose brain is developing abnormally, in that it is developing fewer than the usual number of cortical neurons and synapses. If it continues on its present developmental path, its cerebral cortex will be underdeveloped in certain regions, so that its cognitive capacities will never be higher than those of a chimpanzee.

Most people, I believe, want to say that all three of these fetuses are potential persons. I have conceded that this is true in the case of the Normal Fetus, but the claim is more contentious in the cases of the Fetus with a Chemical Deficit and the Fetus with Cerebral Deficits. On what basis might it be claimed that these latter two fetuses are potential persons?

One response is simply that these fetuses are both the sort of entity that normally becomes a person. If they never actually become persons, that is simply because of the absence of some condition necessary for the actualization of the potential (the chemical or certain cerebral structures that failed to develop). But to point out that these two fetuses are entities of a kind whose normal members tend to become persons is not to show that they have the potential to become persons. It is only to note that *normal* members of the kind have that potential. But *these* two members of the kind are not normal members. And their abnormality is precisely that they lack something that is necessary for them to become persons.

It seems a truism that, in order for X to have the potential to become a Y, it must be *possible* for X to become a Y. It seems to make no sense to say that X is a potential Y if it is literally impossible for X to become a Y. Yet there are forms and degrees of possibility. There is a sense in which it is impossible in the midst of a severe drought for a seed to become a plant; yet there is another sense in which it is clearly possible for the seed to become a plant: all that is necessary is that it should be supplied with water. It is this second kind of possibility that is necessary for potential, for we accept that the seed has the potential to become a plant, even when there will in fact be no rain. Similarly, in a time of famine the probability may be zero that a normal fetus will become a person, yet we accept that it is possible for it to become a person and thus grant that it is a potential person. Perhaps we should treat the case of the fetus with a chemical deficit in the same way, claiming that its lack of the necessary chemical is compatible with its having the potential to become a person in the same way that the normal fetus's lack of nutrition in a time of famine is compatible with its being a potential person.

Is it similarly possible for the fetus with cerebral deficits to become a person? The difference between this fetus and the fetus with a chemical deficit does not seem significant: the one lacks a certain chemical necessary for normal functioning of the brain; the other lacks certain tissues in the brain that are necessary for normal functioning. Yet the claim that it is possible for the fetus with cerebral deficits to develop the cognitive capacities necessary for personhood seems deeply problematic.

Compare the case of a child born without eyes a thousand years ago. Did this child have the potential for sight? I think most people would find it hardly credible to suppose that it did. Now imagine a child born without eyes in a world in which eye transplants are routinely performed. This second blind child clearly has the potential for sight. Certainly if he receives a transplant and is thereby enabled to see, that demonstrates that all along he had the potential to see. Next suppose there were a form of genetic therapy that, if administered to the fetus with cerebral deficits, would cause it to grow the cerebral tissues necessary for normal cognition; and suppose that the growth of these tissues would be identity-preserving. If such a therapy existed, it is clear that the fetus with cerebral deficits would have the potential to become a person, just as the child born without eyes would have the potential for sight if the technology existed for the transplantation of eyes.

Notice, however, what this implies. Suppose that we accept that a child born without eyes a thousand years ago did not have the potential for sight, but that a relevantly similar child born in a world in which eye transplants are performed would have that potential. If this is what we believe, it seems that we should also believe that the fetus with cerebral deficits does not have the potential to become a person in a world, such as ours, in which cerebral augmentation is not possible, but that it would have that potential in a world in which cerebral augmentation could be achieved through genetic therapy. But if there is no intrinsic difference between the fetus with cerebral deficits in our world and the fetus in the world in which cerebral augmentation is possible, the difference in their potentials cannot be a matter of their intrinsic properties. The basis for ascribing to the one fetus the potential to become a person must be wholly extrinsic. Hence its potential to become a person cannot be a basis for moral status, for it is not grounded in its intrinsic properties.

One might adopt a more radical view. One might hold that, as long as it is *physically possible* for the fetus with cerebral deficits to develop the cognitive capacities that are constitutive of personhood in a way that is identity-preserving, that fetus counts as a potential person. And surely it is physically possible for such a fetus's brain to develop further in a way that would give it the relevant capacities. If, as seems likely, a genetic therapy is ever devised that can promote cerebral growth in fetuses that would otherwise be profoundly cognitively impaired, that will decisively show, on this view, that all along fetuses with cerebral deficits have had the potential to become persons. It is just that our science has so far been insufficiently sophisticated to enable us to elicit it.

According to this view, moreover, the basis of the fetus's potential is not extrinsic. The potential is not supplied by the genetic therapy. It is present in fetuses with cerebral deficits that live and die long before the advent of the therapy. For what the potential essentially consists in is an intrinsic receptivity to an identity-preserving transformation into a person. This is a fact about the fetus itself: that it is the sort of thing that can in principle be transformed into a person while continuing to exist.

There are, however, two objections to this understanding of the fetus's potential. First, because it is virtually impossible to identify the full range of identity-preserving transformations that it is physically possible for an entity to undergo, we can in practice have only a limited appreciation of any given entity's potentials. Second, and more important, if it is physically possible, through some as-yet-undiscovered form of genetic therapy, to augment a defective fetus's brain in a way that will enhance its future cognitive capacities, it is surely physically possible to achieve the same result in an animal—for example, a dog. If, therefore, we claim that a fetus with cerebral deficits is a potential person on the ground that it is physically possible for its brain to develop in ways that would be identity-preserving and would overcome or repair the deficits, we must concede that a dog is a potential person for the same reason. And if we claim that the fetus's potential to become a person is a basis for moral status (because it is grounded in a suitably intrinsic receptivity to transformation), we must concede that a dog has an equivalent status, other things being equal. Since, however, no one would (or should) accept that dogs are potential persons with a moral status appropriate to their nature as such, we must abandon the broad conception of potential that implies that they are.

One might seek to distinguish between the potential of the fetus with cerebral deficits and that of a dog by claiming that the way the genetic therapy would work would be to stimulate some dormant gene that the fetus has but a dog lacks. But even if that were true, all it would mean is that the form of genetic therapy necessary to transform a dog into a person would have to be different: it would have to work, not by stimulating a preexisting but dormant gene, but by inserting a gene that would have the same function. There is no reason to suppose that this would be physically impossible.

There is, I believe, no basis for claiming that the fetus with cerebral deficits has the potential to become a person that does not also imply that a dog has that potential. (Recall that the fact that such a fetus is a member of a kind whose normal members are potential persons does not entail that it is a potential person. And for any mechanism that could cause the fetus to develop into a person, there should be an analogous mechanism whereby a dog could be transformed into a person.) If that is right, we should abandon the ambition to include fetuses with cerebral deficits within the category of potential persons. Perhaps we can settle for the more modest conclusion that the normal fetus (and perhaps even the fetus with a chemical deficit) is a potential person.

What we require, it seems, is a distinction between *intrinsic* and *extrinsic* potential, where intrinsic potential to become a Y involves more than mere receptivity to being transformed into a Y in an identity-preserving manner. (Recall that such a distinction seemed necessary earlier, in section 5.1 of chapter 2.) For surely the normal fetus's potential to become a person is in some sense intrinsic, while any potential that a dog might have to become a person is wholly extrinsic. If we can draw the distinction in a way that is principled and that provides an intuitively plausible division of the various cases, we can then claim that it is not the potential to become a person that is the basis of moral status, but the *intrinsic* potential to become a person. It might be argued, for example, that the developed fetus is worthy of respect because it has the intrinsic potential to become a person.

How is the distinction between intrinsic and extrinsic potential to be drawn? One suggestion is that X has the intrinsic potential to become a Y if all it requires from the outside in order to become a Y is its normal environment. In its normal environment—namely, the womb with its various amenities—the normal fetus can develop into a person. Hence it has the intrinsic potential to become a person. The same is not true, of course, of a dog. This view also explains how it can be that an individual can have the potential to become a Y even if the probability is zero that it will actually become a Y. A seed has the potential to become a plant even in a time of drought, because the drought is an abnormal condition. In its normal environment, which includes periodic rainfall, the seed would become a plant. (In this connection, consider the claim of Rabbi Elliot N. Dorff, quoted in the *New York Times,* that embryos "have no legal status whatever in Jewish law when they are outside the womb, because they have no potential for becoming a human being."[5] According to this view, an embryo created in vitro is not a potential human being even if it will actually become a human being if it is implanted in a surrogate womb. If that implication strikes us as implausible, we can explain the mistake by appealing to the view that an entity's potential is determined by what it can become in its normal environment. According to this view, the embryo is a potential human being if it can become a human being when situated in its normal environment, which is the womb. The fact that it will not become a human being if it remains outside the womb is irrelevant.)

I have been deliberately vague about a certain element in this understanding of intrinsic potential. In order for X to have the intrinsic potential to become a Y, must it be the case that, when placed in its normal environment, it *will* become a Y, that it is *likely* to become a Y, or that it is merely *possible* that it will become a Y? Jeffrey Reiman, from whose analysis of the concept of potential I have borrowed the notion of a normal environment, insists on the second of these three options. He claims that, "if the normal environment were such that zygotes did not *usually* develop into human beings, they would not be potential human beings."[6] From this, together with the observation that "fewer than one third of conceptions result in live births," he draws the conclusion, which he welcomes, that "the newly conceived zygote is [not] even a potential human being."[7] I will not dispute the truth of this conclusion, since much depends on exactly what one means by "human being." But if, as seems clear, Reiman accepts that *some* zygotes do in fact become human beings (in the identity-preserving sense), it is doubtful that he can consistently claim that these zygotes were never potential human beings. It would seem to be more reasonable to claim that it is at least sufficient for X to have the intrinsic potential to become a Y if it is possible for it to become a Y in its normal environment, with no external intervention beyond what is part of that environment.

But now a more embarrassing question arises. What constitutes an entity's normal environment? It seems that what counts as normal varies with, among other things, time and technology. A hundred years ago, the normal environment was such that it was not possible for babies born with certain heart conditions to become adults. With the advent of transplant technology, the environment changed in a way that now makes it possible for babies with the same defects to become adults. It seems to follow, on the proposal we are considering, that babies born a hundred years ago with certain heart defects did not have the intrinsic potential to become adults, whereas babies born now with the same defects do have that intrinsic potential. But it is clearly incompatible with the notion of intrinsic potential to suppose that an entity's intrinsic potential varies with the state of technology. It is the essence of intrinsic potential that it is independent of wholly extrinsic factors.

Of course, all potential—including intrinsic potential—requires certain external conditions for its realization. If there is such a thing as intrinsic potential, the potential of a seed to become a plant is surely a paradigm example. Yet the seed requires water, nutrients from the soil, carbon dioxide in the atmosphere, and sunlight in order to realize this potential. The challenge is to determine *how much* of what is necessary in order for X to become a Y can come from external sources compatibly with X's having the *intrinsic* potential to become a Y.

Since personhood is a matter of the possession of certain capacities, let us focus on the potential for having a certain capacity, such as the capacity to see. An intuitively appealing suggestion is that X has the intrinsic potential to have the capacity for sight only if X has an inherent tendency, or is internally programmed, to develop the physical basis for sight, given an environment in which this tendency or program can operate. If, however, the physical basis for the capacity to see (for example, the eyes or the relevant parts of the brain) has to be added from the outside (for example, through an eye transplant or a brain graft) in order for X to have the capacity to see, X has only an extrinsic potential to be able to see. According to this proposal, the normal fetus has the intrinsic potential to see, for it is genetically programmed to develop eyes and a brain with a visual cortex. But a baby born without eyes has at most the extrinsic potential to see, for it must be externally supplied with eyes, which are part of the physical basis of sight.

Attractive though it is, this proposal contains a good deal of indeterminacy. The distinction between intrinsic and extrinsic potential is based on the contrast between an internally programmed tendency to develop the physical basis for a certain capacity and the external addition of the physical basis for that capacity. But consider again the fetus with a chemical deficit. Its internal program does not provide for the production of the chemical necessary for higher cognitive functions. Is the chemical it needs analogous to a vital nutrient—that is, something that can be regarded as external to the physical basis of the capacities constitutive of personhood—or is the chemical a part of the physical basis of personhood? It is unclear how this question should be answered, but the answer will determine whether, according to this proposal, the fetus's potential to become a person is intrinsic or extrinsic.

Or consider the fetus with cerebral deficits. If genetic therapy could stimulate the growth of new brain tissue that would enable the fetus to develop the capacities constitutive of personhood, would that mean that the fetus had the intrinsic potential to become a person? In support of an affirmative answer, one could claim that the physical basis of personhood—the brain—would be developed from within rather than being supplied externally. Yet it could also be argued that the program for the development of critical parts of the brain would have an external source: the genetic therapy. Whether this contention is plausible might depend, in turn, on whether the therapy would activate a preexisting but dormant gene or whether it would supply the gene and thus the program itself.

It is important to remind ourselves that our concern here is with potential as a basis of moral status. Yet it is hard to see how an entity's moral status could depend on considerations of this sort. Let us, however, press on. There are several other problems with this attempt to distinguish between intrinsic and extrinsic potential. The case of the fetus with cerebral deficits reveals a critical ambiguity in the proposed understanding. Suppose the fetus receives the therapy and its brain is stimulated to develop new tissues in which the capacities essential for personhood will eventually develop. Prior to receiving the therapy, its potential to become a person was, intuitively, extrinsic. As I have noted, it is not clear that the proposed way of drawing the distinction can capture that. But now there is a further question. After the therapy has been applied and the fetus's brain has grown new tissues, is its potential to become a person intrinsic or extrinsic? It seems that, according to the proposed understanding, its potential must now be intrinsic, for the physical basis for the capacities constitutive of personhood is now in place. It no longer needs to be supplied externally, but merely requires the usual forms of stimulation and support (nutrition, contact with people, exposure to language, etc.) in order for the relevant capacities to develop. If that is right, the application of the therapy has converted the fetus's potential from extrinsic to intrinsic. If only intrinsic potential is a basis for high moral status, the therapy has profoundly altered the fetus's moral status. But if what is relevant to status is potential, and if it was equally true both before and after the therapy that the fetus was going to become a person, is it really plausible to suppose that its moral status is radically altered at the point at which its potential shifts from extrinsic to intrinsic?

Let us run the process in reverse. Suppose a normal fetus suffers brain damage that destroys various areas of the brain necessary for the development of certain cognitive capacities necessary for personhood. When this happens, the fetus loses its intrinsic potential to become a person and thus, presumably, its moral status as a potential person. But suppose the relevant areas of the brain can, and will, be restored via genetic therapy. And suppose that enough of the fetus's brain would remain unaffected that the same mind would persist throughout: thus the processes of loss and regeneration would both be identity-preserving. Is it really plausible to suppose that during the interval between the occurrence of the brain damage and the restoration of the relevant tissues, the fetus's moral status is significantly lower, even though the fact that it will eventually become a person is unaffected by the processes that change the character of its potential from intrinsic to extrinsic and then to intrinsic again?

These brief remarks should indicate both how difficult it is to draw a distinction between intrinsic and extrinsic potential and also how problematic it is to treat that distinction as critically relevant to an individual's moral status. Let us assume, however, that we have a clear distinction between intrinsic and extrinsic potential and that it implies that, while the normal fetus's potential to become a person is intrinsic, that of the fetus with cerebral deficits is extrinsic. In that way, the distinction avoids the implication that the existence of a genetic therapy for cognitive enhancement would give dogs an intrinsic potential to become persons. Potential derived from this source would, we can assume, count as extrinsic.

It is obvious that even the normal fetus's intrinsic potential to become a person requires considerable external input for its realization. In the absence of physical protection, nutrition, and, later, exposure to language and culture, and so on, even a normal human fetus will not become a person. There are, indeed, many forms of intrinsic potential that must be elicited by human intervention. It seems, for example, that the potential for language is intrinsic in human beings, but a human child will not realize this potential unless it is exposed to language by other people. It is possible, therefore, that certain forms of intrinsic potential may pass unrecognized and may therefore never be elicited. Suppose that we were to discover that this has hitherto been the case with dogs. Suppose that we were to discover that dogs have the intrinsic potential for self-consciousness and rationality but that until now we have failed to recognize this because the potential has never been realized. For suppose that, in order to elicit this potential, it is necessary for someone to cultivate and nurture the relevant cognitive capacities through an intensive and highly structured program of "cognitive therapy." Only through years of patient work, taking virtually every waking moment of the dog's life from earliest puppyhood on, can the relevant mechanisms latent in the dog's brain be activated and developed. For the first few years there are no perceptible results (which is part of the explanation of why the process was not discovered earlier), but after five or six years, dogs subject to this program develop cognitive capacities comparable to those of a normal four-year-old human child.[8]

Suppose that all this were true. What we would have discovered is that, on any remotely plausible conception, dogs have the intrinsic potential to become persons. Assuming we were to discover this, ought we to conclude that all dogs have a high moral status—in particular, that all dogs are above the threshold of respect, so that killing a dog is just as wrong as killing a person, if other things are equal? Indeed, ought we to conclude that we and our forebears have been guilty of monstrous wrongs to dogs, who have always been within the scope of the morality of respect though we have been unaware of it? I doubt that anyone would draw these conclusions. While we would (or should) accept that respect would be owed to any dog whose potential to become a person had been realized, the knowledge that all dogs had this potential would not require us to reassess our estimation of the actual worth of all those dogs whose potential was never cultivated or never would be cultivated. But if we would not accept that all dogs, in these circumstances, would be worthy of respect, we do not really believe that the intrinsic potential to become a person is a basis for respect, or for high moral status generally.

To drive home the point, we can consider a variant of this example. Suppose that the plasticity in the canine brain that allows for this intrinsic potential is transient unless it is exploited; thus, unless the intensive cognitive therapy is begun within the first year of a dog's life, the potential fades and is unrecoverable. In this respect it would be analogous to the human capacity for language acquisition, which steadily diminishes after the first few years of life—except that in this case the potential would not just diminish, but would vanish altogether. If this were the case, all puppies would intrinsically be potential persons, but those that failed to receive the therapy within a year would lose the potential and therefore, presumably, the moral status that goes with it. Puppies would initially be within the scope of the morality of respect, but those that failed to receive the therapy would then drop below the threshold of respect even though, as adult dogs, their actual psychological capacities might be more highly developed than those of puppies that had so far retained their intrinsic potential. This, I believe, is utterly implausible.

6.3. Potential, Cognitive Impairment, and Animals

Even if a human fetus has the intrinsic potential to become a person, that does not affect its moral status. It does not make it worthy of respect. In fact, it seems morally irrelevant whether an entity's potential is intrinsic or extrinsic. An entity's potential is simply what it can become through the full range of possible transformations that would be identity-preserving. We do not need to quibble about different forms and degrees of possibility. The real relevance of possibility is practical. For the important question in each particular case is not how X's potential affects its moral status but how strong a moral reason, if any, there is to try to realize X's potential. And this may be affected by "how possible" it is to realize or to elicit the potential. (The possibility of an eye transplant, for example, would be remote if they were rarely performed and seldom succeeded even when they were.)

If dogs had the potential to become persons—whether through genetic therapy that would stimulate the growth of new cerebral tissues or through cognitive therapy that would activate mechanisms latent in the dog's brain—the crucial question would be how important it would be, morally, to try to ensure that dogs became persons. I believe that the strength of one's moral reason to try to realize X's potential to become a Y depends in great measure on the strength of X's time-relative interest in becoming a Y. (There are, of course, many other considerations that are relevant—for example, one's relation to X, the costs one would be likely to incur, the possibility of undesirable side effects, the probability of success, and so on. But these considerations come into play only if there is a reason to try to realize the potential that is grounded in X's own time-relative interest in its realization. Otherwise, these other considerations simply do not arise.)

How strong a moral reason one has to try to realize X's potential to become a Y is, it seems, completely unaffected by whether the potential is intrinsic or extrinsic.

Consider, for example, two children, one whose ability to see has been thwarted from birth by the presence of microbes that block the action of the optic nerve, and another born without eyes. It is reasonable to suppose that the first of these children has the intrinsic potential for sight, since it possesses a complete visual apparatus whose functions are externally impeded, while the second child's potential for sight is extrinsic, since a critical component of its potential visual apparatus has to be externally provided. Yet it is obvious that, if other things are equal, there is just as strong a moral reason to try to realize the second child's potential as there is to realize that of the first.

To repeat: the important question raised by an individual's potential is how much it matters, for the individual's own sake, that he should fulfill that potential— that is, that he should become what it is possible for him to become, or have what it is possible for him to have. In the case of abortion, the moral importance of the fetus's potential is therefore entirely captured by the Time-Relative Interest Account. Whatever reason there is to ensure the realization of the fetus's potential to become a person is subsumed by the reason to respect its time-relative interest in continuing to live. The good of becoming or being a person is one dimension of the good that its future might contain and that it has a present time-relative interest in having. I argued earlier, however, that its present time-relative interest in having the goods of its own future is relatively weak, given the virtual absence of psychological connections between itself now as a fetus and itself later as a person. What this means is that it matters comparatively little, for the fetus's own sake now, whether it realizes its potential or not.

Consider three possible scenarios. Consider first a fetus with cerebral deficits in a world in which there is no possibility of cognitive enhancement. This fetus, if it lives, will be severely cognitively impaired. Its time-relative interest in continuing to live is, therefore, considerably weaker even than that of the normal fetus. For not only would its future contain substantially less good than that of a normal fetus, but also, if its psychological capacities are abnormally low even at this early age, it will be less closely connected to itself in the future psychologically than the normal fetus.

Second, consider a fetus with cerebral deficits that has the potential to become a person (perhaps because a genetic therapy exists that could enhance its cognitive capacities in an identity-preserving way). If this potential would never in fact be realized, its existence may make little difference to the morality of abortion. For the strength of the fetus's time-relative interest in continuing to live seems to depend on the character of the life that it would be likely to have, not on the character of a life that it could conceivably have but in fact will not. (One qualification is necessary here. It may matter *why* the fetus would not realize its potential to become a person.

It would seem illegitimate for a pregnant woman to defend her decision to have an abortion by claiming that the life her child would have if it were to live would be of low quality, when the reason it would be so is that *she* would refuse to provide her child with the therapy it would need in order to have a better life.)

Third and finally, consider a fetus with cerebral deficits whose potential to become a person would be realized, or would be very likely to be realized. In that case its time-relative interest in continuing to live would be comparable in strength to that of a normal fetus; but that would still be relatively weak.

My claims about these cases presuppose that, if an abortion is performed, the only time-relative interest that would be opposed to the action is that of the fetus at the time. For the abortion itself would effectively preclude the existence of any later time-relative interests. But suppose, for whatever reason, that abortion was not an issue. Suppose that a fetus with cerebral deficits was going to live and that the only question was whether to administer the genetic therapy that would enhance its cognitive capacities, thereby enabling it to become a person. How strong would the moral reason be to administer the therapy? How important is it that the fetus should realize its potential to become a person rather than living its life as a nonperson?

In practice, the interests of the fetus's parents will be strongly engaged in favor of administering the therapy, as will those of any others who might be required to help meet the costs of caring for an individual who would be severely cognitively impaired. But let us put these considerations aside. Alternatively, we might imagine that the parents are wealthy activists on behalf of the disabled who believe that it would be unjustly discriminatory, or would implicitly devalue the lives of the cognitively impaired, to insist that their child should have genetic therapy for cognitive enhancement. Our question might then be whether there would be a moral objection to their not providing the therapy when they would have ample means of doing so. The important question, in short, is whether—and, if so, to what extent—it is important, for the sake of the fetus itself, that it should realize its potential to become a person.

The obvious response, suggested earlier in the section on prenatal harm, is that we must be guided not just by the fetus's present time-relative interests but also by those time-relative interests that it will have in the future that might be affected by whether or not it fulfills its potential. A baby born with a neurological defect that, if untreated, would later prevent it from being able to walk has a present time-relative interest in later being able to walk; but that time-relative interest may be comparatively weak because of the relative weakness of the psychological relations that would bind the baby to itself in the future. But when it becomes older, and closely psychologically related to itself in the future, its time-relative interest in being able to walk may be quite strong (assuming that adaptation does not occur, or occurs only incompletely). It is therefore an important reason to enable the baby to realize its potential and that to fail to do so would be to doom to frustration its later, stronger time-relative interests.

Perhaps a similar claim can be made on behalf of the fetus with cerebral deficits. This, in fact, is one case in which adaptation will assuredly not occur. A severely mentally retarded adult will certainly not prefer his actual life with severe cognitive impairment to the life he might have had if the impairment had been corrected. For the severely retarded adult will lack the cognitive resources to entertain *any* preferences about his life as a whole. But whatever the explanation is of why the fetus's cerebral deficits ought, if possible, to be corrected, it is clear that the commonsense view is that there is a strong moral reason to enable the fetus to realize its potential to become a person. There is, however, a problem here—one that many people will not be inclined to take seriously, though it is, in my view, a serious problem indeed. Again, suppose that the fetus with cerebral deficits lacks a certain gene that directs the growth of various areas of the brain necessary for the cognitive capacities that are constitutive of personhood. If the gene is introduced via therapy, it will stimulate the growth of the relevant areas and the fetus will eventually become a person. Next imagine, as I suggested earlier, that the insertion of a functionally equivalent gene into the body of a canine fetus would stimulate the growth of comparable cerebral tissues, thereby causing the dog eventually to become a person—that is, a being with capacities for certain minimum levels of self-consciousness, rationality, and autonomy. It seems that whatever reasons we have for administering the therapy to the fetus with cerebral deficits that appeal in some way to its own good would apply equally to administering the therapy to the dog. Their potential, after all, appears to be the same: both would rely on the same form of identity-preserving genetic therapy in order to be enabled to become persons.

Of course, extrinsic considerations, such as effects on other people, would normally weigh heavily in favor of administering the therapy to the human fetus but would not do so in the case of the canine fetus. But if we put those considerations aside for the moment and focus just on the reason we would have to administer the therapy *for the sake of the individual who would receive it,* it is difficult to see why we would have more reason to administer it to the fetus with cerebral deficits than to a canine fetus. (Let us assume, for the sake of argument, that a dog with human intelligence could have a life that would be well worth living even in a society in which it would be a freak, would have no acceptable mate, and so on. In short, let us put those contingent problems aside, as well.)

I know of no one who believes that it would be morally important to enable canine fetuses, or even adult dogs, to become persons if it were possible to do so.

There are also, I think, relatively few people who accept that there is comparatively little moral reason, for a defective fetus's own sake, to give it a genetic therapy that would enable it to become a person rather than a severely retarded adult. But there seem to be no intrinsic properties that differentiate the human fetus with cerebral deficits from a canine fetus in a way that would make it important to realize the extrinsic potential of the human fetus but not that of the canine fetus.

It is worth emphasizing the nature of the problem we face. We must adopt one of the following three options:

1. We can accept that there is no strong reason, for a dog's own sake, to enable it to become a person; that there is no significant intrinsic difference between a dog and a human fetus that, if unaided, will develop cognitive capacities no higher than those of the dog; and that there is therefore no strong moral reason, for the defective fetus's own sake, to enable it to become a person rather than a severely retarded adult.

2. We can accept that it is morally important that a fetus with cerebral deficits should be enabled, if possible, to become a person; that there is no significant intrinsic difference between such a fetus and a dog; and, therefore, that there is a strong moral reason, for dogs' own sakes, to enable them, if possible, to become persons rather than retaining the cognitive capacities characteristic of dogs as they are now.

3. We can argue that there is an important intrinsic difference between a dog (or other animal) and a cognitively impaired human fetus that explains why, even if both have an equal extrinsic potential to become a person, we have a strong moral reason in the case of the fetus—but not in the case of the animal—to enable it to fulfill its potential to become a person.

As I have noted, both of the first two options are highly counterintuitive; therefore virtually everyone will want to adopt the third. But it is highly problematic. The problem is to identify a relevant intrinsic difference; but, as I tried to argue at length in section 2.2 of chapter 3, there is in fact no relevant difference to be found. There are no intrinsic differences of psychological capacity or potential, and therefore no difference in capacity for well-being. The only intrinsic differences are physical: differences of physical constitution and morphology traceable to, or equivalent to, the fact that the human fetus and the canine fetus or adult dog are members of different biological species. And these differences are without moral significance. That a human fetus with cerebral deficits has certain physical properties that a canine fetus lacks provides no reason for thinking that it is more important to realize its potential than it is to realize the equivalent potential of the canine fetus.

One way to proceed is to consider why there appears to be little or no moral reason to enable an animal to become a person via cognitive enhancement. It is hard to deny that, if a dog were to receive a genetic therapy that would enhance its cognitive capacities in an identity-preserving way, thereby enabling it to become a person, that would be good for the dog. For it is hard to deny that its capacity for well-being would thereby be expanded and that there would be a high probability that its life as a whole would be better—by as much as the lives of persons are typically better, or more worth living, than the lives of animals. These considerations fail to impress us, however; we do not accept that the fact that an animal's life as a whole would be better if it were to become a person provides a reason to enable it to become a person. Of course, our failure to be impressed might be just the result of prejudice; for there is certainly no shortage of that in our beliefs about the morality of our treatment of animals. Yet our response is consistent with the tendency of my argument in this chapter, which has been to move away from considering the effect that one's action has on the value of an individual's life as a whole and to focus instead on the effect one's action has on the individual's time-relative interests.

One striking reflection is that it does not seem that it would be a *misfortune* for a dog to retain its own low cognitive capacities rather than to become a person. This may seem odd. How could it not be a misfortune for an individual to fail to receive a great benefit? A moment's reflection reveals, however, that there is really nothing odd about this and that certain conditions must be met in order for a missed benefit to count as a misfortune. It would, for example, be good for me to discover a vein of gold in my back yard worth millions of dollars. But it is not a misfortune for me that there is in fact no vein of gold there.[9] It seems, however, that the explanation of why it would not be a misfortune for a dog not to become a person is different from the explanation of why it is not a misfortune for me to fail to discover gold on my property. For there is an important difference between the two cases.

I noted just now that the tendency of my argument has been to replace the concern for individuals' interests, or for the value of their lives as wholes, with a concern for their time-relative interests. And it is where time-relative interests are concerned that the difference between the two cases lies. Whatever else is true, I have a strong egoistic reason for wanting to own large amounts of gold. But someone who cares about a dog for its own sake would seem to have little or no reason to want, for the dog's own sake now, for it to become a person—even if its becoming a person would mean that its life as a whole would be better. Another way of making this point is to note that there is no point in the dog's life at which it would have a serious time-relative interest in becoming a person. Even assuming that the transformation would be identity-preserving and that being a person would be a very great good, the nature of the transformation would be so radical as to exclude certain conditions of egoistic concern. I have argued that, in addition to physical and functional continuity in certain areas of the brain, psychological continuity is among the conditions of egoistic concern—not in the sense that it is *necessary* in order for egoistic concern to be rational, but in the sense that the *degree* to which it is rationally appropriate to be egoistically concerned about oneself in the future varies, other things being equal, with the degree to which one would be psychologically continuous with oneself in the future. This, I believe, applies in the case of animals as well. For conscious animals are, like ourselves, essentially minds; therefore the conditions of identity and of egoistic concern are the same for animals as they are for us. But if this is right, the psychological distance between a dog now and itself as it would be if it were to become a person would be too great for the dog to have a serious time-relative interest in being thus transformed. And this, I suspect, is the main reason why it would not be a misfortune for a dog to fail to become a person: it has no time-relative interest that would thereby be frustrated. Even though the prospect of becoming a person would be a prospect of a great good, a dog simply cannot be related to that good in a way that makes it important for it to have or to achieve it.

To make this point intuitively clearer, one might imagine the prospect of becoming like a god. Imagine the possibility of becoming vastly more intelligent and developing a vastly richer and deeper range of emotions, including emotions of which one cannot now form any conception. One would be as different from oneself now, in terms of psychological capacities, as one is now from a dog (or, more to the point, as different from oneself now as a dog would be from itself if it were to become a person). One would be, in short, so utterly psychologically remote from oneself as one is now that one may now have little or no egoistic reason to want to become that way. Even if the transformation would be identity-preserving and would lead to a state that would be clearly superior to one's present state, it would be too much like becoming someone else—and, of course, losing oneself in the process—to be very desirable from an egoistic point of view.

I have argued that the psychological distance between a normal fetus and the person it might later become is too great for it to have a strong time-relative interest in realizing its potential to become that person. I have suggested, furthermore, that the same is true, mutatis mutandis, of a dog with the potential to become a person, and of a person with the potential to become a god. But if this is right, the same must be true of a fetus with cerebral deficits that has the potential to become a person. Like a normal fetus, the fetus with cerebral deficits cannot have a strong *present* time-relative interest in becoming a person. For the psychological relations that would hold between itself now and itself much later, when it would be a person, are too weak. But notice that the fetus with cerebral deficits will, as long as it remains retarded, *always* be distantly psychologically related to itself in the future. In this respect it is like an animal rather than a normal fetus. Its relation to itself in the future will always be comparable to the relation that a normal fetus bears to itself in the future, or the relation that an animal bears to itself in the further future. This is because the mental life of the fetus with cerebral deficits will, as long as it remains retarded, never develop much beyond that of a fetus or an animal. Even as the fetus with cerebral deficits develops and grows, therefore, there will never be a point at which it will have a strong time-relative interest in being a person rather than remaining what it is: a severely cognitively impaired human being.

Because of this, the reasoning that may condemn many forms of prenatal injury, and may support the correction, when possible, of fetal impairments, does not apply in the case of the fetus with cerebral deficits. For this reasoning appeals to the time-relative interests that a fetus will *later* have. The reasoning is that, in the case of a fetus *without* cerebral deficits, it is wrong, if other things are equal, to inflict an injury that causes disability, or to fail to correct a condition that causes disability, because this will frustrate the strong time-relative interest that the individual will later have, when he becomes a person, in having certain abilities rather than being disabled (assuming that adaptation does not occur). But the fetus with cerebral deficits is different. It is relevantly like an animal in that, even as it develops physically, it will remain psychologically cut off from itself in the future and thus will never have a strong time-relative interest in being or becoming a person. Thus we cannot appeal to any later time-relative interest it will have in being or becoming a person in order to defend the view that it is important for it to become a person. Like an animal that fails to receive a genetic therapy that would enable it to become a person, the fetus with cerebral deficits never has a strong time-relative interest that would be frustrated by its failure to become a person.

If this is right, it suggests that, just as it is not a significant misfortune for an animal that could become a person to fail to do so, so, too, it is not a serious misfortune for the fetus with cerebral deficits if it fails to become a person. While it may be a serious misfortune for either to have a level of well-being well below the higher levels of which it is capable, it is not a significant misfortune, in itself, for either to have limited cognitive capacities or a limited range of well-being. Individuals who are not persons are not necessarily unfortunate for that reason.

It seems, therefore, that we cannot defend the commonsense intuition about the fetus with cerebral deficits by appealing to its time-relative interests. If we are guided by a concern for time-relative interests, we will have little reason, apart from that deriving from a concern for the time-relative interests of others, to try to ensure that a fetus with cerebral deficits, or even a congenitally severely cognitively impaired adult, is transformed into a person, if that becomes possible.

The problem, of course, is that these conclusions about fetuses with cerebral deficits and congenitally severely retarded adults are highly counterintuitive. Almost no one would accept them. And there is worse to come. The case of the fetus with cerebral deficits is parallel to cases involving prenatal injury, except that it involves allowing an individual to be harmed rather than causing it to be harmed. Thus the claims that I have made about the case of the fetus with cerebral deficits should also apply to a case in which one causes a normal fetus to have cerebral deficits. Consider:

Prenatal Retardation. Unless she takes a certain drug, a pregnant woman will develop a moderate disability. The drug would, however, cause the fetus she is carrying, which she intends in any case to put up for adoption, to be severely mentally retarded. Her present interest in not having the disability is stronger than the time-relative interest the fetus presently has in becoming a person rather than being retarded (which must be comparatively weak because of the weakness of the prudential unity relations), and indeed is stronger than any time-relative interest the fetus will ever have in being or becoming a person. She therefore takes the drug.

Intuitively, the woman's action seems clearly wrong. But how can we explain why it is wrong?

It is worth repeating why her interests may outweigh the combined present and future time-relative interests of the fetus. This fetus, like every other normal fetus, has only a very weak present time-relative interest in realizing its potential to become a person. And if it is caused to have cerebral deficits sufficient for severe retardation, it will *never* have a significant time-relative interest in being a person. If, therefore, the woman is guided only by a concern for its time-relative interests, both present and future, she will have only a weak moral reason not to cause this normal fetus to be retarded rather than allowing it to become a person. This will be true even if *doing* what is against an individual's time-relative interests is significantly worse than *allowing* what is worse for the individual's time-relative interests to occur. For this asymmetry can yield a strong objection to causing the fetus to become retarded only if its *being* retarded would be a seriously adverse condition. But, as long as we focus only on its time-relative interests, there is no reason to suppose that that is true.

This, therefore, is another form of prenatal injury that cannot be adequately objected to by appealing to the fetus's present and future time-relative interests. But the explanation of why the appeal to time-relative interests will not work in this case is different from that in cases involving adaptation. It is not that the fetus with cerebral deficits may later rationally prefer its life with retardation; it is, rather, that its cognitive capacities do not allow for the possession of *any* significant time-relative interests, except perhaps ones that are both negative and concerned only with the immediate future, such as a time-relative interest in the avoidance of great suffering now or in the near future.

It is important to note that what seemed to be the best solution to the problem of adaptation cannot apply in the case of Prenatal Retardation. That solution was to claim that, because prenatal injury harms the victim when he is a person, it comes within the scope of the morality of respect. Because of that, it is not a sufficient justification for the infliction of prenatal injury that the interests it serves outweigh those it frustrates. In the case of Prenatal Retardation, however, the fetus that is caused to be severely retarded is thereby prevented from ever becoming a person. The act that we wish to condemn has the effect of preventing itself from coming within the scope of the morality of respect.

One option is, of course, to appeal to what in section 5 of this chapter I called the Criterion. Both the cases with which we are now concerned—the fetus with cerebral deficits and the normal fetus that might be caused to have cerebral deficits— are cases in which the fetus will exist in all the possible outcomes of one's choice; therefore, according to the Criterion, one ought to be guided by a concern for the effect that one's choice will have on the value of its life as a whole. Since a fetus would have a substantially better life if its cognitive capacities would be those of a person rather than comparable to those of an animal, an appeal to the Criterion supports the common intuition that one has a strong moral reason to administer the genetic therapy to the fetus with cerebral deficits and, if anything, an even stronger reason not to cause a normal fetus to have cerebral deficits. But the Criterion is problematic in various ways. It seems, in its application to cases of this sort, to presuppose that identity is what matters—that is, that identity is the basis of egoistic concern. This is not only implausible in itself, but is also incompatible with the argument I have advanced concerning abortion. Even more important for present purposes, the Criterion does not appear to offer any ground for differentiating between a fetus with cerebral deficits and a comparably endowed animal. If it were possible to enable an animal to become a person, it seems that one would have the same reason to enhance its cognitive capacities as one would have to enhance those of the fetus with cerebral deficits—namely, that this would make its life as a whole much better. The only way to avoid this implication, if one appeals to the Criterion, is to deny that an animal's life would be better if it were to become a person. One would have to deny, for example, that the Superchimp has a better life than a normal chimpanzee. And that is hard to do.

It is tempting to think that it is *obvious* why there is reason not to cause, or if possible to cure, mental retardation in a human fetus, while there is no reason to try, if possible, to enhance the cognitive capacities of an animal. The explanation, it might be thought, is simply that mental retardation in a human being is a pathological condition, a defect or impairment, while the possession of comparable cognitive capacities by an animal cannot be regarded as a defect or disability, for it is entirely normal. A retarded human being is therefore unfortunate in a way that a normal animal is not. It is clear, however, that this explanation involves an implicit appeal to what is normal for the members of a particular species as a standard of evaluation—that is, it simply resurrects the Species Norm Account. And although this account may fairly accurately reflect common ways of thinking about these matters, it is vitiated by its attribution of decisive evaluative significance to an evaluatively neutral artifact of biological taxonomy—namely, species categories. As the example of the Superchimp demonstrates, what counts as fortune or misfortune is not determined by species membership.

The fundamental problem is to understand how the exact same intrinsic state could be bad or unfortunate for one individual but acceptable or even fortunate for another. It is obvious that this is often the case. A person who suffers brain damage that reduces him to a condition of contented idiocy, with cognitive capacities and a mental life comparable to those of a contented dog, is clearly in a dreadful condition. It may not be dreadful *experientially*—that is, it may not be dreadful because of the subjective character of the individual's experiences—but it is dreadful nonetheless *for this individual.* But the same state would not be dreadful for a dog. It might, indeed, be a comparatively fortunate state for a dog. Thus the explanation of why this condition is bad for the former person cannot be that it is intrinsically bad, in the way that suffering is intrinsically bad. The condition is bad only in a certain context, against a certain background, or relative to some norm or standard. The Species Norm Account claims that it is bad for the former person because it is bad by comparison with the range of conditions possible for normal human beings— that is, because it is at the low end of the scale of states that are possible for one endowed with psychological capacities that are normal for members of the human species. But while it seems right that a condition must be evaluated by comparison with what is possible given a certain set of psychological capacities, it seems a mistake to suppose that the relevant capacities are those typical of the members of the individual's own biological species. In the case of the Superchimp, for example, how it is faring depends not on how its condition compares with the condition of typical members of its species but on how its condition compares with what is possible for it, given the psychological capacities that are constitutive of its own actual nature.

These reflections led me, in section 5.1 of chapter 2, to consider an account of fortune and misfortune that I called the Peak Capacity Account. According to this view, how well or badly off an individual is depends on how its condition or level of well-being compares with the spectrum of states of well-being accessible to it, given the peak psychological capacities it has so far possessed. This explains why the person who suffers brain damage is unfortunate: his condition is very bad by comparison with the range of states that were possible for him when his psychological capacities were at their peak. But the Peak Capacity Account conflicts with intractable intuitions about retardation. Recall the case, also presented in section 5.1 of chapter 2, of the Brain-Damaged Individual. In this case, a newborn infant suffers brain damage that arrests its psychological development at its present level. Most of us strongly believe that this infant has suffered a misfortune and that, as it grows, its condition will be an unfortunate one (despite the fact that it does not have and never will have a strong time-relative interest that will be frustrated by its loss). If, however, we assess misfortune relative to the range of well-being made possible by the peak psychological capacities that an individual has achieved, the infant's condition may never count as unfortunate at all. For it may well fare, both now and in the future, as well as possible relative to the highest capacity for well-being that it has ever possessed.

What I have called the Intrinsic Potential Account was intended to remedy the deficiencies of the Peak Capacity Account. It seems that what is unfortunate about the newborn infant that suffers brain damage is that for most of its life it will fare very poorly relative to the range of well-being that it once had the intrinsic potential to achieve. This reflection prompted me to propose that whether a being is well or badly off depends on how its level of well-being compares to the range of well-being made possible by the highest psychological capacities it has actually achieved *or* that it had the intrinsic potential to achieve. This is the Intrinsic Potential Account.

This account allows that the Brain-Damaged Individual is unfortunate, because its level of well-being will forever fall dramatically short of the higher levels it once had the intrinsic potential to achieve. Thus it explains how it can be a misfortune to suffer cognitive impairment even if the victim never has more than a marginal time-relative interest in avoiding retardation or becoming a person. It therefore has the resources to condemn the woman's taking the drug in Prenatal Retardation. And it offers its explanation of the misfortune involved in cognitive impairment by evaluating an individual's condition by comparison with what the individual's own nature or constitution makes possible rather than by reference to characteristics typical of the individual's species. Thus it also allows that the Superchimp is unfortunate in its brain-damaged condition, since its level of well-being then falls well short of the levels it was once capable of achieving.

Yet, as I noted in chapter 2, the Intrinsic Potential Account seems incapable of supporting our intuition in the case of the Fetus with Cerebral Deficits. Because of its congenital cerebral deficits, this fetus lacks the intrinsic potential to become a person; therefore the Intrinsic Potential Account cannot deem its failure to become a person a misfortune; nor can it, therefore, support our intuitive conviction that it is important, for the fetus's own sake, to administer to it a genetic therapy that would cause it develop the areas of the brain that it congenitally lacks.

There is, moreover, another, equally disturbing problem with the Intrinsic Potential Account. Recall that earlier, in section 6.2 of this chapter, I sketched a scenario in which dogs are discovered to have the intrinsic potential to become persons—a potential that has until now remained undiscovered because it requires intensive external stimulation to be elicited. If this were to happen—that is, if dogs were discovered to have this potential—the Intrinsic Potential Account would imply that we have all along been mistaken in believing that dogs are not, in general, unfortunate beings. According to the Intrinsic Potential Account, what we would have discovered is that dogs have all along been unfortunate because the levels of well-being they have actually achieved have consistently fallen well below the levels that they have had the intrinsic potential to achieve. In this respect they are comparable to a human being who suffers brain damage in early infancy, except that they retain a potential that continues unrealized, whereas the infant's potential goes unrealized because it is lost. The dogs and the Brain-Damaged Individual are equally pitiable because they are condemned to live at a level far below that which they have or once had the potential to achieve. These implications, however, strike most of us as utterly implausible. While we believe that an infant that suffers brain damage would be unfortunate, we would not conclude that dogs are, and have always been, unfortunate if we were to discover that they have the intrinsic potential, which they have never realized, to become persons. The Intrinsic Potential Account delivers the wrong conclusion in this case.

I must end this section inconclusively. I began by suggesting that the strength of one's moral reason to facilitate the realization of an individual's potential is determined primarily by the strength of the individual's time-relative interest in becoming what it has the potential to become or having what it has the potential to have. Whether the individual's potential is intrinsic or extrinsic seems not to matter. I was immediately confronted, however, by an apparent counterexample: the fetus with cerebral deficits. If it were possible to enable this fetus eventually to become a person—for example, by administering a genetic therapy that would cause it to develop the missing areas of its brain—it seems intuitively that one would have a moral reason of considerable strength to do so. Yet this fetus has at present only a very weak time-relative interest in becoming a person and, as long as it remains severely cognitively impaired, it will *never* have more than a weak time-relative interest in being or becoming a person. The Criterion, I noted, supports the commonsense intuition in the case of the fetus with cerebral deficits, but it seems to presuppose the mistaken view that, in this case at least, identity is the basis of egoistic concern;

and, more importantly, it appears to imply that there would be equal reason to administer a genetic therapy for cognitive enhancement to an animal.

The various accounts of fortune (that is, of what it is for an individual to be fortunate or unfortunate) appear to fare no better. The Species Norm Account does distinguish in the desired way between the fetus with cerebral deficits and an animal with comparable intrinsic potential, but it does so in a way that is arbitrary. It implies that the fetus is worthy of cognitive enhancement, while the animal is not, simply because the fetus is a member of the human species. Because it arbitrarily makes fortune dependent on species norms, the Species Norm Account has wholly implausible implications in the case of the Superchimp.

The Peak Capacity Account supports the view that there would be little or no reason to provide cognitive enhancement for animals but, by parity of reasoning, fails to support the view that there would be a strong reason to provide genetic therapy for the fetus with cerebral deficits. Indeed, because it implies that it would not be a misfortune for a fetus or neonate to suffer severe brain damage, it offers no basis for objecting to *causing* a fetus or newborn infant to become severely retarded. The Intrinsic Potential Account, by contrast, implies that it can be a misfortune to lose the potential to become a person; hence it can condemn the act of causing a normal fetus to have cerebral deficits, as the woman does in Prenatal Retardation. It also supports the view that there would be little or no reason to provide cognitive enhancement for an animal; but, like the Peak Capacity Account, it cannot justify our intuition that there would be a strong reason to provide genetic therapy for the fetus with cerebral deficits. And it has implausible implications in the case in which dogs are discovered to have the intrinsic potential to become persons.

It is worth noting that the Intrinsic Potential Account draws a distinction that is not captured by an exclusive focus on time-relative interests. It implies that both the Brain-Damaged Individual and the fetus in Prenatal Retardation that is caused to have cerebral deficits are unfortunate because they fare poorly relative to the kind of life they had the intrinsic potential to have. Yet it also implies that the fetus with cerebral deficits may hardly be unfortunate at all. As I noted in section 5.1 of chapter 2, this may initially strike us as arbitrary. One reason why this may be so is that, at every point, the Brain-Damaged Individual's time-relative interest in becoming a person may be no stronger than that of the fetus with cerebral deficits. Similarly, the Intrinsic Potential Account implies that if dogs had the intrinsic potential to become persons (even if intensive "therapy" were necessary to elicit it), they would be unfortunate to remain ordinary dogs. But it also implies that dogs as they actually are would not be unfortunate not to become persons, even if it were possible to enable them to do so via genetic therapy. In both cases, however, the dogs would have an equivalent time-relative interest in becoming persons.

This discrepancy would be minimized if the Intrinsic Potential Account were to acknowledge that both the Brain-Damaged Individual and dogs with intrinsic potential would be only slightly unfortunate. And this seems possible. As I noted earlier, animals and human beings whose psychological capacities never rise above those of animals seem psychologically too insubstantial to be the victims of *tragic* misfortune. Thus, as I also noted, the Intrinsic Potential Account must recognize that it is a substantially more serious misfortune to fare badly relative to levels of well-being one is or has been *capable* of achieving than it is to fare badly relative to levels of well-being one has, or had, only the intrinsic *potential* to achieve.

The problem with this response, however, is that it applies equally to the fetus in Prenatal Retardation that is knowingly caused to be severely retarded. If the Intrinsic Potential Account can recognize only that this individual suffers a slight misfortune, it fails to provide the basis of a strong condemnation of the woman's act.

It is important to realize that the problem here is quite general. It is not just a problem for the Intrinsic Potential Account of fortune or for the view that, within the morality of interests, our concern should be with time-relative interests rather than with interests. There do not seem to be any considerations that plausibly explain and justify our intuitions about these various cases. We believe, for example, that there would be a significant moral reason to employ genetic therapy to enable the fetus with cerebral deficits to become a person but that there is no corresponding reason to enable an animal with comparable psychological capacities to become a person. Yet there seems to be no fundamental difference between their intrinsic natures (hence we cannot claim that the fetus is above the threshold of respect while the animal is below it), they both have the same extrinsic potential to become a person, they each have an equal (and quite weak) time-relative interest in realizing their potential to become a person, and their lives as wholes would both be better if they were to become persons. They are distinguished only by their species membership, and that seems an insufficient basis for claiming that it is very important for one, but not the other, to become a person. Similarly, we believe strongly that the woman acts wrongly in Prenatal Retardation. The Intrinsic Potential Account offers an explanation—namely, that her act causes her child to fare poorly relative to the sort of life it had the intrinsic potential to have. Yet there seems to be nearly as strong a reason to provide genetic therapy for the fetus with cerebral deficits as there is not to cause a normal fetus to become retarded. Hence it is unlikely that the appeal to potential can be the full explanation of why the woman's act is so objectionable.

These reflections may compel us to reconsider our understanding of the importance of cognitive enhancement in the case of congenitally severely mentally retarded human beings. While it is incontestably important to correct (and, a fortiori, not to cause) severe cognitive impairments in human fetuses and infants, the foregoing discussion calls into question the assumption that it is important to do so *for the sake of the fetus or infant.*

It may be that the main reason that people in general have to correct the impairment of a fetus with cerebral deficits has to do with the interests and concerns of human beings other than the fetus itself. ("People in general" embraces all those who might be affected by whether the impairment is corrected other than those who are specially related to the fetus. The latter presumably have a much stronger reason to care about the fetus for its own sake; hence any reason there would be to correct the impairment for the fetus's own sake will apply with considerably greater force to them—for example, the fetus's biological parents—than to others.) Our reason—that is, the reason that people in general have—is similar to the reason we have to ensure that, if a human being is going to come into existence, it should be one with normal cognitive capacities rather than a different one that is severely retarded. While it is preferable that an individual with normal cognitive capacities should exist, it is not better *for that individual* to exist than not to exist. It is not for that individual's sake that we ought to ensure that he exists. Rather, our reason to ensure that the one individual exists rather than the other may be primarily that that is better for *us*—that is, for people in general.

Of course, another relevant consideration is *impersonal:* it is simply a better outcome—that is, the world is a better place overall—if the individual with higher capacities (and therefore, presumably, a better life) exists. This is the better outcome even if there is *no one* for whom it is better. Similarly, it is impersonally better if a fetus with cerebral deficits has those deficits corrected. In neither case, however, can impersonal considerations provide a complete account of our moral reason for bringing about the better outcome. Just as it is impersonally better to cause a human being with higher cognitive capacities to exist rather than one with lower capacities, so it is impersonally better to have a child rather than to breed an animal. But surely breeding an animal rather than having a child (if one cannot do both) is less objectionable (if it is objectionable at all) than causing a severely retarded human being to exist rather than a person with normal cognitive capacities. Similarly, it would also be better impersonally if an animal were enabled to become a person; but, as we have seen, no one believes that we would have a significant moral reason to transform an animal into a person if that were possible, though most believe that we would have a strong moral reason to enable a fetus with cerebral deficits to become a person. If these cases cannot be differentiated on impersonal grounds, it is likely that a regard for our own interests is a significant part of our reason to bring an individual with higher capacities into existence rather than a different individual with lower capacities, and also a significant part of our reason to correct cerebral deficits in a fetus.

NOTES

1. A view of this sort is defended in Reichlin (1997).
2. Similar distinctions are drawn in Stone (1987) and Buckle (1988).
3. Parfit (1994), 38.
4. Singer (1993a),153.
5. Wade (1999).
6. Reiman (1999), 65; emphasis added.
7. Reiman, 65 and 66.
8. There is an echo here of Michael Tooley's example in which kittens, if injected with a certain chemical, will eventually develop into persons. The difference is that the source of the kittens' potential is extrinsic. See Tooley (1973), 86.
9. Compare Draper (1999).

REFERENCES

Buckle, Stephen. 1988. Arguing from potential. *Bioethics* 2: 227–253.
Draper, Kai. 1999. Disappointment, sadness, and death. *Philosophical Review* 108: 387–414.
McMahan, Jeff. 2002. *The Ethics of Killing*, 302–329. New York: Oxford University Press.
Parfit, Derek. 1994. Persons, bodies, and human beings. Unpublished.
Reichlin, Massimo. 1997. The argument from potential: A reappraisal. *Bioethics* 11:1–23.
Reiman, Jeffrey. 1999. *Abortion and the Ways We Value Human Life.* Lanham, MD: Rowman and Littlefield.
Singer, Peter. 1993a. *Practical Ethics.* 2nd ed. Cambridge: Cambridge University Press.
Stone, Jim. 1987. Why potentiality matters. *Canadian Journal of Philosophy* 17:815–30.
Tooley, Michael. 1973. A defense of abortion and infanticide. In Joel Feinberg (ed.), *The Problem of Abortion*, 51–91. 2nd ed. Belmont, CA: Wadsworth.
Wade, Nicholas. 1999. Embryo cell research: A clash of values. *New York Times,* July 2:A11.

CHAPTER NINE

Abortion and the Margins of Personhood

MARGARET OLIVIA LITTLE

I. Introduction

When a woman is pregnant, how should we understand the moral status of the life within her? How should we understand its status as conceptus, as embryo, when an early or again matured fetus? According to some, human life in all of these forms is inviolable: early human life has a moral status equivalent to a person from the moment of conception.[1] According to others, such life has no intrinsic status, even late in pregnancy.[2] According to still others, moral status emerges when sentience does. Until the fetus is conscious—a point somewhere at the end of the second trimester,[3] it has no moral status at all; after it is conscious, it does.[4]

But for a great many people, none of these views suffice. It is something rather more moderate that marks their intuitions. For many people, the human life at stake in early stages of pregnancy is not the moral equivalent of a paradigmatic person: if one somehow had to extinguish the life of an embryo in vitro to save a five-year-old child, the choice would be clear. On the other hand, even early abortion involves a morally sober loss: contraception is preferable to abortion on grounds of morality, not just public health. Most clearly, the fully matured fetus has the same level of moral considerability as does a newborn: birth does not mark a change in intrinsic moral status. In short, what a great many people believe is a *graduated* view of embryonic and fetal status: even at early stages of pregnancy, developing human life has an important value worthy of respect; its status grows as it does, increasing gradually until, at some point late in pregnancy, the fetus is deserving of the very strong moral protection due newborns.

I think this is exactly right, and in the present essay I sketch the outlines of such a view. I begin by considering why it has been difficult for philosophical theories to give more nuanced views of embryonic and fetal status. Discussion of abortion and the status of early human life has been dominated by two traditions, natural law on the conservative side, Enlightenment models on the liberal.[5] I believe that each has important insights to offer but that those insights are better understood when we start not with an all-or-nothing conception of moral status, but with a genuinely developmental picture of it. Part anticipatory and part achieved, moral status comprises a number of interweaving stages each leading to and giving way to the next.

I then consider the implications such a view has for our public understanding of legal regulations around abortion. As many have noted, the legal status of abortion cannot be settled by determination of fetal status alone: so long as such life resides in a woman's body, living in and off of her resources, abortion laws implicate women's fundamental rights of bodily dominion. Added to this is the question of fetal viability—not because the emergence of viability changes the fetus's intrinsic status, but because it implicates what opportunities the fetus has independent of the woman, and hence what restrictions we may place on efforts of hers that would interfere with those changes. Considered together, I'll argue, these factors underwrite a liberal but shifting view of abortion. Early in pregnancy, abortion should be unrestricted, not because the embryo and early fetus have no value, but because pregnancy asks an enormous amount of a woman, and she is in the best position to judge whether it is a price that can be paid. As pregnancy continues, it takes more justification decently to abort, but the pregnant woman is still the proper authority for making decisions about whether that justification is reached. Late in pregnancy, the fetus's status and viability solidify; abortion—an act that aims at the death of the fetus rather than just bringing about an early end to gestation—is a grave affair that should be reserved for unusual cases involving the health or life of the mother.

This is a view of abortion that many, at least, will find reasonable. It is also a view that explicitly acknowledges a genuine, if growing, moral status to early human life. Sometimes, those concerned to emphasize the importance of women's bodily dominion—and to balance what may legitimately be seen as a tendency on the part of some to highlight the fetus over the woman—have tended to downplay the issue of fetal status altogether. Hoping to remain neutralist, they are silent or vague about the status of developing human life. As one who is deeply committed to protecting legal access to abortion, I find this a profoundly flawed strategy. It ends up doing a deep disservice both to the maturing fetus and to the experiences of pregnant women and abortion providers; more than that, I'll be arguing, it threatens to undermine the very real arguments that exist for minimizing detailed state regulation of even late pregnancy and birth.

II.

According to one tradition, early human life is inviolable from the moment of conception. Sometimes described as the sanctity of human life doctrine, the position states that moral status is independent of developmental stage, accomplishments, or exercisable capacities. There are two main avenues to this view.

One is found in the natural law tradition. Grounded in Aristotelian metaphysics as it was taken up and inflected by Aquinas,[6] the view is, of course, committed to a theological worldview; it is also committed, though, to the idea that Aquinas's work revealed a "natural law" that is accessible to reason without reliance on religious premises.[7] According to advocates of this position, inviolability attaches not to specific accomplishments or stages, such as rationality, any more than it attaches only to adolescents or adults rather than infants. Instead, moral status attaches to the substance sortal of human being, and early human life is already that. To end the life of the embryo is thus to deprive one of us of the good of life—a profound and fundamental wrong.

Of course, one cannot simply assert that a given substance has full moral status as such; what is it, then, in virtue of which this one does? Most agree that species membership does not suffice: that a creature has a particular genome seems neither necessary nor sufficient for moral status.[8] The answer, according to some, is that full moral status belongs to life that carries the biological potential for rationality.[9] It is not just that the human embryo *could* become rational—that a special elixir could change a cat into a rational creature does not now give it moral status.[10] The claim, instead, is that having the potential for rationality in one's *nature* confers a status such that the good for such a creature presses always and already on us with the force of a creature who now is rational.

The question many will ask, though, is why. Having now the potential for a capacity is not usually thought to provide one with the benefits that possession of the capacity would bring. Having the potential for moral status is not itself immediately prescriptive; one may wonder why the whole is granted a status by virtue of its peak achievement. At its most powerful, the view traces instead to the fundamental conviction that inviolability is an *essential* rather than accidental feature.[11] Other moral statuses may come and go, but inviolability is the sort of moral status that attaches, if it does at all, to the identity of the creature, and hence must come into and go out of existence as the creature does: if ever inviolable, then always inviolable. Added to a view that we are essentially human organisms, it follows that even the earliest moments of the human organism carry an inviolability equal to its matured stage.

The view is certainly a coherent one. It is also, of course, precisely what the gradualist denies. To the gradualist, it is just as fundamentally intuitive that moral status is a *stage* sortal; it is just as fundamentally intuitive that status is precisely the sort of thing that can emerge and shift over the life of a biological organism. The question, then, is whether the essentiality claims key to the conservative position retain their plausibility independently of controversial commitments to a soul or to the broader metaphysical commitments of the natural law tradition.

A second avenue to the conservative conclusion is one based on the value of the goods held in anticipation for the creature. Don Marquis gives the argument its most famous expression.[12] In an argument meant to bypass controversial metaphysical commitments, he argues that the wrongness of ending embryonic life can be based on reflection about what is wrong with killing someone.[13] One important piece, at least, of why it is wrong to kill someone is that doing so deprives him of a future that we ourselves are committed to thinking of as valuable—namely, a "future like ours."[14] But human embryos and fetuses also have such futures stretching out before them, whatever their current lack of capacities. To end the embryo's life is to rob it of this future. Just so long as we agree that a future like ours is a good worth protection, so, too, we must be committed to the view that ending embryonic life is a serious wrong.

The first indication that there is a problem with the view is that, according to its logic, it is worse to end the life of a one-week embryo than that of a five-year-old child. The badness of death is judged by the extent of future lost, after all; and the loss of future is greater the earlier life is ended.[15] For many, though, such an outcome is highly implausible, raising the question of whether Marquis's argument puts the cart before the horse. Certainly, part of what is wrong with killing a paradigmatic person is the loss of future life inflicted on her, but that loss may constitute the basis for a prohibition in part because she is a creature that already counts, by independent criteria, as having moral status.

A second problem presses on the idea that the embryo "has" a future in the sense required by the argument. Claiming independence from the idea of an embryo's potential or nature, Marquis instead relies on the idea of the future it would have enjoyed but for the interference of the aborting woman.[16] As Frances Kamm points out, however, at least for early pregnancy, that comparison is a misleading one.[17] Until viability, the fetus *has* no trajectory independent of the gestational assistance the woman provides. Abortion ends the life of the embryo or fetus, to be sure, and often by active means; but some killings, as she puts it, share the formal features of a letting die, which is that they leave the creature no worse off than they would have been absent the woman's help to begin with.[18] At least early in pregnancy, we might say, it is not clear that one should describe ending gestation as depriving the embryo of its future rather than continuing gestation as helping to provide it with one.

Those who resist the idea of inviolability from the moment of conception most often look to a very different tradition—the tools and categories of the Enlightenment. Purposefully distanced from specific religious traditions and skeptical of "human" as a parochial category, these views tend to eschew the idea of reasoning from membership in any natural kind, biological or metaphysical: what matters for moral status is an *achievement* the individual has reached, and the achievements at issue are achievements of the *mind*.

On the most restrictive view, the achievement in question is that of rationality.[19] If natural law looks to Aquinas, here the historical anchor is Kant: our value is located in our possession of a will, in our status as self-legislators.[20] This approach looks to a different element of why killing is wrong—namely, it is a violation of our *autonomy*, the dominion we have as beings capable of self-governance.

While rationality is clearly a deeply important grounding of moral status, though, the limitations of claiming it as a necessary condition for strong moral protection are also clear. If cats are out on this view, so, too, are our young children and failing elders. A theory that grants status to non-autonomous humans only by polite extension is a limited theory, indeed.

More common, then, is the idea of locating the relevant capacity in a broader psychological achievement, namely, sentience.[21] The badness of death is located in the radical way in which it sets back a creature's interests, and interests are understood as something one can *take* an interest in—hence the core importance of consciousness. The claim is not that one has moral standing only while sentient, of course: our interests, once underway, can extend to what happens to us while asleep or even after death. The claim, instead, is that creatures that have never *been* sentient cannot be harmed, for harm is found in a setback of interests, and no interests have gotten underway until sentience arrives on the scene.

This view has its own challenges. First, having insisted that interests are tied at core to the notion of a point of view, one may wonder why bare sentience suffices for status. Why are the first flickers of consciousness robust enough to ground the form of moral status that issues protection in continued life, rather than just introducing a possible evil, namely, experiential suffering, that one should not inflict? Faced with this concern, some *idealize* the contents of interests: David Boonin, for instance, argues for an idealized desire account of interests, according to which one can have an interest in matters about which one has no knowledge, appreciation, or, indeed concept.[22] If idealization can be this ambitious, though, it begins to put pressure on the claim that sentience is necessary for status: if things so far outside our ken can count as factors in our interest, one might wonder why we need any "ken" to begin with.

Others, agreeing that genuine interests require more than mere sentience but skeptical of such thoroughgoing idealizing moves, respond instead by raising the bar on the form of subjectivity that creatures must have in order to earn strong moral protection against killing. Several argue, for instance, that *self-awareness* is needed: one must have attitudes toward the world and self to count as having interests in attaining goods, such as continued life, rather than interests in avoiding immediate experiential evils such as pain.[23]

The concern for these theories is that, having raised the bar this high, it does not look like one that newborns surmount. And indeed, some of these theorists bite the bullet: infanticide may be problematic for contingent reasons, but that is all.[24] If we feel distress at the prospect of ending a newborn's life, there is nothing intrinsic to that life in virtue of which distress is warranted. Once again, such a view is logically possible, but it will seem to many to have gone wrong: if self-awareness does not ground full protection for infants, it is a very good reason to think that such considerations do not exhaust the bases we look to in determining moral status.

Jeff McMahan has recently given a particularly sophisticated and particularly strongly psychologically based view of moral status.[25] McMahan has a very strong allegiance to sentience: according to his view, we are essentially embodied minds; hence we never existed as embryos or presentient fetuses.[26] Once sentience is on the scene but before the threshold of autonomy is reached, moral protection for continued life is only as strong as are the organism's "time-relative interests"—that is, the value of the organism's future interests, judged in both quantity and quality (how much and how good a life it would have), discounted by the degree to which those future goods now matter to the creature.[27] They are discounted, more specifically, as a function of how psychologically unified and connected the creature is with that future.[28]

Applied to embryos and fetuses, the view ends up with a rather startlingly minimal status for early human life. Until the fetus is sentient, it has no status; more than that, concern for it is something akin to a category mistake, like mistaking the clay for the statue. Once sentience emerges, one of us exists; but because fetuses have so little psychological connection with their potential future, they are owed very little in the way of moral protection. Given that change is not appreciable until quite some time after birth, even newborns merit little.

III.

On the above options, we face a stark choice. On the first view, early human life is, from the very first, inviolable; early miscarriage is, in intrinsic terms, as profound as the loss of a child. On the second view, early human life has no status until sentience: from the perspective of intrinsic status, abortion is the moral equivalent of contraception until consciousness emerges—likely not until after the midway point of gestation. And for those, like McMahan, who extend status by only modest increments to the matured fetus and newborn, protection is minimal all along.

Such starkness is a reflection of the bifurcating starting points of the options. Roughly speaking, the conservative tradition states that anticipatory factors are sufficient for full moral status. Ensconcing them in a metaphysical normative essence, status is found in features appreciable from a whole life perspective, with no indexing to what the life has thus far become. Roughly speaking, the liberal tradition states that status is a matter of achievement. Emphasizing the importance of mindedness, it finds the factors relevant to status (and sometimes identity) in reflection on the form of life the creature has when its death is considered.

But many of us, struck by the gradual development from fertilized egg to growing fetus to newborn, have something more like binocular vision when it comes to contemplating moral status. Part anticipatory and part achieved, status is something that emerges and increases as the balance between potential and actualization shifts. The early stages of human life are not equivalent in moral import—in the pulls and tugs, the mandates and constraints—that later life presents to us; it is not yet one of us. On the other hand, the human embryo or early fetus is not just any living organism, properly characterized in full abstraction from what it could become: it is, as it were, on its way to becoming one of us. What it is and what it would become if nurtured sit side by side; neither alone offers the full story.

Warren Quinn offers a view that takes seriously this approach to thinking about early human life.[29] Like a house under construction, he argues, the embryo and early fetus are best understood as not yet a full human person, but as already developing into one.

He sets forth two different ways this thought can be unpacked. The first is a variant on distinguishing stages relevant to status.[30] As he points out, there is a sense in which "human being" can itself be considered a stage in the life of the human organism. A modest enough stage, it is nonetheless subsequent to our very earliest months. Just as a house is not present, though a pile of bricks is, until a certain level of function has been reached, so too the human being emerges when the most fundamental systems of the fetus—the basic capacities both metabolic and minded—are in place. But this does not have to mean, he points out, that considerability is utterly lacking until this stage has been reached—as though early abortion represents nothing of moral import. There is already an organism extant with a good. The prescriptivity of this good increases as its status does, explaining why, if all abortions represent loss, later ones involve the death of an entity with more significant claims on us.[31]

The second view, which Quinn calls the "process" view, takes the gradualist suggestion more literally. Here, "human being" returns to the familiar category of a substance rather than stage sortal—it is the kind of thing we most fundamentally are, but it is a substance that comes into being only gradually.[32] On this view, that is, the human being is always and already there from the start, but only in partial existence. The embryo and early fetus already exist as an organism in empirically determinate form, of course, just as a house in the process of being built already exists in fully determinate form as a "construction." In both cases, though, the entity is more fundamentally understood by reference to another substance—human being and house, respectively—that it is coming to be. "Organism," like "construction," is what Quinn calls a "mock generic,"[33] a sortal we use to mark a determinate reality that, in a further sense, is best understood as a different substance—human being and house—that is gradually coming on the scene.

On either view, the good of the early human life has a claim on us, but not a full one. On the first view, it is there in a mitigated way because it is there only as the good of the organism as such, rather than the good of a human being: given that the life, if it developed, would be such a valuable one, its continued life carries a prescriptive force, but not yet at the level of prescriptivity that would be issued by the good of a human being. On the second view, the good is partly prescriptive because the being to which the good belongs, namely, one of us, is only partly present. On both views, the importance of sustaining the life is in part determined by what it has the potential to become, and in part by what it has already managed to be.

While Quinn's central concern is to make room for the gradualist enterprise rather than to defend a specific point at which full status emerges, he notes that, on both versions, a key point of being more fully one of us is plausibly the point at which the matured fetus's capacities to learn are on board.[34] More than mere consciousness but nothing as ambitious as self-awareness, such a stage marks the point at which the life can take in and respond to the world.[35] An element of mindedness, then, has some importance for Quinn, but for a different reason than for Enlightenment-based thinkers: it is not because prenatal life has no status until it is significantly minded, since its value is present even before, nor again because the emergence of this capacity brings in some complete set of human interests, fully present and idealized, since many of these are yet to be developed. Such mindedness is relevant, rather, because it marks the point at which a human being in general is more robustly on the scene.

Details aside, Quinn's fundamental insight is that moral status need not be a one-size-fits-all concept: some aspects of status may be present even as other aspects arrive later. At some point, a key common denominator emerges, when the human organism has the fundamental protections of a "right to life." Even before this point, though, the life has value, and its status continues to shift after that point is reached.

Indeed, the variegated nature of moral status (variegations that again can ride atop the fundamental, strong form of protection signaled by a right to life) is familiar enough when we think of the developmental story that continues after birth. As the infant emerges into the world, its psychological connections emerge as more coherent, and if all goes well, a subject emerges—viewing, wanting, representing, exerting and manipulating, taking in, querying. Here we see the process of moving from a human being to a *subject*, and a subject to a *self*, with attendant changes in how we must treat the being. One's stewardship for the future interests that the infant cannot yet glimpse must gradually give way to appreciation of, and growing constraint by, the contemporaneous interests and preferences of the child.

Continuing further, if all goes well, the young child starts to respond to reasons: initial forays are made into structuring the world by what is and is not done. This, too, is a gradual process; the apparatus of normative engagement is tested and tried on; the toehold of accountability and of normative powers—the ability to bind oneself, to be held responsible, to demand, forgive, and claim one's due—emerges. Here is the beginning and gradual emergence of an *agent*, a creature with the ability to will, a creature in possession of values and commitments, not just interests. These are changes that, once again, alter how we may treat the entity, as paternalistic concern for its welfare must increasingly defer to its own autonomous choices of will. Nor is all of this a mere progression or sequence in which one stage simply replaces another. It is, instead, quite literally a developmental picture, with prior stages maturing into the next stage. And often in cantilevered fashion: it is in meeting the needs of one stage that we introduce the next need—meeting the need for the breast in order to satiate and calm over time introduces oneself as an object the infant now wants and needs to ground its sense of continued existence. It is also one often marked by what we might call "proleptic engagement": it is by treating the young as if they already were in the next stage that we help usher them into it. It is by treating the infant as a creature capable of learning that we help it become more robustly a creature that can learn; it is by treating a young child as a fledgling agent that we help it turn into one.[36]

On this approach, the gradual coming to be of a *human organism*, with a biological good that can be aided or thwarted, gives way to the gradual coming to be of a *human being*, with its far more significant considerability, which gradually becomes a *self*, with its interests and preferences, which gives way in turn to the gradual coming to be of an *agent*, with will and commitments. Four different economies of considerations, the prescriptivity of which each emerges gradually, largely supplanting the prior, in a partial replacement of each. The interests that come with self, the exercises of normative authority that come with agency, each have nascent forms and themselves increase in strength, inflecting how we value and reason about one another in early stages of life.

IV.

This approach offers a very different picture of the moral status afforded for life inside the womb, one that increases in strength as the life develops more fully. Even at early stages, human life has a value worthy of respect. Miscarriage or abortion represents *loss.* Not just a loss for those with hopes of a child, but the loss of a distinct life that had a good in at least the organismic sense and that was, as it were, on its way to becoming one of us. Contraception is preferable to abortion: if life is not to be developed into a person, better that it not be created. Love for such a life may not be required; but nor, if it does emerge, need it be some sort of category mistake. It can be love of this creature now (an organism that, if the pregnancy continues, will turn out to have been the beginning stages of one's child), and proleptic love for the child it would become.

On this view, later abortion is more serious than earlier abortion, even before sentience has emerged. As the fetus's status increases, it has stronger claims for protection and assistance. If women and abortion providers regard abortion at twenty-two weeks as far different from early abortion, that is, it is understandable: by twenty-two weeks, the fetus is far more developed as a human being along many dimensions, even if not in minded terms. The further one goes into a pregnancy, the more justification it takes to decently end a pregnancy. And finally, at some point within the third trimester, the matured fetus becomes equivalent in intrinsic moral status to a newborn. Its claims for protection and assistance, stated as such, are the same as those of a newborn.

Superimposed on this graduated view of intrinsic moral status is determination of fetal viability—of the point at which others can reasonably and meaningfully sustain the fetus's life if only it can be safely delivered from the pregnant woman. "Viability," of course, is a bright-line idea masking a continuum of probabilities and complexities— how good the chances of survival, how brutal the interventions, how sober the risks of catastrophic impairment, how enormous the resources to assist to relative independence.[37] But when the fetus is robustly viable, this has important implications for the status of aborting. Not because it has anything to do with the fetus's intrinsic status: the two are conceptually and materially independent. (If I become uniquely dependent on your blood supply after a strange illness, that does not change my status as a full rights bearer.) But viability is highly relevant to the status of abortion, and for the reason we saw earlier when talking about Marquis and Kamm.[38] The act of aborting is conceptually liminal, as we might put it, between killing and letting die. Whether it is more like the latter is a function in part of whether the fetus has a hopeful trajectory independent of the woman's gestation. When the fetus has no opportunities that the act of aborting would forestall, abortion is properly viewed less as interference and more akin to a letting die, to a removing of life-sustaining assistance. The woman may of course face responsibilities (from modest to strong, depending again on how much status the life has accrued) to continue providing the assistance. The point is that questions about the legitimacy of abortion of previable embryos and fetuses can be contained to more local issues of balancing potential responsibilities to help with the burdens and invasions of doing so. But when the fetus has opportunities independent of the pregnant woman, then the act of aborting (as opposed to, say, early delivery) forestalls realization of those opportunities and must be justified, if it can be, in light of that more demanding metric.

When considering the moral and legal status of abortion, then, we must consider the status of the fetus as well as its outside opportunities. What we must also, and crucially, consider, whatever the stage of the pregnancy, is what its continuation means for the woman. This, of course, is the other variable fundamental to assessing the moral and legal status of abortion. Whatever the status of early human life, it does not develop on its own. It develops by way of enormous infusion of resources of the woman, living in and off of her body, transforming its every physical system in the process. Put bluntly, it takes a great deal of work to turn early human life *into* something of full moral status. Gestation, to state the obvious, is not just any form of help: it involves the use of one's very body; its continuation can implicate every corner of a girl or woman's life. That such life has a value worthy of respect means there are reasons—of increasing strength across the pregnancy—to offer that infusion; but its costs, judged both as burdens and intimacies, can be substantial, and deeply context dependent, grounded in what the pregnancy means in the narrative context of the woman's life.

Together, these variables yield a shifting picture of abortion. In the first trimester, the intrinsic moral status of early human life is modest, the burden of continuing deep, and the fetus has no trajectory independent of the woman's gestational assistance. The profound and ongoing nature of the assistance implicate rights of bodily dominion; further, given that the life is not yet a child, abortion rights at this stage have a leg in the rights of reproductive decisional privacy. What continued pregnancy asks prospectively of the woman, in short, is enormous; to legally require a woman to continue gestating when these three conditions are met would arguably be to require more than we require of any other citizen. A constitutionally protected right of access to abortion, then, is a core protection for women's status as citizens; and early abortion, while regretful, can be regarded as a decent and, indeed, potentially honorable action.

If the pregnancy continues and the fetus develops into the second trimester, increasing fetal status means that it takes greater justification decently to abort. But good reasons there well may be. While earlier abortion is clearly preferable, there are nonetheless considerations that may lead women decently to abort in this trimester. If the fetus's status evolves, so too may the woman's circumstances: a smooth first trimester may turn into a second trimester with overwhelming nausea and waves of fatigue; a rocky marriage ends and the woman's partner leaves her. Or again, women living in chaotic households or impoverished circumstances find they can only in the second trimester confront, decide, and make arrangements for an abortion they would have chosen earlier under better circumstances. Or again, news of significant disability comes to light only after the first trimester. Whatever we might say about the care of premature infants born with such conditions, the finding of profound abnormality in the middle stages of pregnancy brings its own issues, both because the fetus's status, while substantial, is not yet equivalent to a newborn, and because of what it means to have one's body carrying, attached to, and sustaining a fetus with a profound impairment.[39]

As viability approaches, all these considerations become more freighted. Given that others now can help this life, decisions about its disposition are no longer fully contiguous with the woman's decisions about her body and life. Especially when robust viability precedes full moral status (a gap that will only increase with further technology), a gray zone emerges in which decisions over the life of the fetus hover between the private and the public.

In the third trimester, matters change significantly. Status and viability solidify. Others can help; the fetus has opportunities independent of the gestating woman. And they are interests of a creature with full moral status. Our interest in the fetus emerges as substantive, both because its intrinsic status solidifies and because we now can help to do the work of sustaining and developing it if it can be delivered safely from the woman. In particular, the distinction between *aborting*—a medical procedure that involves killing the embryo or fetus—and *ending gestation*—procedures that include early induction or delivery—emerges as central: restrictions on killing may be justified even where requirements that the woman provide continued use of her body are not.

But this is not to say that issues of bodily dominion evaporate—even in the third trimester, even when the fetus has full moral status. So long as a woman remains pregnant, with deeply intertwined physiologies, the fetus's presence in her body implicates her health, life, and bodily integrity in ways that can be profound. More than that, getting the fetus *out* implicates the same. Birth is not just a matter of opening a door; quite literally entwined, the fetus's placenta is burrowed into the walls of the uterus (as anyone who has witnessed a woman bleed out during delivery can attest). Further, whatever the responsibilities of a pregnant woman to the matured fetus, and they are surely profound, there are specific elements of bodily dominion that the fact of pregnancy ought not compromise, such as the right of a citizen not to be compelled to undergo surgery for another's benefit.[40] If women should not have an unrestricted right to kill their matured fetuses, decisions about whether and how to end a pregnancy and deliver a baby are ones that may still be appropriately regarded as up to her.

In short, there are still profoundly important issues around the legal regulation of abortion even in the third trimester, not because the status of the matured fetus is insignificant, but because of the very significant policy-based concerns with state regulation of conduct during pregnancy and birth. Law is perforce crude; abortion legislation that goes beyond broad statements of the sorts of reasons we regard as legitimate for abortion, such as protecting the health and life of the woman, risk intrusion into details best left to the woman and her medical team. Whether, when, and how to regulate abortion in the third trimester depends on many factors: how often we think that individuals, in the absence of detailed state regulation, will act egregiously; whether softer forms of social management, such as medical professional codes, substantially obviate the need for state action; how much a given state entity can be trusted to understand and respond to the real-world difficulties and nuances that hard cases are going to involve.

If women's advocates resist detailed regulation of abortion in the third trimester, such as those limiting abortion methods, it is not because they think the fetus's residence inside the woman gives her absolute dominion over its fate but because they are mindful of the crudeness of regulation. Because the rather singular event of getting one person out of another's body, when the former is quite literally entwined with the latter, implicates a broad range of medical and bodily integrity issues that the state may be ill-posed to second-guess or enforce. Because medical decisions at the very beginning of life, like those at its very end, are the subject of judgments and emergencies that the courts and legislatures may be ill-placed to regulate by algorithm. Because life has tragedies, and those living in and with those tragedies may be better placed than the courts to decide what to do in their face.

To be clear, then, *no one* thinks that in the third trimester, women have a positively protected indiscriminate interest in ending the fetus's life, as though we should defend a de jure right to feticide for whatever reason at any time. Instead, concerns about abortion regulation late in pregnancy are concerns about the difficulties of specifying and balancing those issues, given the realities of pregnancy, in the real world. Women need not be granted a right to elective abortion—that is, abortion independent of considerations of the woman's health and life—in the third trimester, but details of medical need or method may not be ones best demarcated by legislative bodies.

Attending to considerations such as these also helps to explain why one might reasonably resist or worry about laws that categorize fetuses as persons. It is sometimes argued that, if a matured fetus has a moral status equivalent to newborns, as we should agree, then we should subsume them under the legal concept of "personhood" or, again, "unborn child." But this would be to go badly wrong. Kinds are not just names; they are summary concepts that bring with them wholesale patterns of reasoning, precedent, and the like. The matured fetus is the same as a newborn in intrinsic status, but regulating the body is different from regulating the custody of a child. The category of "person," like the category of "child," was made with physically individuated and separated persons in mind; these are sortals animated by the enterprise of regulating human social interactions.[41] They are, in a phrase, not designed with fetuses in mind. This doesn't mean that fetal status does not matter; it means that it needs to be developed in a theory that is adequate to the, shall we say, unique conditions under which it lives. Fetuses are not natural persons, not because they have no moral status, but because the fetus deserves a theory of its own.[42] Not because the fetus has a lesser intrinsic moral status than the newborn, as though its location inside and attachment to the pregnant woman dilutes its import, but because legal personhood is a concept that has a pragmatic life of its own, and one which, developed to deal with other scenarios, may not extend well to those who reside in another's body.

Notice now that, if all of this is a key reason why regulation of even third-trimester abortion must be done with care, it is also a key reason why silence or vague gestures about the status of early human life is so dangerous. Late in pregnancy, when full moral status and viability converge, a key premise in arguing for minimal state regulation of abortion is that women are in fact unlikely to seek, or physicians to provide, abortions at this stage. But this premise is hard to maintain if those relying on it never speak of or endorse the consideration that accounts for that reticence: the belief that matured fetuses have lives that should not be taken except in extreme circumstances. If women's advocates cannot acknowledge the moral status of a matured fetus, it will be difficult indeed to appreciate why pregnant women can be trusted to do so.

Rationales around rights and restrictions to abortion really are different across pregnancy. In early pregnancy, the embryo and early fetus have more modest status; ending pregnancy is more about ending assistance than about interference; the bodily integrity issues involved in continuing gestation and birth compared to early abortion are profound. The rights at stake for the pregnant woman are rights of reproductive decisional privacy, equality, and protection against the state compelling continued bodily assistance and birth. By the third trimester, robust fetal status and robust fetal viability converge: others could sustain this life; the woman's actions affect its substantive chances. Critical issues of bodily dominion remain, but they shift to the difficult and complex issues of balancing the needs of the fetus with its location. In between the first and third trimesters, abortion is, well, just that—in between.[43] As women and abortion providers alike attest, decisions here are decisions full of ambivalence and difficulty, burdens and grief—just what we might expect on a gradualist picture.

NOTES

1. BARUCH BRODY, ABORTION AND THE SANCTITY OF HUMAN LIFE: A PHILOSOPHICAL VIEW 116–22 (1975); John Finnis, *The Rights and Wrongs of Abortion: A Reply to Judith Thomson*, 2 PHIL. & PUB. AFF. 117, 144–45 (1973); Patrick Lee & Robert P. George, *The Wrong of Abortion*, in CONTEMPORARY DEBATES IN APPLIED ETHICS 13 (Andrew I. Cohen & Christopher Health Wellman eds., 2005).

2. PETER SINGER, PRACTICAL ETHICS 96–99, 186–88 (2d ed. 1993); Michael Tooley, *A Defense of Abortion and Infanticide*, in THE PROBLEM OF ABORTION 51, 51–52 (Joel Feinberg ed., 1973); Mary Anne Warren, *On the Moral and Legal Status of Abortion*, 57 MONIST 43, 57–59 (1973).

3. *Brain activity* arises much earlier, but *sentience* emerges with the development of organized brain activity of the form EEGs capture. One review of the science puts this development at somewhere between twenty-four and twenty-eight weeks gestational age. *See* DAVID BOONIN, A DEFENSE OF ABORTION 107–09 (2003).

4. BOONIN, *supra* note 3, at 115–27; JEFF MCMAHAN, THE ETHICS OF KILLING: PROBLEMS AT THE MARGINS OF LIFE 267–80 (2002); *see generally* BONNIE STEINBOCK, LIFE BEFORE BIRTH: THE MORAL AND LEGAL STATUS OF EMBRYOS AND FETUSES (1992); Elizabeth Harman, *The Potentiality Problem*, 114 PHIL. STUD. 173 (2003).

5. *See supra* notes 1, 2, 4 and accompanying text; *infra* notes 7, 10 and accompanying text.

6. *See generally* SAINT THOMAS AQUINAS, SUMMA THEOLOGIAE (Timothy McDermott ed., 1989). For a recent and excellent defense of natural law, see ROBERT P. GEORGE, IN DEFENSE OF NATURAL LAW (2001).

7. *See generally* Lee & George, *supra* note 1.

8. *See, e.g.*, David DeGrazia, *Moral Status, Human Identity, and Early Embryos: A Critique of the President's Approach*, 34 J.L. MED. & ETHICS 49 (2006).

9. Burleigh T. Wilkins, *Does the Fetus Have a Right to Life?*, 24 J. SOC. PHIL. 123, 123–27 (1993).

10. The example of the cat is Tooley's. Tooley, *supra* note 2, at 86–88.

11. Lee & George, *supra* note 1, at 16–19.

12. Don Marquis, *Why Abortion is Immoral*, 86 J. PHIL. 183, 189–90 (1989).

13. *Id.*

14. *Id.*

15. *See* RONALD DWORKIN, LIFE'S DOMINION: AN ARGUMENT ABOUT ABORTION, EUTHANASIA, AND INDIVIDUAL FREEDOM 86–87 (1993); MCMAHAN, *supra* note 4, at 165–74; DeGrazia, *supra* note 8, at 54.

16. *See* Marquis, *supra* note 12, at 192.

17. F.M. KAMM, CREATION AND ABORTION: A STUDY IN MORAL AND LEGAL PHILOSOPHY 22–27, 84–87, 130–32 (1992).

18. *Id.* at 22–27.

19. Joel Feinberg, *Abortion, in* MATTERS OF LIFE AND DEATH 183, 190 (Tom Regan ed., 1980).

20. IMMANUEL KANT, GROUNDWORK OF THE METAPHYSICS OF MORALS 52–54 (Mary McGregor ed. & trans., Cambridge Univ. Press 1997) (1785).

21. Many are in this camp. *See supra* note 3.

22. *See, e.g.,* BOONIN, *supra* note 3, at 64–84.

23. *See generally* Tooley, *supra* note 2.

24. *See, e.g.,* McMAHAN, *supra* note 4, at 170–71, 338–43.

25. *Id.* at 232–40, 275–76.

26. *Id.* at 66–69.

27. *Id.* at 165–74.

28. *Id.*

29. Warren Quinn, *Abortion: Identity and Loss, in* MORALITY AND ACTION 20 (Warren Quinn ed., 1993). For a discussion of human beings as "emergent beings" see Joan C. Callahan, *The Fetus and Fundamental Rights*, COMMONWEAL, Apr. 11, 1986, at 203, 205. Influenced by McMahan's time-relative interests view, but freed from the assumption that entities must be sentient in order to have interests, David DeGrazia defends a view that is consonant with the idea that organismic good strengthens in prescriptivity as it develops. *See generally* David DeGrazia, *The Harm of Death, Time-Relative Interests, and Abortion*, 38 PHIL. F. 57 (2007).

30. Quinn, *supra* note 29, at 26–27.

31. *Id.* 45, 51.

32. *Id.* at 30–35.

33. *Id.* at 34, 36.

34. *See id.* at 37.

35. As a friend of mine who is an obstetrician noted to me, this stands in stark contrast to radically premature infants, twenty-four weeks or so, in the neonatal intensive care unit, for whom touch itself can so overwhelm the systems that it leads to cardiac arrhythmias.

36. My thanks to Mark Lance for this last point. For a discussion of speech acts that institute normative status in anticipatory form see REBECCA KUKLA & MARK LANCE, "YO!" AND "LO!": THE PRAGMATIC TOPOGRAPHY OF THE SPACE OF REASONS ch. 8, soc. 1 (Harvard Univ Press 2009).

37. *See* Norman Fost, David Chudwin & David Wikler, *The Limited Moral Significance of "Fetal Viability,"* HASTINGS CENTER REP., Dec. 1980, at 10 (describing the ways in which viability is itself a gray concept).

38. *See supra* notes 12, 17 and accompanying text.

39. The documentary *Severina's Story* follows the case of a Brazilian woman carrying an anencephalic fetus denied access to abortion by the legislature until her third trimester. DVD: SEVERINA'S STORY (Debora Diniz & Elaine Brum 2004) (on file with author).

40. *See In re A.C.*, 573 A.2d 1235, 1249–51 (D.C. 1990) (en banc) (holding that an individual has the right to accept or reject medical treatment, and that the court may have to act

as a surrogate and substitute its judgment when an individual is unable to make an informed decision).

41. Elizabeth Anderson emphasizes issues about moral status as a marker of inclusion in society in the context of the animal rights debate. *See* Elizabeth Anderson, *Animal Rights and the Value of Nonhuman Life, in* ANIMAL RIGHTS: CURRENT DEBATES AND NEW DIRECTIONS 277 (Cass R. Sunstein & Martha C. Nussbaum eds., 2004).

42. Catharine A. MacKinnon, *Reflections on Sex Equality Under Law*, 100 YALE L.J. 1281, 1314 (1991) ("As it is, the fetus has no concept of its own, but must be like something men have or are: a body part to the Left, a person to the Right. Nowhere in law is the fetus a fetus.").

43. My thanks to Elizabeth Anderson, in email correspondence, for this way of putting the point.

CHAPTER TEN

Revisiting the Argument from Fetal Potential

BERTHA ALVAREZ MANNINEN

Background

One of the most famous, and concurrently one of the most derided, arguments against the morality of abortion is the argument from fetal potential. This argument maintains that the fetus' potential to become a human person and enjoy the valuable life common to human persons entails that its destruction is *prima facie* morally impermissible. It is important to note here that the term *person* is used here in the strict philosophical sense; it is not meant to denote any and all human beings, as it is normatively used, but rather any being, human or nonhuman, that has the mental capacity to be rational, self-conscious, autonomous, and a moral agent.

One of the reasons that this argument is so interesting is that it is simultaneously ridiculed by some philosophers and lauded by others. Many who reject the argument do so because they believe that it results in what is often called the "sperm/ova problem": if we regard the potential of a fetus to become a person as a morally relevant reason against killing it, we must also hold the same of human gametes, who also possess the potential to become persons. For example, Bonnie Steinbock writes:

> The strongest objection to the argument from potential is that it seems to make contraception, and even abstinence, prima facie morally wrong. If the objection to abortion is that it deprives the zygote of a "future like ours," why, it may be asked, cannot the same complaint be made of contraceptive techniques that kill sperm, or prevent fertilization? Why don't gametes have "a future like ours"? . . . so if abortion is seriously wrong because it kills a potential person, then the use of contraceptives is equally seriously wrong. In using spermicide, one commits mass murder![1]

L.W. Sumner makes a similar accusation:

> As far as the potentiality argument is concerned, abortion and contraception are both wrong, both equally wrong, and both wrong for precisely the same reason.[2]

Conversely, other philosophers hold that the argument from potential is significant because it is the only thing that explains the stewardship that adult human beings have in regard to human neonates. Newborn infants lack the psychological maturity to possess goals, aims, beliefs, or purposes. This does not, however, exclude them from the moral community. The reason why it does not is because we realize that infants have the potential to develop these conscious goods, and it is this potential that, as Jim Stone argues, grounds the infant's interest in growing up and realizing that potential.[3] Every single semester that I teach the issue of abortion in class, I put up a picture of two cells that look striking similar, almost identical. I then reveal to my students that one is a skin cell, and the other is a fertilized egg at the zygotic stage of development. "Do they have the same moral status?", I ask them. When I scratch my arm and kill skin cells, is my action as morally problematic as abortion? My students always answer that the two cell types are morally different; that the zygote is of a different status than my skin cells. In defense of this distinction, they always give the same reason: the zygote, if implanted into a uterus, has the potential to become a baby who will then become a person, whereas my skin cells do not. Since the vast majority of my students, in my seven years of teaching, share this intuition, I think that it is an intuition that is worthy of being explored rather than cavalierly dismissed.

The term "potential" as it is being used in this essay is not meant to describe mere *possibility*, i.e., X has the potential to achieve Y does not just mean X may possibly attain Y. If that were what was meant by potential, it would be very weak indeed. A seed would not just be a potential flower or plant, but also a potential food or a potential material for an art project. A kitten would not just be a potential cat, but also a potential delicacy at some restaurant, or a potential fur coat. Rather, potential, in the way I am using it here and the way I assume most advocates of the argument from potential use the concept, refers to, as Stephen Buckle puts it, a certain being's "potency . . . the power it [actually] possesses in virtue of its specific constitution"[4] to grow into a being of a certain sort. That is, X is a potential Y if X possesses the power to become Y; that X *will* become Y, if it lives long enough. In this way, a caterpillar is a potential butterfly (since it possesses the power to become a butterfly; it *will* become a butterfly if it lives long enough), as a child is a potential adult. A fetus is a potential person in this way; a fetus may not just *possibly* become a person, it *will* become a person, if its growth is unfettered and if it lives long enough.

With this introduction in mind, I can proceed to stating the goal of this paper, which is two-fold. First, I will criticize the classical arguments proffered against the importance of fetal potential, specifically the arguments put forth by philosophers Peter Singer and David Boonin, by carefully unpacking the claims made in these arguments and illustrating why they are flawed. I will argue that both Singer and Boonin assume that possessing actual person-hood is a necessary condition in order to be accorded the right to life, but it seems that this is the very issue at hand and the very claim that those who argue in favor of the importance of fetal potential will challenge and subsequently reject.

Second, I will maintain that a fetus potential can be salient when it comes to the morality of abortion, but that its proper place cannot be found until we first address a very important and difficult issue: the question concerning personal identity, and when the fetus becomes the type of being who is relevantly identical to a future person. I will illustrate how we cannot begin to tackle this perennial applied ethics issue without first addressing the metaphysical quagmire of personal identity, for where one stands on this metaphysical issue may greatly influence when one thinks potential begins to matter when it comes to the human fetus.

Against Singer and Boonin
What Is Wrong with the Classical Objections Concerning Fetal Potential?

John T. Noonan uses a version of the argument from potential in order to provide one of many reasons why he deems abortion morally impermissible.

> If a fetus is destroyed, one destroys a being already possessed of the genetic code, organs, and sensitivity to pain, and one which had an eighty percent chance of developing further into a baby outside the womb who, in time, would reason . . . once conceived, the being was recognized as man because he had man's potential.[5]

For many philosophers, the argument from potential is considered invalid, either because the argument rests on a logical mistake or because it is misapplied in the abortion debate. Individuals who argue in the first manner maintain that the logical mistake comes in asking us to treat a potential X as if it is an actual X. Particularly, it asks us to treat a potential person, the fetus, as if it were already an actual person. However, the argument goes, how we treat a being ought to depend on its *actually possessed* properties, rather than on its *potentially possessed* ones. For those who would counter that an exception should be made for the life of the fetus because the right to life is somehow different and deserves to be extended to the fetus in virtue of its potential to become a person, the second objection applies. That is, given that potential Xs are never treated as actual Xs simply in virtue of their potential, there seems to be absolutely no reason to extend this special treatment to fetuses. As Paul Bassen writes: "Nowhere outside the abortion debate itself is there a precedent for supposing that future prospects can create a present sake."[6] Therefore, although a standard human fetus possesses the potential to become a person and hence enjoy the kind of life typical to persons, this alone, the argument goes, does not create an obligation to protect the fetus as it exists currently.

It seems to me that those who argue against the moral relevance of fetal potential (whom I will call "anti-potentialists") do not really comprehend the role that their opponents give to the potential of the fetus. The fault of this misapprehension lies on both sides, for those who argue that the potential of the fetus does play a significant role when determining the morality of abortion (whom I will call "pro-potentialists") have not adequately clarified their position in light of the objections offered by anti-potentialists. It is my objective in this section to detail the anti-potentialists' concerns and propose some methods that the pro-potentialist can use in order to respond to these concerns.

Let us begin by outlining the standard argument against the moral permissibility of abortion given the purported moral relevancy of the fetus's potential.

— **Premise 1:** All innocent persons have a moral right to life.
— **Premise 2:** Since all innocent persons have a moral right to life, all potential innocent persons also have a moral right to life.
— **Premise 3:** The human fetus is a potential innocent person.
— **Conclusion:** The human fetus has a moral right to life.

For both anti- and pro-potentialists, premise one is uncontroversial, and premise three ought not to pose much of a problem either, since it is a biological claim rather than a moral one. Indeed, the standard human fetus, barring any unfortunate accident, will grow into an infant, child, and adult, and therefore will enjoy the life of a standard human person. The controversy, then, seems to lie in premise two: why is it true that the right to life of an innocent person ought to extend also to the fetus given its potential? How should premise two be defended?

Peter Singer presents a scathing objection to premise two because he does not think that an adequate defense of it is possible.

> There is no rule that says that a potential X has the same value as an [actual] X, or has all the rights of an X. There are many examples that show just the contrary. Pulling out a sprouting acorn is not the same as cutting down a venerable oak. To drop a live chicken into a pot of boiling water would be much worse than doing the same to an egg. Prince Charles is the potential King of England, but he does not now have the rights of a king.[7]

David Boonin offers the following analysis, and subsequent rejection of, premise two.

> Perhaps the simplest argument from potentiality is one that rests on a general assumption of the following sort. Potential possession of a right entails actual possession of a right . . . [the argument's] major assumption rests on a logical error. It is certainly not true of properties in general that if a given individual potentially has a given property, then the individual already has this property.[8]

As anti-potentialists regard it, any argument from potential commits the error of maintaining that for all things X, if X is a potential Y, then X ought to already be treated as an actual Y. Particularly, when it comes to the role of potential in the abortion debate, the argument commences with the uncontroversial premise that all innocent persons have a right to life. From this, the argument implicitly accepts the generalization expressed above. Since all actual innocent persons have a right to life (as premise one asserts), and since any potential person ought to be treated as an actual person (as entailed by the above generalization), a potential person also ought to possess the right to life. The fetus can certainly be substituted for the X variable, since a fetus is a potential person. Thus, the fetus also has a right to life.

At first blush, it does seem that Singer and Boonin present valid criticisms of this argument: it does not seem to follow that potential Xs are to be treated like actual Xs merely in virtue of their potential. Indeed, there are various examples that illustrate just the opposite. Prince Charles and Prince William are both potential kings of England. Notice that they are not just *possibly* the future kings of England (as perhaps Prince Harry is); if they live long enough, both Charles and William *will*, respectively, become the king of England in the future. However, this potential does not accord them the rights of kings while they are princes. Medical students, although potential physicians, do not possess the same rights (or responsibilities) as actual physicians do.[9] Children, although potential adults, do not possess the same rights as actual adults; for example, they cannot vote or drink alcoholic beverages. As these examples illustrate, beings are treated in accordance with their actually possessed properties, not their potentially possessed ones.

In light of this, the pro-potentialist seems to be making a mistake in logical reasoning, or at the very least asking us to make an exception when it comes to the human fetus without justification. But, as Singer puts it: "We should not accept that a potential person should have the rights of a person, unless we can be given some specific reason why this should hold in this particular case."[10] Singer argues that, when it comes to the right to life, it is essential that an individual be able to perceive of herself as a continuing entity existing over time so that she may be capable of desiring continued existence. In order to possess this conceptual capacity, the being in question must be a person.

> [T]he desire relevant to possessing a right to life is the desire to continue existing as a distinct entity. But only a being who is capable of conceiving herself as a distinct entity existing over time—that is, only a person—could have this desire. Therefore only a person could have a right to life . . . an individual cannot at a given time—say, now—have a right to continued existence unless the individual is of a kind such that it can now be in its interest that it continue to exist . . . since no fetus is a person, no fetus has the same claim to life as a person.[11]

Since the fetus never meets this necessary requirement, no fetus can ever be classified as a person, and its mere potential to one day be one does not ground a right to life now: "if [the requirements for personhood] are the grounds for not killing persons, the mere potential for becoming a person does not count against killing."[12]

It is in Singer's response that we can begin to see a possible line of defense for the pro-potentialist. Notice premise two again.

— **Premise 2:** Since all innocent persons have a moral right to life, all potential innocent persons also have a moral right to life.

Now, also take notice of the different examples that are given by both Singer and Boonin in order to challenge the truth of premise two: Charles and William, although potential kings, do not have the same rights as an actual king. Medical students, although potential physicians, do not have the same rights as actual physicians. Children, although potential adults, do not have all the same rights as actual adults, for example they lack the right to vote or drink alcoholic beverages. (This is my own example, although Boonin makes the broad argument that there are some rights and responsibilities that adults have that children do not.) Thus, in order to be consistent with these examples, fetuses, although potential persons, are not persons yet and so ought not to be accorded a right to life.

What do all these examples have in common? What these examples all share is that the rights that are mentioned (the rights of the king of England, the rights of a physician, and the right to drink and vote) are such that it is sufficient that one meet an actual condition (of being a king, a physician, or an adult) in order to attain the corresponding right *and also that it is necessary that one meet this condition.* That is, it is necessary that one actually *be* the king of England in order to have the rights of the king of England, which is why neither Charles nor William possesses these rights currently. It is necessary that one *be* a physician in order to have the rights of a physician (which is why potential physicians do not have these rights, no matter how close to graduation they are). In our society, it is necessary that one be an actual adult in order to have the right to vote and drink alcoholic beverages. *This* is the reason why potential does not count in these examples. If it is *necessary* to actually have a certain property in order to have a certain right, then it follows, of course, that potentially having this property cannot bestow that right upon an individual, for the individual simply does not meet the necessary requirement. Singer assumes that being a person is sufficient *and necessary* in order to have a moral right to life, and so he concludes that the pro-potentialist is mistaken if she thinks that having the potential to be a person can secure such a right. And Singer is correct, *if* it were also the case that being an actual person is a necessary condition for being accorded a moral right to life.

But I suspect that this is *exactly* what the pro-potentialist would (and should) contest. The pro-potentialist can agree that there are indeed cases where potential Xs are not to be treated as actual Xs solely in virtue of their potential, but she can also argue that this rule is not categorical. When it comes to the right to life, the pro-potentialist ought to question a much more fundamental assumption that is implicit in the anti-potentialist's argument: *Why* should being an actual person be a necessary condition for possessing a right to life? Singer's reasoning for this is un-satisfactory. He argues that self-consciousness, a mental capacity attributable only to persons, is necessary in order to be able to conceive of oneself as a distinct entity that exists over time, which in turn allows one to have the capacity for the requisite desire in order to possess a moral right to life: the desire for continued existence. In other words, Singer argues, *pace* Michael Tooley, that one must be capable of desir-ing continued existence in order to have an interest in, and thus a moral right to, continued existence.[13] I will illustrate the flaws of this argument below, but suffice it to say, for now, that the pro-potentialist should be wary of accepting this argument for why being a person is a necessary condition for possessing a moral right to life.

Perhaps, the pro-potentialist may argue, there are certain reasons why we bestow the right to life upon an actual person that may also apply to a potential person (and indeed there are, as I will argue below), thereby undermining the anti-potentialist's implicit assumption that it is necessary that one be an actual person in order to have a right to life. In other words, the pro-potentialist can agree that it is indeed true that potential Xs cannot have the same rights as actual Xs *providing that it is also the case that it is necessary that one be an actual X in order to have those rights*. However, the pro-potentialist can simply reject the thesis that it is necessary that one be a person in order to have a right to life (although being a person is certainly sufficient for such a right) and argue, instead, that the fetus's potential somehow suffices to ex-tend to it a right to life.[14] Singer's and Boonin's examples will not convince the pro-potentialist that a fetus lacks a moral right to life because they are assuming a crucial premise that the pro-potentialist already rejects, if only tacitly.

When Potential Is Morally Relevant

The task that the pro-potentialist now faces is to explain why the fetus's potential is a morally relevant characteristic that justifies extending to it a right to life. I believe that this can be done. What I want to do now is refute Paul Bassen's point that "[n]owhere outside the abortion debate itself is there a precedent for supposing that future prospects can create a present stake"[15] by discussing examples that seems to run contrary to this assertion.

THE MORAL RIGHT TO HEALTH INSURANCE

Despite the rising costs and ailing benefits in our health care system, many would agree that all human beings, no matter how young, how old, or how sick, have a moral right to health insurance and the guarantee of health care. The Universal Declaration of Human Rights upholds this right in Article 25:

> Everyone has the right to a standard of living adequate for the health and well-being of himself and of his family, including food, clothing, housing and medical care and necessary social services.[16]

In our society, then, most would maintain that currently ill individuals have a moral right to health insurance because having such insurance constitutes a great benefit for them and depriving an ill individual of medical insurance constitutes a harm. To deprive actually ill individuals of health insurance would make it increasingly difficult for them to get the treatment they need to alleviate their illness. In a society such as ours that seeks to protect the well-being of its citizens, the right to health insurance and subsequent medical care is certainly vital in order to achieve such protection.

In addition, *potentially* ill individuals, like my child or myself, also have a moral right to health insurance. But why do we accord this latter group health insurance, even though they are not *actually* sick? Because possessing health insurance, even in the absence of an impending illness, also constitutes a great benefit for potentially sick people and a deprivation of health insurance also constitutes a harm for potentially sick people.

Both actually sick people and potentially sick people possess what Joel Feinberg would call a "welfare interest" in continued health. Welfare interests are very basic or foundational interests; interests which, if thwarted, can result in an entire collapse of one's whole matrix of interests. Without continued health, the ability one has to fulfill other interests in life will be compromised. While I have an interest in continuing to work, raising my children, and taking care of my home, I would fail to realize any of these interests if my interest in health were thwarted. As Feinberg notes: "[a]ll the money in the world won't help you if you have a fatal disease . . ."[17] Welfare interests, which include the interest in continued health, are "the very most important interests a person has, and cry out for protection, for without their fulfillment, a person is lost . . . an invasion of a welfare interest is the most serious . . . harm a person can sustain."[18]

Although a discussion concerning the exact purpose and nature of moral rights is beyond the scope of this essay, it suffices to say that one function of moral (and legal) rights is to protect people's interests, especially the very important and foundational ones. Actually sick individuals have a moral right to health insurance because it reasonably guarantees health care, and this, in turn, helps to protect their welfare interest in continued health. This is also what having health insurance provides for potentially sick individuals. Possessing health insurance gives potentially sick people peace of mind and a guarantee that when they do actually get sick medical treatment will be available for them. For consider what would occur if potentially ill people had to wait until they were actually sick to start the process of obtaining health insurance. By the time all the paperwork is completed and the monetary costs of premiums have exchanged hands, the illness will have probably taken a turn for the worst, and this, of course, would impede their respective welfare interest in continued health. So the very fact that people are potentially sick is a sufficient reason to extend health coverage to them now, even though there is no actual illness impending. Of course, a potentially ill person does not have the moral right to actual medical *treatment* while she is just potentially sick; she has this particular moral right only when she becomes actually sick. This is because being actually sick is a necessary condition to receiving actual medical care, since medical care does not serve any beneficial role to someone who is only potentially sick and a deprivation of medical care would not harm someone who is only potentially sick, only to those that are actually sick (e.g., there is no point in a doctor wrapping my arm in a cast if it is not broken in the first place). What a potentially sick person has a moral right to, even in her healthy state, is the guarantee that when she does become ill, health care will follow, and this is precisely what health insurance provides for the potentially sick person.

The welfare interest in continued health seems to be a wholly objective interest, rather than a subjectively mediated one. By this I mean that it is not necessary that a person actually desire continued health, or even possess the capacity to desire continued health, in order to possess an interest in it. An infant with a heart defect, for example, surely has an interest in a life-saving operation to repair her ailment, even though the infant lacks the cognitive capacities necessary to be capable of desiring the operation. While an infant cannot *take* an interest in her continued health (i.e., she is incapable of desiring her continued good health, since she lacks the capacity to even understand what "health" means), she surely *has* an interest in her continued health. It is because we recognize the importance of preserving the well-being of members in society, even if they are too rudimentary in their capacities to actually take an active interest in their health, that we extend a moral right to health care to the actually sick and the potentially sick. Whether one possesses the actual property of being sick, or whether one merely potentially possesses that property, having a moral right to health insurance helps to secure one's important welfare interest in continued health, which, in turn, helps the development and well-being of members of our moral community in a variety of ways.

THE MORAL RIGHT TO AN EDUCATION

As a professor, I am exposed every day to the effects of sub-par education, especially when it comes time for students to turn in papers and their poor writing abilities become painfully apparent. This illustrates that being deprived of a good education works against the interest of a person. Thus, all *actually* rational agents have the moral right to a decent education because such an education hones their rational abilities and enriches their mind. To deprive a rational agent of an education constitutes a harm for her, since it deprives her of the opportunity to cultivate her rational faculties. To provide a rational agent a decent education, of course, constitutes a great benefit.

A very young, not fully rational, child, also has a moral right to a decent education even though she is not currently the rational agent she will become in the future. In fact, young children rarely practice many of the subjects that are taught to them at their young age; rather they come to exercise such knowledge sometime later in life. As R.J. Gerber puts it, "[T]he careful education tendered to the young in our society suggests that we do, in fact, prize human potential for what it may actually receive in the distant future."[19] For example, there is very little a child of ten can do with her knowledge concerning long division or multiple digit multiplication. (Indeed, they are keen enough to pick this up to a certain extent when they cry: "When will I ever use this in real life?") If pressed, neither parents nor teachers may think that the child is deriving such benefits from these facets of education currently. Rather, it is the child's *potential* as a future rational being that grounds her *current* interests in learning more complex mathematics. Therefore, it is indeed a good thing to allocate to her, indeed to all children, a moral right to a decent education, even though the fruits of such an education may not make themselves manifest until much later; to not do so runs the risk of impeding the child's capacities as a rational agent and thus stifles her well-being.

The interest in a good education may not be as foundational as the interest in continued health (for many people do live their lives and pursue other interests even in absence of a good education), but it is a very important interest nevertheless, and it is an interest that, also, is wholly objective rather than subjectively mediated. That is, even if a young child begs and screams not to go to school (as I often did as a child), we do not thereby conclude that she has forfeited her moral right to an education. Furthermore, an autistic child, or a child afflicted with Down syndrome, may not have an actual desire for an education and may even, because of limited cognitive capacities, wholly lack the capacity to possess such a desire. Yet if that education helps her advance her limited abilities so that she may become reasonably self-sufficient in the future, then she does *have* an interest in the type of education that would benefit her even if she cannot *take* an interest in it. This all illustrates, again, that the interest in obtaining an education really is an objective, rather than a subjective, interest.

Consider the current market for educational infant toys. Many parents shower their children with educational toys from infancy (the Baby Einstein and Leap Frog collections attest to the fact that there is a viable market in this area), given the parents' desire to cultivate and nurture their child's innate rational abilities from early life. Even the best possible pet owners, in contrast, do not expose their cats or dogs to such educational toys simply because these nonhuman animals lack the potential to achieve a rational mind and so the animals would derive absolutely no benefit from this exposure in any way. This is why, I suspect, there are no Baby Einstein or Leap Frog collections for puppies or kittens. This certainly attests to the fact that we treat beings with certain potentials (e.g., the potential for rational agency or autonomy) differently than we treat beings that lack such potential. As L.W. Sumner notes:

> It is not astonishing that someone who values rationality should care for creatures who will be rational in the future as well as those who are rational at present. Protecting the lives of the potentially and actually rational are merely two different means of promoting rationality.[20]

OTHER INSTANCES WHEN POTENTIAL MATTERS

To depart from the subject of rights briefly, consider moral education. We teach our very young children to say "please" and "thank you," to share their toys, to say that they are sorry when they have done something wrong. When we ask this of a two-year-old now, we do not do so because she is receiving current benefits from such moral education. A two-year-old will probably not learn an immediate lesson about the importance of sharing or politeness when we make her share her toys or express gratitude, rather we do so because of her potential as a future moral agent, and her potential in this area certainly affects how we treat her *now*. Indeed, if one sides with Aristotle on this matter, it is imperative that we bestow moral education upon our children from a very early age, even though they may not be current moral agents, because this will make a crucial difference towards their becoming virtuous individuals in the future: "It is not unimportant then, to acquire one sort of habit or another, right from our youth; rather, it is very important; indeed, all-important."[21] That is, a child's potential to become a moral agent grounds a present interest in being exposed to moral education.

Finally, consider a young child that displays a keen ability to play a musical instrument. Her music teacher tells you, her parent, that she has the potential, if that potential is cultivated, to become a fantastic pianist or violinist. Her potential to be a great musician creates a current interest in being given the best music lessons that are within your financial means to acquire. If the child is deprived of such lessons, and as a result never cultivates or realizes her potential, then it can be said, quite rightly, that the child has been harmed, and that she would have greatly benefited had she received those lessons. The child's *potential* grounds a *current* interest in music lessons, and her potential also grounds the extent that she is harmed if she is deprived of those lessons (i.e., if her potential to become a phenomenal musician was great, then she was more harmed by being deprived of those lessons in comparison to some other child who had very little, if any, potential in the area of music).

The point of these examples is to illustrate that Bassen was simply incorrect when he claims that future prospects do not create a present sake, for all of the above examples indicate otherwise. A being's potential can certainly play a pivotal role in deciding how she should be treated or, more precisely for the topic at hand, what moral rights should be allocated to her. While it is true that a potential X cannot be given the rights of an actual X *in certain instances* (when being an actual X is a necessary condition in order to have specific rights), this is not a universal rule, as the above examples illustrate. Potentially possessing a property may be sufficient for entailing an interest in some moral right if possessing that moral right constitutes a benefit for the individual that potentially possesses that property and a denial of that moral right constitutes a harm (e.g., it is not necessary that one actually be sick in order to possess a right to health insurance; potentially possessing the property of being sick is sufficient for entailing a moral right to health insurance, since possessing this right constitutes a benefit, and its denial constitutes a harm, for the potentially sick as well as for the actually sick). From this we can arrive at the following generalization:

THE MORAL RELEVANCY OF POTENTIAL PRINCIPLE

A potential X may be granted the same moral rights as an actual X in virtue of its potential if its potential generates an interest in such a moral right; that is, *if possess-*

ing the moral right constitutes a benefit for the potential X and a denial of the moral right constitutes a harm.

It is important to stress the caveat that the potential X must both benefit from the extension of the right of an actual X and also be harmed by its denial. This is because someone may argue that extending the rights of an actual king onto a potential king may indeed benefit him, for I am sure both Charles and William would benefit from the rights and benefits the current queen possesses. Potential physicians, medical students, would certainly benefit from being treated as actual physicians, and so someone may argue that this is sufficient grounds for extending the rights of actual physicians onto them. But in these examples, the potential Xs would not be harmed by a denial of these rights, and so there is no pressing need to accord them these rights when they are still in their potential state. This is not the case for the examples I mention that do warrant extending the rights of actual Xs onto potential Xs. In these cases, a subsequent harm would befall the potential Xs if denied the rights of actual Xs while still in a potential state. The same goes for a right to life. As I will argue below, not only is extending the right to life onto a potential person a benefit to him, but its deprivation is also a very grave harm, as it would be for an actual person.

Moral rights (and legal rights as well) exist for the *very purpose* of protecting the well-being and welfare of individuals. While I certainly do not have a moral right to anything whatsoever that is in my interests (e.g., I may have an interest in obtaining the money in your wallet, but this does not grant me a moral right to the money in your wallet), moral rights are there to, at the very least, protect our very important welfare interests—the interests that would result in a serious harm if violated. Of course, the respective interests in continued health and continued existence are two of the most important welfare interests there are, and so it can be argued that our moral right to health care and our moral right to life are grounded upon the premise that these integral welfare interests are to be protected as much as possible for all the members of our moral community. If possessing a potential property can make a being a proper subject of harm in virtue of that potential, then this should suffice to extend to her a moral right that would protect her interest in not being harmed and helps to ensure her welfare.

The interest in continued existence is quite possibly the most important welfare interest any individual possesses. As Feinberg writes:

> Indeed, there is nothing a normal person . . . dreads more than his own death, and that dread, in the vast majority of cases, is as rational as it is unavoidable, for unless we continue alive, we have no chance whatever of achieving those goals that are the ground of our ultimate interest.[22]

Contra Singer, there seems to be no reason to hold that only actual persons have an interest in continued existence. Singer argues that one must possess the capacity to desire continued existence in order to have an interest in it. Not only does this render fetuses incapable of possessing this interest, it renders infants and very young children (e.g., toddlers) incapable as well, since they too lack the conceptual capacity necessary to desire continued existence (and Singer is infamous for his argument that, because of this reason, there is nothing intrinsically morally impermissible about infanticide).

Certainly, however, this flies in the face of common sense. Most of us hold that infants and young toddlers certainly do have a welfare interest in continued existence, despite their lack of personhood and therefore their inability to desire continued existence. That is, many of us hold that the interest in continued existence is a wholly objective, rather than a subjective, welfare interest. A terminally ill infant, for example, certainly possesses a welfare interest in continued existence, which in turn grounds a *prima facie* moral right to procure a life-saving operation. It would be dubious, to say the least, to argue that it is permissible to let an infant die, when her defect can be easily repaired, on the grounds that she has no interest in the operation or her continued existence because she is utterly incapable of desiring it. As Stone puts it: "An infant need not desire a welfare to have one."[23]

Yet I submit that the reason they have such an interest is strictly in virtue of their potential to become persons. If an infant was afflicted with some horrible defect that rendered her incapable of ever growing past the mental age of a few months old, many would hold that her interest in continued existence would vanish or at least would be rendered so weak it would almost be negligible. This is so because death would not harm her as much, if at all, when she has no hopes of ever mentally evolving past a few months old; we would be depriving her of very little by allowing her death, whereas we would be depriving a healthy infant of much more if we killed her, given the enriching life typical to persons. The welfare interest in continued existence is wholly objective rather than subjective, but when it comes to nonpersons, such as infants and young toddlers, their welfare interest in continued existence is based on their potential to become persons and live the rewarding life common to persons. That we usually regard the killing of healthy infants as murder, and that we seem to have no moral qualms or objections against bestowing medical treatment upon infants so that they can continue living their lives and realizing their potential, illustrates that potential does matter. At least when it comes to infants, their potential to become persons certainly influences their *current* welfare interest in continued existence, which, in turn, grounds an interest in medical care and leads to the moral (and legal) judgment of infanticide as a form of murder. (There does seem to be a problem with this claim when we consider whether a mentally disabled infant, who will never really grow to have the robust mental capacities of a person, has an interest in continued existence. My claim does seem to, *prima facie*, entail that they lack such an interest, and this may indeed pose a problem given that mentally disabled individuals who are not persons, nevertheless, may experience a life of subjective, although perhaps rudimentary, pleasures. The best response I have for this problem, at the moment, is the following. It is the case that mental disabilities come in degrees, and some individuals with mental disabilities approximate personhood more than others. The strength of the interest in continued existence that a disabled infant possesses may run parallel to how closely she can approximate personhood in the future. As abovementioned, if she has a disease that rendered her unable to ever surpass the mental age of a few months old, her interest in continued existence would seem to be much weaker than the interest in continued existence that a healthy infant possesses. Here, I can appeal to Marquis and his "future-like-ours" view. Perhaps an interest in continued existence is only as strong as how much an infant's future is "like ours," i.e., like a person's. I do want to point out, however, that if we do want to argue that even rudimentary subjective pleasures are sufficient to establish some robust interest in continued existence, we should be willing to grant this interest to all nonhuman animals who experience rudimentary subjective pleasures, lest we concede to speciesism.)

Thus, potential can be relevant when it comes to ascribing present interests to some beings in some situations. We can now restate the pro-potentialist's argument as follows:

— **Premise 1:** All innocent persons have a moral right to life.
— **Premise 2:** Since all innocent persons have a moral right to life, all potentially innocent persons also have a moral right to life.
— [*Justification for premise 2*: A moral right to life would constitute a benefit for a potential person as well as for an actual person, and its denial would constitute a harm for a potential person as well as for an actual person].
— **Premise 3:** The fetus is a potential innocent person.
— **Conclusion:** The fetus has a moral right to life.

This is the justification I believe a pro-potentialist ought to give in defense of premise two. The pro-potentialist can argue that the anti-potentialist's rejection of premise two is a result of his tacit assumption that only actual persons can qualify as bearers of a moral right to life, a claim that the pro-potentialist rejects. As the above examples are meant to illustrate, it seems perfectly justified to treat a potential X as an actual X *if* the potential X has an interest in such treatment; *if* doing so constitutes a benefit for the being in question and a denial of that treatment constitutes a harm. It is my potential to become sick that grounds my current interest, and my moral right, to health insurance even though I am not actually sick; it is a young child's potential to become a rational and moral agent that grounds her current interest in academic and moral education, even though she may not currently be a rational or a moral agent. In all these instances, the potential being possesses some sort of current or actual interest in virtue of her potential, and thus a moral right can be properly bestowed upon her, in virtue of her potential, in order to protect that interest and, in turn, her well-being and welfare.

So, we have seen that, at times, potential matters and that at other times it does not matter. Does potential matter when it comes to how we ought to treat or regard the human fetus? I think that an argument in the affirmative has best been made by Jim Stone in his articles "Why Potentiality Matters" (1987) and "Why Potentiality Still Matters" (1994). Stone argues that the human embryo or fetus is a being that is intrinsically determined, due to its biological nature, to become a being whose life contains a set of great conscious goods. That is, the embryo's biological nature as a member of the species *Homo sapiens* is of the type that contains its own causal powers that lead to, as Stone puts it, the embryo "mak[ing] itself self-aware."[24] Because the embryo's biological nature is "sufficient to realize self-awareness, social interaction, and the possibility of moral stature," this alone grounds the embryo's claim to "care and protection."[25] Stone's main premise in his argument is that

> [a]nything benefits from having the good which it is its nature to make for itself. I submit that we have a prima facie duty to creatures not to deprive them of the conscious goods which it is in their nature to realize.[26]

Because the embryo or fetus has a biological nature that, if left to its natural progression, will result in a great good for the embryo or fetus, there is a basis for grounding an interest in continued existence to the embryo or fetus: the embryo or fetus has an interest in continuing to function and realizing its biological nature, a nature that typically brings with it a set of conscious goods that are valuable to possess.

If Stone is right, then the human embryo or fetus possesses a welfare interest in continued existence because its potential as a future person tells us something about what the embryo or fetus is *now*. A fetus's potential is a marker of what it is in its biological nature to achieve, and this, in turn, grounds a welfare interest in continuing life so that it may achieve these conscious goods. Thus, a fetus's potential informs us about what type of future it has *now* and so the type of future of which it is deprived if not allowed to achieve the conscious goods that it is part of its nature to achieve. As Stone writes:

> . . . [I]f the developmental path determined by the creature's genetic constitution leads to a conscious good for her the creature has an *actual* interest in growing up.

It is true for her that growing up is a benefit and not growing up is a harm. A creature's present interests are relevant to her rights; therefore potentiality matters.[27]

Thus, the fetus's potential can play an important role in the abortion debate. The fetus's potential to become a person indicates what type of future life it will come to possess if allowed to grow up, and this, in turn, grounds a *current* interest in continued existence so that the fetus may realize that future. This interest may be protected by extending to the fetus at least a *prima facie* moral right to life.

I can foresee two possible objections to my argument, the second of which can serve to segue into the next section of this essay. The first objection is the following. Perhaps I should view my obligation to give my child a good academic and moral education as an obligation to the adult the child will become, rather than to the child at her present state. That is, if I deprive my child of an education *now* there will be a future person, my child *qua* adult, who will be substantially worse off than she would have been had I given her a proper education. Similarly, if I deprive my gifted child of music lessons now, the real victim is not the current child, but rather the adult the child will become who was deprived of the opportunity to become a wonderful musician. Thus, my offspring's potential does not serve to render her *qua* child a victim, but rather her *qua* adult a victim if her potential is not realized. Potential, therefore, does not ground any *current* interests at all. By the same token, the fetus's potential for personhood does not ground any *current* interest for the fetus. The real subject of harm is the future person, who does not actually come into existence if the fetus is aborted.

This leads to the second objection. I can harm the future person that the fetus becomes if I do something now against the fetus, for example, I can administer to a pregnant woman a drug that would result in the fetus's eyes not developing correctly, thereby blinding the future person that develops from the fetus. That is, once the fetus is born there is an individual (the subsequent infant, child, and adult) who is substantially worse off than she otherwise would have been had the development of her eyes not been interfered with while in the fetal stage. But notice, the objection continues, that this is not what happens when we are talking about abortion. If a fetus is aborted, what we are doing is *preventing* the existence of a future person rather than partaking in a current action that will result in a harm for a future person. Thus, when we abort the fetus, we are really harming no currently existing being and we are doing nothing but preventing the existence of a future being. Whereas if we thwart the development of a fetus's eyes, we are, thereby, truly harming someone: the future person that will be blinded as a result, granting that the fetus is allowed to be born and grow up.

The upshot of these two objections is essentially the following: the reason I have to worry about bestowing proper education or medical insurance upon my child in virtue of her potential is because there will be a future being that would be a victim of that deprivation. However, no such future victim exists if the fetus is killed. So, potential matters in the first set of cases I have described because we are dealing with the welfare of a future individual that will suffer as a result of the current child's deprivation. But if I kill a fetus now and stop it from realizing its potential, then there will be no such individual that will be harmed in the future.

Although the two objections are related, I will discuss each one of them distinctly in turn. When it comes to the first objection, which holds that my obligations are really to my offspring *qua* adult rather than my offspring *qua* child, and thus potential really does not ground *current* interests after all, I offer the following two responses. First, once a being exists that can be identified with a future being that experiences conscious goods in her future, then realizing that future is in the *current* being's interest, and not just in the interest of the future being she will become, because that future does not belong to some random other; rather that future is *her* future, and a being has an interest in realizing a future that is full of great conscious goods for her. Indeed she has a welfare interest in such a future, for without being allowed the opportunity to live out her life, any other possible interest she may possess is thwarted. The adult human person and the infant or child from whom she emerged *is the same individual* and thus, it makes little sense to discuss them as if they were two separate entities. As Michael Lockwood puts it: "The infant that [I] once was *had*, I want to say, a strong prospective interest in developing further, seeing that the kind of life [I have enjoyed] constitutes a great benefit, and that the infant and later [me] *are one and the same individual*."[28]

Second, even if I grant that the proper subject of my moral obligation is to my offspring *qua* adult, rather than to my offspring *qua* child, this really makes no practical difference in how I treat my child who is currently at a young stage because, again, *they are the same individual; they share an identity relation*, and therefore I could not fulfill my obligation to my adult offspring without, in a sense, "going through" my young offspring. If I have an obligation to my adult offspring to ensure that she is an educated person, I cannot fulfill this obligation without educating her as a child. If I have a moral obligation to ensure that my offspring grows into adulthood so that she can experience a valuable life, then I cannot fulfill this obligation without ensuring that her welfare interest in continued existence is respected throughout all the stages of her life.

The second objection can be read in two ways. If the fetus is *not yet identical* to any future person, if there is no identity relation between the currently existing fetus and some future person, then it is true that all abortion does is deprive a possible person from coming into existence rather than harming a currently existing individual. Unless one wants to declare contraception or abstinence *prima facie* morally wrong, however, it must be conceded that there is no obligation to bring possible people into existence. Yet, if the fetus shares an identity relation with a future person so that the person's life constitutes the fetus's future, then the objection is not at all effective. It would be tantamount to arguing that it is morally impermissible to harm a future person by inflicting a current damage that will affect her in her future state (e.g., blinding a fetus so that the future person will suffer from blindness), but that harm can be circumvented by ridding the world of the being altogether; a being that *already exists*, an *actual* being, who would grow up to experience all the conscious goods common to the life of persons. If this is correct, however, then I am hard-pressed to find any reason why killing a being would ever constitute a moral harm against it, unless we reduce the moral harm of killing a person to simply thwarting her desire for continued existence, which would render the interest in continued existence a subjective, rather than objective, interest. It certainly seems dubious to argue that we can evade the future victimization of a being by killing the being now, an individual that actually exists and whose future you are taking away, so he will not exist in the future when harm may have taken place. I do not evade the moral wrongness of blinding my baby by killing her so that she will not have to suffer from being blind. If anything, I do nothing but add much insult to injury.

But notice that the whole discussion demands that we antecedently answer the question of personal identity. If the fetus is nothing more than the material precursor to an actual human life, so that there is really no identity relation between the currently existing fetus and a future person, then abortion would be tantamount to birth control in the sense that it only prevents the existence of an individual. However, if one thinks that the fetus already *is* the same individual as the future person, then killing the fetus is not preventing the existence of anyone, it is, rather, killing someone that already exists and as such is tantamount to killing an infant or a young child who would have, if not killed, grown into a person. For example, because Sumner holds that the attainment of sentience is such a pivotal threshold for a fetus to cross, he argues that

[e]arly (prethreshold) abortions share the former category with the use of contraceptives, whereas late (post-threshold) abortions share the latter category with infanticide and other forms of homicide . . . after the [fetus crosses the] threshold [of sentience] there is such a creature, and its normal future is rich and full of life. To lose that life is to sustain an enormous loss.[29]

For Sumner, human life begins to exist in all relevant ways, in a way that grants what he calls "moral standing" to the fetus, upon the acquisition of the capacity for sentience and consciousness. It is at this point, then, that potential begins to matter for Sumner, for now there is a being with moral standing that stands to gain from that potential developing and concurrently stands to lose from that potential being frustrated. Before then, however, there is no such being; all that exists before then is a merely possible being, according to Sumner.

I will take it as a given that we are under no moral obligation to respect the interests of only possible people simply because possible people can, at best, have only possible interests. If an individual life has not yet come into existence, if it is only a possible being, then we cannot speak of respecting *actual* interests. Therefore, we cannot address the issue of the moral importance of fetal potential until we first address the issue of personal identity. That is, we must first determine when a being begins to exist who is identical to a future person, thereby making it the case that the current individual possesses an actual welfare interest in not being killed so that she can realize her potential to become that person.

When Does Fetal Potential Become Morally Relevant?
THE NECESSITY OF ADDRESSING THE ISSUE
OF PERSONAL IDENTITY

Potential certainly seems to matter, and it certainly seems to matter when it comes to the human fetus if one thinks that the fetus is a being that is identical to a future being who will experience the conscious goods typical to persons and thus has an interest in realizing those goods. Does this mean that my argument leads to a rather conservative position against abortion? It may or it may not; this question cannot really be answered until we first address the question of personal identity. In other words, the answer to this very complex practical moral problem has its roots in the intricate metaphysical issue of when a being's identity begins to exist. Jim Stone captures this importance quite well when he asserts that "[a] human creature's moral right to life begins when he does."[30]

When does potential matter? I would like to adopt Michael Lockwood's claim that "[a] potential for X generates an interest only where there is some individual for whom the development of the potential for X constitutes a *benefit*."[31] That is, in order to discuss meaningfully the benefits of realizing a being's potential, the being in question must be more than a purely possible being, since possible beings can, at most, have only potential interests and not actual ones. That is, the being must *actually exist* in order to possess a current and *actual* interest in realizing that potential. (This does not mean that the being must exist *right now* in order to have some sort of interest. As Lockwood argues, the actual existence of this being can be understood in a tenseless fashion, a being that exists at any time, either past, present or future. If we know that a being is going to certainly exist in the future, then we can certainly thwart its interests now by doing something that will be detrimental for him in the future).[32]

One reason it is so important to stress that potential only begins to matter when there is a being in existence of whom the realizing of that potential would constitute a benefit is because doing so allows a response to the sperm/ova problem. Although both a sperm and an ovum each possesses some potential, if united, to produce a being who will grow up to become a person, neither of them possess the potential on their own. At conception, the sperm and the ovum lose their numerical identity and together give rise to a wholly new being: a being that possesses the genetic constitution of the sperm and the genetic constitution of the ovum, but is not identical to either. Gametes produce a new being, but neither of them, themselves, are this new being and so the being who would come to benefit from the realization of potential does not exist before the gametes unite. Don Marquis, for example, argues that before conception takes place, there does not yet exist a subject to whom we can attribute a valuable future. Gametes themselves do not possess a valuable future because they cease to exist upon fusion and a new ontologically distinct being, the zygote, begins to exist.

> Prior to conception there is no individual that is the same individual as the later human being that has, or would have had, a valuable life. Individual identity does not survive fusion or fission, whether contraception, amoeba reproduction, or brain bisection are the examples.[33]

Stone also holds to a similar view.

> The sperm and the egg cannot both be identical to the adult human being, nor can that creature be identical to the adult human being, nor can that creature be identical to just one of them. . . . Both the sperm and the egg can produce something which has the potential of becoming an adult human being, but neither the sperm nor the egg has that potential itself.[34]

The kind of potential harbored by gametes to become persons is of a different type than the potential harbored by infants, children, and perhaps even fetuses. In order to more clearly distinguish between these two different types of potential, Stone denotes them differently. There is what he calls "strong potential," which is identity-preserving potential. If A has the strong potential to become B, then "A will produce B if A develops normally and the B so produced will be such that it was once A."[35] Then there is what he calls "weak potential," which is nonidentity-preserving potential. To say that A has the weak potential to become B is to say that

A can help in the production of B, but A itself will not become B. That is, A is "an element in a causal condition that produces B and, further, the matter of A will be (or will at least help produce) the matter of the B."[36] A child, for example, has the strong potential to become an adult person because the adult and the child are *the same individual;* they have an identity relation. Gametes, on the other hand, have only the weak potential to become an adult person because their respective matter will help produce the future adult, but neither of them is already the individual that will become that adult. There is no identity relation between an adult person and the gametes that produced her, if for no other reason than because they are numerically different: gametes are two distinct beings in their own right while the adult human is a single distinct being.

It is strong potential that matters when it comes to this issue. Since a child has the strong potential to become an adult, that adult's life already forms part of the child's *current* interests in growing up, since it *his* future that we are talking about. Gametes, however, do not possess an identity relation with that future being and so the best we can do is discuss the *possible* interests of the *possible* individual that *may* come into fruition *if* the gametes unite. There is no actual interest yet because there is no actual subject yet, and thus no subject of whom the realization of potential would constitute a benefit. Once an individual begins to exist that is the same individual as a later being, then we can meaningfully say that there is an individual currently in existence that would benefit from being allowed to develop that potential. When all we have are gametes, there is no subject yet in existence that would benefit from being allowed to grow up, and, therefore, there is no such victim yet that is being deprived of that opportunity. As Stone writes:

> If we kill the fetus we deprive her of a welfare she would have otherwise have realized for herself. The sperm and the egg, on the other hand, can never have these properties even though they can produce something which can. If we kill them there is no good of which they are deprived.[37]

So when does there begin to exist a subject that is identical to a future being, so that realizing that future being's life grounds a current interest in that subject growing up? The answer to this question will determine when strong potential begins to exist and thus when there is a current actual interest in continued existence. I will not endorse any one view of personal identity here, since defending one view is a long and complex thesis in its own right, and would take us beyond the scope of this essay. Instead, what I will do is offer a brief survey of three accounts of personal identity in order to illustrate how pivotal the question is before we can find the proper place of potential when it comes to attributing to a fetus a welfare interest in continued existence.

ANIMALISM

Animalism is the philosophical view of personal identity, famously defended by Eric Olson,[38] that states that people continue to exist over time so long as their numerically distinct organism continues to exist. According to this theory, you are essentially a human animal, you persist as long as your organism does, and you come into existence whenever your numerically distinct organism comes into existence. According to some philosophers, however, this does not occur until approximately fourteen days post-fertilization, when the cells in the zygote no longer divide into identical daughter cells, and when multiple ontologically distinct zygotes can no longer emerge (which is how multiple births come to be). For example, the philosopher and theologian Normal Ford argues that "it would be hard to admit the presence of an individual human being in the zygote if, in principle, it could lose its ontological identity whenever twinning occurs in the course of development."[39] Furthermore, Karen Dawson writes:

> . . . the individual created at fertilization may not remain the same throughout life. The simplest demonstration of this is identical twinning which is possible for about 12 days after fertilization. In this process the original zygote ceases to exist. Conversely, during this time it is also possible for two zygotes derived from the independent fertilization of two eggs to fuse forming a chimera—the one individual resulting from two fertilization events.[40]

According to animalism, then, we begin to exist not when our unique genetic code comes into existence, not at conception, but rather when our numerically distinct organism begins to exist, at approximately fourteen days post-fertilization, when division is no longer possible and thus where there is irreversible biological identity. After this time, however, we have a distinct human animal that is identical to a future human animal that will live the type of life common to persons. Thus, according to animalism, human identity begins rather early in pregnancy. Coupled with the ethical considerations of potential outlined above, such a view of personal identity *may* lead to a rather conservative view on abortion because there is an identity relation between what is now an embryo (the fertilized egg after two weeks), and the subsequent person the embryo will become in virtue of the fact that they are the same human animal. According to someone who holds to animalism, the embryo has the strong potential to become that adult, and thus the embryo, and the subsequent fetus, can be properly ascribed an interest in continued existence. (I want to emphasize the term *may* because it is still possible to maintain that the fetus has a welfare interest in continued existence, in virtue of being the same human animal as a future person that will live a valuable life, but still hold that abortion is morally permissible. The reason for this is that it has yet to be established whether the fetus's interest in continued existence trumps a woman's right to bodily autonomy. This is an entirely separate question, however, and, other than briefly mentioning it again below, it is not an issue that I will deal with in this essay. Moreover, it does not necessarily follow that the beginning of an identity relation with a future person entails the beginning of moral status. For example, David DeGrazia separates the two in his recent book *Human Identity and Bioethics*.⁴¹ Although he does endorse a version of animalism in his book, he does not argue that moral status begins whenever numerical identity begins.)

PSYCHOLOGICAL CRITERION ACCOUNT OF PERSONAL IDENTITY

Animalism, however, is rejected by many. Some philosophers argue that personal identity is intimately correlated in some sense with possessing some sort of mental life, although many differ as to how robust that mental life must be in order to establish an identity relation. The view that we are essentially *persons*, and thus that we come into existence as persons, persist as persons, and die when we lose our personhood, is called the Psychological Criterion Account of Personal Identity. For example, Mary Ann Warren argues that:

> personal pronouns like "we" refer to people; we are essentially people if we are essentially anything at all. Therefore, if fetuses and gametes are not people, then we were never fetuses and gametes, though one might say that we emerged from them. The fetus which later became you was not *you* because you did not exist at that time . . . [s]o if it had been aborted nothing whatever would have been done to you, since you would have never existed.⁴²

Notice that Warren also makes the assumption that a being must exist, in some way, before she can be the proper subject of harm or benefit. If we were never identical to a fetus, if, in fact, we came into existence gradually as our personhood gradually arose, then abortion would not have harmed *us* because we had not yet existed in the fetal stage. In this sense, Warren may perhaps agree with Lockwood that the realization of potential is only morally relevant when there exists a being of whom the realization of that potential constitutes a benefit. But, according to Warren, no such individual yet exists at the fetal stage because the fetus is not identical to any future person who experiences life. Thus, there exists no one, at the fetal stage, who would benefit from the realization of potential. Peter Singer, who also maintains that it is necessary to be an actual person in order to have an interest in continued existence and a moral right to it, also seems to espouse a similar view of personal identity. He writes:

I am not the infant from whom I developed. The infant could not look forward to developing into the kind of being that I am, or even into any intermediate being, between the being I now am and the infant. I cannot even recall being the infant; there are no mental links between us.[43]

Singer seems to hold that in order for there to be an identity relation between the infant from whom I developed and myself currently, the infant must have been able to conceive of herself as a future person and must have had the capacity to "look forward" to becoming that future person. In other words, self-consciousness, in addition to memory retention, seems to be a necessary condition, according to Singer, for possessing any type of significant mental links that could establish an identity relation. Like Warren, therefore, Singer seems to be arguing that an identity relation between past and future stages of a self can only come into being once personhood arises, for only persons possess self-consciousness in the robust fashion that Singer believes is requisite for an identity relation.

The plausibility of the Psychological Criterion Account is not the subject of this paper, and so I will neither defend nor criticize it. What is important to see, however, is the upshot of accepting this theory when it comes to the question of the importance of fetal potential. If we are essentially persons, and thus we do not really begin to exist until there is a person on the scene, fetuses, then, possess only the weak potential to produce persons, i.e., their matter will contribute to the making of a future person, but they will not *become* persons themselves. On this view, then, fetuses lack identity-preserving potential. Although Stone disagrees with the Psychological Criterion Account himself, he succinctly sums up the consequences of holding to such a view.

> Warren's view is that the being which realizes self-awareness is a person; a person comes into being when it realizes self-awareness; hence a person was never a fetus or an infant. It follows that the fetus, like the sperm, produces a numerically different entity which is the thing that thinks and feels, so the fetus has no welfare of its own.[44]

Therefore, according to this view, potential never counts throughout the fetal stage and no fetus ever has an interest in continued existence. Of course, this also leads to the conclusion that any potential that a neonate possesses is also nonidentity-preserving potential, since neonates are not persons yet. Thus, killing a neonate does not deprive her of her future simply because she has no such future yet, since she is not yet identical to any future person. This would make the killing of a neonate intrinsically morally negligible, since all we are doing is preventing a future person from coming into existence, rather than killing an actually existing one, which is a position that Warren herself admits to.[45]

EMBODIED MIND ACCOUNT OF PERSONAL IDENTITY

This account of personal identity also holds that possessing some sort of mental life is necessary for identity to exist and persist over time. However, the degree of mental complexity that is requisite is nowhere near the robustness that the Psychological Criterion Account requires. According to the Embodied Mind Account, a human being begins to exists in all the ways that matter, in a way that allows her to be identified with a future being, when she gains the capacity for conscious awareness sometime during fetushood (at approximately mid-gestation). Jeff McMahan is one such defender of this view.

> I suggest that the corresponding criterion for personal identity is the continued existence and functioning, in nonbranching form, of enough of the same brain to be capable of generating mental activity. This criterion stresses the survival of one's basic psychological capacities, in particular the capacity for consciousness. It does not require continuity of any particular *contents* of one's mental life.[46]

Michael Lockwood also seems to adhere to this theory, although he does not refer to it by this title. Nevertheless, he argues that

> [w]hat our identity actually consists in, I suggest, is, once again, whatever as a matter of scientific or metaphysical fact, normally underlies these more superficial continuities and provides the deep explanation for them; and from a purely secular standpoint I should have thought that the overwhelming most favored candidate was a continuity of organisation within those parts of our brain that directly sustain those activities we think of as mental . . . considerations of identity firmly favor the view that before the brain has matured to the point of being able to sustain psychological functions, a human life has yet to begin.[47]

Advocates of this view, then, maintain that no human identity really begins to exist until the fetus becomes capable of consciousness awareness. Before this point, the human fetus possesses a biological life, but not a biographical one. A biographical life occurs once the fetus becomes capable of having some sort of inner mental life, when it becomes a locus of consciousness. Persistence of identity does not necessitate a robust form of self-consciousness or rationality, as the Psychological Criterion Account seems to hold, but it does necessitate at least *some* form of mental life, even if it is a comparatively rudimentary one.

As a result of this view, the fetus's potential begins to matter in terms of attributing to it an interest in continued existence when it becomes the type of being whose brain can sustain the capacity for conscious awareness, for it is here when an identity relation with a future person begins to exist, and thus it is here when we can attribute the life of this future person as rightfully the fetus's future. McMahan holds, therefore, that "just prior to twenty weeks [the approximate gestational age when a fetus acquires the capacity for consciousness awareness], there is no one there to be affected by an abortion. After twenty-eight weeks, the developed fetus is definitely present and would be affected for the worse by an abortion."[48] Along the same vein, Lockwood writes:

> If this is right, then the potential of a human embryo for developing into a [p]erson does not confer on it any right to protection. For it has no brain at all. Consequently, that which would stand to benefit by the development of this potential *does not yet exist.*[49]

What is interesting to notice is that none of the above-mentioned philosophers really denies that potential never matters, not even Warren who perhaps has the most liberal abortion view and who also, not coincidentally I think, pushes identity much further into biological life than is commonsensical. (Most of us do think that there is an identity relation between us as adults and our infant self.) I say this because I suspect that Warren herself would agree with me that in the examples stated in the previous section, potential does seem to matter and does indeed ground interests: it is because a child is a potential moral agent that her current moral education matters; it is because she is a potential rational agent that her current academic education matters. Potential does matter, but the question is *when* does it begin to matter, and it is *here* where disagreements arise. I fully endorse Lockwood's view that "it is potential plus identity that morally counts for something."[50] The disagreement arises when there are conflicting views concerning when personal identity begins to exist. If one thinks that personal identity consists of the persistence of the numerically single human organism, i.e., animalism, then potential counts rather early in gestation, while still in the embryonic stage, whenever irreversible numerical identity is established. If one holds to the Psychological Criterion Account, potential never matters throughout gestation, since personal identity consists in being the same person over time, and a person comes into existence only after post-infancy. The Embodied Mind Account is the middle ground, which states that personal identity begins in mid-gestation, and therefore, for anyone who holds this view, potential may begin to matter only then.

Conclusion

Nothing I have said in this essay necessarily grounds a position that abortion is always morally wrong or unjust (which is why I keep referring to the fetal moral right to life as a *prima facie* right). Even though potential can ground an interest in continued existence for an early embryo or mid-gestation fetus, depending on what theory of personal identity one adheres to, we still have to contend with Thomsonian-like objections which state that a fetus's moral right to life does not entail a woman's obligation to sacrifice her body in order to gestate it for nine months.[51] Nevertheless, I believe I have demonstrated why potential does matter, and I hope to have also illustrated that perhaps the major disagreement about this issue has more of its roots in the metaphysical question of personal identity than has previously been acknowledged.

Even the most basic and pervasive ethical debate, like the abortion debate and the debate concerning the moral relevancy of fetal potential, is intimately connected with underlying metaphysical assumptions, even though these assumptions are rarely discussed amongst applied ethicists. This illustrates that the tendency to divorce "traditional" or "abstract" philosophy from "practical" philosophy is unfortunate and misguided. In this case, we cannot address the issue of when fetal potential becomes morally relevant until we first address the matter of personal identity, and this is a subject that is very thorny indeed. Although I have only given a brief synopsis of three major views, there are many others, each as highly contested by some philosophers as the next. However, by pointing out the underlying metaphysical assumptions in this area of applied ethics, I hope to have at least nudged the debate further in a new and, with any luck, effective direction.

REFERENCES

1. Steinbock B: *Life Before Birth: The Moral and Legal Status of Embryos and Fetuses* New York, NY: Oxford University Press; 1992:63.
2. Sumner LW: *Abortion and Moral Theory* Princeton, NJ: Princeton University Press; 1981:104.
3. Stone J: Why Potentiality Matters. *Can J Philos* 1987. 17(4):821.
4. Buckle S: Arguing from Potential. *Bioethics* 1988. 2(3):233.
5. Noonan JT: An Almost Absolute Value in History. In *The Morality of Abortion: Legal and Historical Perspectives* Edited by: Noonan JT. Boston, MA: Harvard University Press; 1970:51–59.
6. Bassen P: Present Stakes and Future Prospects: The Status of Early Abortions. *Philos Public Aff* 1982. 11 (4):333.
7. Singer P: *Practical Ethics* New York, NY: Cambridge University Press; 1993:153.
8. Boonin D: *A Defense of Abortion* New York, NY: Cambridge University Press; 2003:46.
9. Boonin D: *A Defense of Abortion* New York, NY: Cambridge University Press; 2003:48.
10. Singer P: *Practical Ethics* New York, NY: Cambridge University Press; 1993:153.
11. Singer P: *Practical Ethics* New York, NY: Cambridge University Press; 1993:97, 151.
12. Singer P: *Practical Ethics* New York, NY: Cambridge University Press; 1993:154.

13. Tooley M: Abortion and Infanticide. *Philos Public Aff* 1972, 2(1):37–65.

14. Stone J: Why Potentiality Matters. *Can J Philos* 1987, 17(4):815–830. Stone J: Why Potentiality Still Matters. *Can J Philos* 1994, 24.2: 81–294

15. Bassen P: Present Stakes and Future Prospects: The Status of Early Abortions. *Philos Public Aff* 1982, 11(4):333.

16. United Nations: "Universal Declaration of Human Rights." [http://www.un.org /Overview/rights.html]. Accessed on 27 February 2007.

17. Feinberg J: *Harm to Others: The Moral Limits of the Criminal Law* New York, NY: Oxford University Press; 1984:57.

18. Feinberg J: *Harm to Others: The Moral Limits of the Criminal Law* New York, NY: Oxford University Press; 1984:37.

19. Gerber RJ: Abortion: Parameters for Decision. *Ethics* 1972, 82(2):149.

20. Sumner LW: *Abortion and Moral Theory* Princeton, NJ: Princeton University Press; 1981:101.

21. Aristotle: *Nicomachean Ethics* Irwin, Terence (trans.). Indianapolis, IN: Hackett Publishing Company; 1985.

22. Feinberg J: *Harm to Others: The Moral Limits of the Criminal Law* New York, NY: Oxford University Press; 1984:81.

23. Stone J: Why Potentiality Still Matters. *Can J Philos* 1994, 24(2):293.

24. Stone J: Why Potentiality Matters. *Can J Philos* 1987, 17(4):821.

25. Stone J: Why Potentiality Matters. *Can J Philos* 1987, 17(4):822

26. Stone J: Why Potentiality Matters. *Can J Philos* 1987, 17(4):821.

27. Stone J: Why Potentiality Matters. *Can J Philos* 1987, 17(4):828.

28. Lockwood M: Hare on Potentiality: A Rejoinder. *Bioethics* 1988, 2(4):347.

29. Sumner LW: *Abortion and Moral Theory* Princeton, NJ: Princeton University Press; 1981:200.

30. Stone J: Why Potentiality Matters. *Can J Philos* 1987, 17(4):829 (emphasis in original).

31. Lockwood M: Warnock versus Powell (and Harradine): When Does Potentiality Count? *Bioethics* 1988, 2(3):199 (emphasis in original).

32. Lockwood M: Hare on Potentiality: A Rejoinder. *Bioethics* 1988, 2(4):343–346.

33. Marquis D: Korcz's Objections to the Future-of-Value Argument. *J Soc Philos* 2004, 35(1):57.

34. Stone J: Why Potentiality Matters. *Can J Philos* 1987, 17(4):817.

35. Stone J: Why Potentiality Matters. *Can J Philos* 1987, 17(4):818.

36. Ibid.

37. Stone J: Why Potentiality Matters. *Can J Philos* 1987, 17(4):823.

38. Olson E: *The Human Animal: Personal Identity Without Psychology* New York, NY: Oxford University Press; 1997. Olson E: Was I Ever a Fetus? *Philos Phenomenol Res* 1997, 57.1:95–110

39. Ford N: *When Did I Begin?: Conception of the Human Individual in History, Philosophy and Science* New York, NY: Cambridge University Press; 1988:112.

40. Dawson K: Fertilization and Moral Status: A Scientific Perspective. *J Med Ethics* 1987, 13:176.

41. DeGrazia D: *Human Identity and Bioethics* New York, NY: Cambridge University Press; 2005.

42. Warren MA: Do Potential Persons Have Rights? In *Responsibilities to Future Generations* Edited by: Partridge E. Buffalo, NY: Prometheus Books; 1981:264.

43. Singer P: *Practical Ethics* New York, NY: Cambridge University Press; 1993:97.

44. Stone J: Why Potentiality Matters. *Can J Philos* 1987, 17(4):824.

45. Warren MA: Postscript on Infanticide. In *The Problem of Abortion* Edited by: Feinberg J. Belmont, CA: Wadsworth Publishers; 1984.

46. McMahan J: *The Ethics of Killing: Problems at the Margins of Life* New York, NY: Oxford University Press; 2002:68.

47. Lockwood M: Warnock versus Powell (and Harradine): When Does Potentiality Count? *Bioethics* 1988, 2(3):205, 207.

48. McMahan J: *The Ethics of Killing: Problems at the Margins of Life* New York, NY: Oxford University Press; 2002:277.

49. Lockwood M: Warnock versus Powell (and Harradine): When Does Potentiality Count? *Bioethics* 1988, 2(3):208 (emphasis in original).

50. Ibid.

51. Thomson JJ: A Defense of Abortion. *Philos Public Aff* 1971, 1(1):47–66.

PART THREE

POTENTIALITY
AT THE END OF LIFE

CHAPTER ELEVEN

Are DCD Donors Dead?

DON MARQUIS

Ever since brain death came to be understood in the 1970s as death of the whole human being, organ transplantation has, for the most part, been closely linked to it. The typical donor has been somebody declared brain dead while on life support and while the heart continues to beat, thereby keeping the organs suffused with oxygen. However, because relatively few healthy people—people with suitable organs—have died in just this way, the number of organs available for transplantation has been much less than the number of people needing them. One strategy for making up the difference has been the introduction of "donation after cardiac death" protocols, which provide for vital organ donation from people declared dead on the basis of cardiac death.

The typical DCD case goes like this: The prospective donor, although not brain dead, has suffered extensive neurological damage and is on life support.[1] Following a decision from the person's family, life support is withdrawn and cardiac arrest results. If the heart does not resume beating on its own within two to five minutes, it will never resume beating on its own. In a DCD protocol, after one of these intervals, death is declared. Consent for organ donation has been obtained from the donor or his family, and after death is declared, the donor's organs are removed for transplantation as quickly as possible.

DCD protocols are subject to two major constraints. On the one hand, organ removal must occur as soon as possible after cardiac arrest to prevent organ damage. The point of organ transplantation is to provide the recipient with healthy organs, but because the donor's circulation has stopped, the donor's organs are deprived of oxygenated blood. The longer the deprivation, the more likely organ damage will be. On the other hand, the organs must not be removed so soon after cardiac arrest that the donor is not actually known to be dead. A DCD protocol is justified only if, given the former constraint, the latter constraint can be satisfied. Those who defend DCD protocols believe that both constraints can be satisfied.

Since DCD protocols have won wide support, these arguments have apparently been persuasive. That does not mean they are sound, however. I shall argue that DCD donors are not known to be dead.

Death and Reversibility

An article in the August 2008 issue of the *New England Journal of Medicine* illuminates how the declaration of death in a DCD protocol can be problematic. Mark Boucek and colleagues reported on three successful infant heart transplants performed on the basis of DCD.[2] Boucek's investigational protocol, approved by the ethics committee at his institution, permitted death to be pronounced only seventy-five seconds after cessation of donor cardiac function, much less than the two-minute minimum interval recommended by the Society of Critical Care Medicine.[3]

The shorter interval can be both defended and criticized. On the one hand, the longest reported period between cardiac arrest and autoresuscitation (that is, the resumption of a heartbeat without external resuscitation) in DCD cases has been sixty seconds, and adopting a shorter interval minimizes damage from warm ischemia, therefore maximizing the likelihood that the transplant will work. On the other hand, one might wonder whether the patients were genuinely dead. To begin with, whether there are now sufficient data to justify the seventy-five second interval and whether the data that presently exist—or will exist—can be extrapolated from adults to infants is arguable.[4] This issue can be resolved only after the acquisition of more data, however, and I set it aside, pending the data.

Other issues cannot be set aside so easily. The most obvious starts from an observation about the very term "donation after cardiac death." A "gift of cardiac life" received from someone who has suffered "cardiac death" strongly suggests a contradiction. If the donor's heart is truly dead, then it would not be able to function in the recipient. If the transplanted heart functions in the recipient, then it was not dead when it was still in the donor. If the donor's heart was not dead, then the donor should not have been pronounced dead on the basis of cardiac death. If the donor was not dead, then Boucek's transplant did not accord with the dead donor rule— the axiom of the transplant community that stipulates that vital organs may be taken only from the dead.

This issue can be developed in another way. The orthodox definition of death in this country goes like this:

An individual who has sustained either (1) irreversible cessation of circulatory and respiratory functions or (2) irreversible cessation of all functions of the entire brain, including the brain stem, is dead. A determination of death must be made in accordance with accepted medical standards.[5]

Most cadaver organs have been obtained from individuals who meet the second condition, but not the first. In these people, ventilator-supported respiratory and circulatory functions supply oxygenated blood to potential donor organs. As a result, the warm ischemia that otherwise would cause organ damage is retarded or prevented. The number of brain-dead potential organ donors is far from sufficient to meet the need for transplantable organs, however, and the DCD protocol is designed to generate a source of vital organs from individuals who satisfy the first criterion for being dead, but not the second.

Both criteria for being dead refer not merely to the cessation of a vital function, but to the *irreversible* cessation of that function. Robert Veatch has pointed out that, because the donated hearts in Boucek's transplants actually were restarted in the infant recipients, *irreversible* cessation of cardiac function in Boucek's infant donors plainly had not occurred. Veatch concluded that this consideration could be expanded to an objection, not just to Boucek's transplants, but to any heart transplant from a donor declared dead on the basis of the DCD protocol. He concluded that "it would simply not be possible to perform successful heart transplantation in a manner consistent with the dead donor rule after death pronounced on the basis of cardiac criteria."[6]

Note that Veatch's objection is not primarily to the transplantation itself, but to the declaration of death that, given the dead donor rule, made the transplant morally permissible. This makes it possible to expand Veatch's objection even further than he did. Consider DCD donors who, in addition to successfully donating a heart, also donate other vital organs. One could argue that because cessation of cardiac function was actually reversed in these cases, cessation of cardiac function was reversible. Since cessation of cardiac function was reversible, the DCD donors were not really dead, even though death was pronounced. Since the donors were not really dead, donation of *any* vital organ would, in these cases, violate the dead donor rule.

Veatch's objection can be expanded even more. Consider cases of DCD donation in which the heart is *not* one of the organs transplanted. Boucek's transplants suggest that in such DCD cases, cardiac donation may have been possible. If, in any such case, the heart *could have been* transplanted successfully, then in any such donor, cessation of circulatory function could have been reversed. If cessation of circulatory function could have been reversed, then the donor was not dead and the dead donor rule was violated.

Reflection on Veatch's critique of Boucek's transplants ultimately leads to a critique of any declaration of death in a DCD protocol. The central point is that the donor's loss of cardiac function is, for all we know, reversible. If the cessation of cardiac function is reversible, then cardiac death has not occurred. If cardiac death has not occurred, then there is no basis for a declaration of death. I shall call this objection to the DCD protocol "the reversibility objection."

Boucek's transplants make the reversibility objection vivid. However, the reversibility objection has long been implicit in discussions of DCD protocols. Justifications of the DCD protocol can be understood as responses to this reversibility objection. The DCD protocol is justified only if at least one of these responses is sound. There are two basic kinds of responses, which I shall call "the appeal to permanence" and "the appeal to a norm."

The Appeal to Permanence

The DCD protocol has been defended on the grounds that because the cessation of circulatory function in a DCD donor is permanent, such donors are really dead. John Robertson has defended the DCD protocol by appealing to "commonsense views of death, for the person is not now breathing and never will again."[7] James Bernat, who has defended the orthodox definition of death on many occasions, has argued that we should understand death as "the permanent cessation of critical functions of the organism as a whole."[8] Plainly, the cessation of circulatory and respiratory function in all DCD donors, even in Boucek's infant donors, is permanent. The point of pronouncing death after cardiac arrest only when autoresuscitation is no longer possible is to ensure that cessation of cardiac function is permanent. If irreversibility and permanence are the same thing, then DCD organ donors are dead, or so goes the argument.[9]

Are permanence and irreversibility the same? To say that a patient's medical condition was permanent is to say that after his medical condition was acquired, the patient lived with it his whole life. But a patient might live his whole life with a curable—and, therefore, reversible—medical condition. Many people in developing countries live their entire lives with medical conditions that would have been eliminated had they lived in the developed world. To say that a patient's medical condition was *irreversible*, however, is to say that after the medical condition was acquired, no known intervention *could* have eliminated it. Thus, it might well be the case that a patient's aortic stenosis was a permanent condition of his heart, for after he acquired it he lived with it his whole life, but it does not follow that the patient's aortic stenosis was irreversible, for perhaps the patient could have undergone open-heart surgery and had the stenosis corrected. A condition is permanent if the condition is never actually reversed. A condition is irreversible if the condition never *could* be reversed. In short, irreversibility entails permanence; permanence does not entail irreversibility. Therefore, given the plain meanings of the terms, the permanence of the cessation of circulatory function in DCD donors does not entail its irreversibility. Accordingly, if a patient is pronounced dead solely on the basis of the permanent cessation of circulatory function, then, unless the patient is brain dead, the sufficient conditions for being declared dead have not been met.

An example also shows what is wrong with the appeal to permanence. Suppose that Joe has a heart attack and his circulatory function stops. Fred, a physician standing next to Joe, refuses to perform cardiopulmonary resuscitation on Joe because Joe is a rival for the affections of his love interest. No one else resuscitates Joe. Suppose that cardiopulmonary resuscitation would have been successful, but because it was not performed, cessation of Joe's circulatory function was permanent. Was Fred's refusal to act wrong? Not if we understand the irreversible cessation of circulatory function as equivalent to the *permanent* cessation of circulatory function, for the cessation of circulatory function in Joe was permanent as soon as his circulatory function stopped. On that understanding, Joe was dead as soon as he collapsed, and Fred's failure to perform resuscitation was not wrong, for he had no obligation to resuscitate a corpse. But of course this conclusion is absurd.

Consideration of Boucek's heart transplants provides an additional reason for rejecting the appeal to permanence. The cessation of circulatory function in Boucek's donors was permanent for the very simple reason that the donor heart was removed. In these infants, the cessation of circulatory function was permanent because their hearts were removed, and the removal of their hearts was permissible because the cessation of circulatory function was permanent. This attempt at justification of the DCD protocol wears its circularity on its sleeve.

Since "DCD" actually stands for "donation after cardiac death," should the criterion of cardiac death be the permanence of the cessation of *cardiac* function instead of the permanence of the loss of *circulatory* function? The permanence of the cessation of cardiac function in Boucek's cases is quite incompatible with the success of his transplants! Therefore, if we take for granted the appeal to the permanence of the loss of cardiac function, Boucek's donors were not dead precisely because the transplants were successful.

We may safely conclude that the appeal to permanence cannot justify a death declaration in accordance with the DCD protocol.

The Appeal to a Norm

DCD protocols are most often defended by claiming that, in the context of such protocols, "'irreversible' . . . is best understood not as an ontological or epistemic term, but as an ethical one."[10] According to John Robertson:

Because the patient had issued a prior directive against resuscitation or his family has lawfully requested a do not resuscitate order, no resuscitation after cardiac arrest would be morally and legally acceptable in situations of potential non-heart-beating donation [DCD donation]. Therefore, the patient may legitimately be viewed as having irreversibly lost all cardiopulmonary function when death is pronounced on cardiopulmonary grounds.[11]

Robertson is claiming that because cessation of circulatory function in the donor should not be reversed, the appropriate sense of "irreversible" that applies to the cessation of circulatory function is normative. Therefore, the cessation of circulatory and respiratory functions in the donor is irreversible, and the donor is dead.

Here is a defense of Robertson's view. The normative sense of "irreversible" to which Robertson is appealing is the sense of "can't be reversed," which is the sense of "can't" in "You can't cross the intersection when the light is red!" This sense of "can't" is plainly normative. Of course, unless being hit by a car complicates the analysis, it is physiologically possible to cross the intersection when the light is red, as we all know.

The analysis of Robertson's argument requires a brief detour into the distinction between *dispositional* and *occurrent* properties. Reversible is, in most contexts, a dispositional property, and in this way is akin to soluble, fragile, or flammable. A thing has a dispositional property in virtue of having the capacity to exhibit a corresponding occurrent property under certain conditions. We say that the table salt in your salt shaker is water-soluble, for example, not in virtue of it actually being dissolved in water, but because it has the capacity to dissolve when put in water. We say that something is fragile, not (typically) in virtue of its being actually broken, but because it would break if not handled carefully. We say that kindling is flammable, not (typically) in virtue of its actually burning, but because it has the capacity to burn if ignited. Analogously, we say, in ordinary contexts, that some condition is reversible, not because the condition actually has been reversed, but because the condition is such that it would be reversed under circumstances that could obtain.[12] Thus, soluble is a dispositional property; dissolved is the corresponding occurrent property. Fragile is a dispositional property; broken is the corresponding occurrent property. Flammable is a dispositional property; in flames is the corresponding occurrent property. Reversible is a dispositional property (in most contexts); actually reversed is the corresponding occurrent property.

Now we are in a better position to understand Robertson's argument. Robertson is claiming that, in DCD donors, because the cessation of circulatory function should not be reversed, the context of "irreversibility" is normative, and in this normative context, "irreversible" acquires an ethical meaning. But does "irreversible" acquire an ethical meaning in DCD contexts? One reason to think it does would be that, in general, when moral or legal norms apply, terms that are ordinarily dispositional acquire normative meaning.

Let us test this assumption. Suppose I am examining your gold ring. It would be wrong for me to dissolve the ring by dropping it in *aqua regia*. Because a norm applies in this case, would anyone say that "insoluble" has an ethical meaning and that, therefore, the ring is insoluble in *aqua regia?* Suppose that I am holding a plate of your fine china. It would be wrong for me deliberately or carelessly to drop that plate. Because a norm applies in this case, would anyone say that "not fragile" has an ethical meaning in this case and that, therefore, your fine china is not fragile? In these contexts, in which moral norms apply, "ethical" interpretations of these dispositional terms seem incorrect. Therefore, the assumption that would justify Robertson's inference does not seem to be true. In the absence of this justification, Robertson's claim seems to be merely special pleading.

Is there some other way of defending the view that "irreversible" acquires a normative meaning in DCD situations? In fact, there are arguments that being dead is special, and that the judgment that someone is dead, unlike judging that something is soluble or that something is fragile, does have an ethical meaning. Robert Veatch has defended this view at length.[13] Tom Tomlinson's defense of the DCD protocol appeals to this understanding of what death is:

> [T]he determination of death authorizes many decisions and actions that presume that the deceased has lost most of the interests which she had in life. This is a presumption necessary for supporting the ethical conclusion that our former obligations to protect or account for those interests have ended. If it were the case that her loss of those interests was not reasonably believed to be irreversible, then our obligations to protect those interests could not have ended with the determination of her death. Thus, if death has these ethical implications for the demise of our obligations to the deceased, its determination must include a judgment of irreversibility sufficiently secure to warrant the ethical judgments that follow. A revealing translation of "irreversible" in criteria for determining death, then, is "the possibility of reversal is not ethically significant" and this translation has useful application to the Pittsburgh [DCD] protocol.[14]

Almost everything that Tomlinson says about the irreversibility of death is true. Some examples illuminate his position. When a woman's husband dies, she no longer has the obligation not to marry another individual. If her husband's death were reversible, then this would be problematic. For example, suppose her dead husband came back to life after another year. If she had married another man in the meantime, then she would be guilty of bigamy. Consider another example. The obligation of my children (who are my beneficiaries) to respect my property rights will cease when I die. If my death were reversible, think of the complications that could ensue after they had sold or begun to inhabit my house! Tomlinson is correct: irreversibility is an important part of our concept of death, and death's irreversibility has ethical consequences.

Tomlinson's view of the nature of the relationship between irreversibility and ethical judgment is more problematic. The claim of irreversibility in DCD contexts is based on an individual's, or his surrogate's, right to refuse care—on a moral and legal norm. The irreversibility of death seems different. In the above examples, the ethical importance of irreversibility depends on the actual nature of death. The dependency relation is reversed.

This reversal has an explanation. The notion of irreversible nonexistence is central to our notion of death. Its centrality to our notion of death is based, not on moral norms, but on biological reality, whatever our moral norms might be. Although people can come back from a tough bout with pneumonia, people, as a matter of fact, can't come back from the dead. That is because corpses cannot be reconstituted into living individuals. The fact that corpses cannot be reconstituted into living individuals explains why we have no moral qualms about cremation. Put colloquially, when your life is over, it is really over. Death is, as a matter of fact, an irreversible state. Indeed, death is irreversible nonexistence. (Those who are religious may want to add, "on this earth.")

The ethical significance of this has an explanation. We are essentially living human beings. At the moment of a human being's death, that individual human being no longer exists and never will again. The obligations Fred had to Joe when Joe was alive Fred no longer has to Joe's remains, not because "death" has an ethical meaning, but because a necessary condition of Fred's having an obligation to Joe is that both Fred and Joe exist. Joe's remains are not Joe. Put generally and abstractly, A has an obligation to B only if both A and B exist.[15] This claim is not based on a truth about obligations. Rather, it is basically about statements concerning relational properties. When A is obligated to B, A stands in a moral relation to B. In order for A to stand in *any* relation to B, both A and B must exist. Similarly, statements like "A is taller than B" and "A is to the left of B" can be true only if both A and B exist. Therefore, after an individual transitions into irreversible nonexistence (the colloquial term for this is "dies"), one can no longer have duties to what is remaining because there is no longer a "him" to whom one has duties, and never will be again.

Tomlinson is mostly correct: The death of an individual and our obligations to that individual are connected. However, the connection is this. The fact that a person is dead is the basis for a change in our obligations. The reason is that a necessary condition for having an obligation to someone is that there is someone to have the obligation to. And the reason for this is that a necessary condition for one individual to stand in a relation to another is that there are two individuals. Tomlinson claims (correctly) that the judgment that an individual is dead depends on the judgment that his condition is irreversible. However, he claims (incorrectly) that the judgment that an individual's condition is irreversible depends on our obligation to an individual not to resuscitate him if a DNR order was requested. Tomlinson's argument gets the dependency relation backwards. Therefore, it is unpersuasive.

There is another problem with the appeal to a norm as a basis for the judgment of irreversibility and, therefore, as a basis for pronouncing death. The Tomlinson-Robertson view leads to the consequence that DCD donors should be judged dead on the basis of an appeal to a norm. Consider patients in the television show *ER* who enter the emergency room with no heartbeat and are successfully resuscitated. Such patients, when they enter the emergency room, are in the same physiological state as patients declared dead on the basis of the DCD protocol. As a consequence, there will be many pairs of patients whose bodies are in *exactly the same state*, even though one member of the pair is considered dead and the other alive. But death is a state of a body. Therefore, this consequence of DCD death declarations is unacceptable.

The principle on which this argument is based is important and deserves a bit of comment and explanation. There has been controversy concerning the definition of death in recent decades. Folks who do bioethics have proposed many candidate definitions. Some of the candidates are irreversible loss of higher brain function, irreversible loss of all functions of the entire brain, and irreversible loss of circulatory and respiratory function. For all I know, perhaps someone has argued that a body is dead only when it is no warmer than its surroundings. Perhaps others have argued that only rigor mortis is sufficient for death. It is important to note that all of these candidate definitions, as different as they are, have something in common. They propose to set out the conditions of a human body that justify calling that body dead. They presuppose a general principle concerning death: If an individual is dead in virtue of his body being in state S, then all other individuals in state S are also dead. This principle entails that if DCD donors are dead, then all other individuals whose bodies are in the same state are also dead. Since many individuals in the same bodily state as DCD donors are plainly not dead because they are resuscitated, we may conclude that not all DCD donors are dead. The justification of the DCD protocol in terms of the appeal to a norm therefore fails.

Here is another difficulty with the appeal-to-a-norm defense of the DCD protocol. According to this defense, the obligation to respect a patient's right to refuse medical care makes the condition of the patient irreversible. Consider the following case. An individual is in a severe automobile accident and arrives in the emergency room. You are the emergency room physician. You judge that the patient's blood loss is so great that the patient will soon die unless she receives a blood transfusion. Her surrogates decline the transfusion because the patient is a Jehovah's Witness. You respect the refusal and she dies. You would say, of course: "Her condition was reversible! I wish I could have transfused her!"

If the appeal-to-a-norm defense of the DCD protocol is sound, however, you would be wrong to say that. Robertson seems to be committed to the view that since reversing the patient's condition was not legally or morally permissible, the patient should have been viewed as being in an irreversible condition. This seems clearly incorrect, but this line of reasoning is the same as that used in the appeal-to-a-norm defense of the DCD protocol. Therefore, the line of reasoning used in the appeal-to-a-norm defense of the DCD protocol is unsound.

Many of the arguments given so far against the appeal-to-a-norm defense of DCD death declarations have involved a considerable level of abstraction. Let us return to actual cases and consider Boucek's infant donors. Those who adopt the appeal-to-a-norm defense of DCD death declarations will claim that because the parents of Boucek's infants requested the removal of life supports and because physicians had an obligation to respect that request, the cessation of cardiac function in those infants was irreversible. This certainly seems false. The cessation of cardiac function in Boucek's infants was not irreversible, either in a physiological sense or in an ethical sense. The cessation of cardiac function could actually be reversed because the transplants were in fact successful, and the cessation of cardiac function ought to have been reversed for the sake of the lives of the transplant recipients. It follows that surrogate refusal of resuscitation in DCD cases is not sufficient to underwrite the irreversibility of cardiac function. According to the appeal-to-a-norm defense of the DCD protocol, surrogate refusal of resuscitation in DCD cases is sufficient to underwrite irreversibility. Therefore, the appeal-to-a-norm defense of the DCD protocol is unsound.

Objections to Robertson's argument are regularly dismissed by proponents of the DCD protocol on the grounds that the obligation to respect the wishes of the patient or his family "is everywhere accepted in medical ethics."[16] This defense of the argument commits the straw man fallacy. Rejecting Robertson's argument is quite compatible with respecting the wishes of the family or the patient. The mistake in Robertson's argument is the inference from that obligation to the conclusion that the proper meaning of "irreversible" for the purpose of death declarations is normative.

It is useful to put the above points in context. What was above called "the reversibility objection to the DCD protocol" might seem to some to have force. According to the appeal-to-a-norm defense of DCD death declarations, normative considerations bequeath a normative meaning to "irreversibility." The point of that appeal is to rebut the reversibility objection. Is the appeal-to-a-norm defense a bit of special pleading because of the need for more transplantable organs, or can it be justified?

How should we go about answering this question? We can look at contexts involving what we would say about other (ordinarily) dispositional properties when moral norms apply. We can also look at other medical contexts in which moral norms apply, to see what someone would say about reversibility in them. Considering these other contexts is important because justification involves, either explicitly or tacitly, appeal to what is more general than that which is justified.

The analysis in this essay has shown that both of the standard justifications for DCD determinations of death are unconvincing. We have good reasons for supposing that the reversibility objection to the DCD death declaration is sound. When a DCD donor is declared dead, it is not known that he has suffered irreversible loss of circulatory and respiratory functions. Therefore, given the standard legal definition of death, the basis for declaring DCD donors dead does not obtain. Furthermore, because DCD donors are not brain dead, they are not known to be dead at all.

Removing Vital Organs

The analysis presented here does not, by itself, entail that removing vital organs from the kinds of individuals falsely declared dead on the basis of a DCD protocol is wrong, however. It implies something more complex. It implies that either (1) donation after cardiac death is unethical because, as far as is known, the dead donor rule is violated, or (2) the dead donor rule should be either jettisoned or carefully qualified or fudged. Neither alternative seems appealing. If donation after cardiac death is unethical, then a procedure that saves many lives ought to be halted. Rejecting or revising the dead donor rule seems to involve the wrongful ending of innocent human life.

A number of strategies might be offered to justify the moral permissibility of violating the dead donor rule in narrow circumstances. For example, Franklin Miller and Robert Truog have argued that withdrawing life support from patients with devastating neurological injuries with the valid consent of surrogates should be understood as the ethically permissible killing it really is. They have gone on to defend the inference that removing vital organs from the same kinds of patients with the valid consent of surrogates is no different in principle and is another instance of ethically permissible killing.[17] James Bernat has argued that, although there is a "mismatch" between a permanence standard and an irreversibility standard for declaring death in DCD cases, a permanence standard is an "acceptable compromise."[18] Jerry Menikoff has pointed out that even though the dead donor rule is violated in DCD cases, removing livers and kidneys from these not-yet-dead donors does not kill them. This is because removing their life supports, not removing their livers and kidneys, is the cause of their deaths. They do not live long enough to die from liver or renal failure.[19] Menikoff's point might be used to argue that exceptions to the dead donor rule may be made when the principle that apparently justifies the rule does not apply. The relevant principle is that intentionally killing one innocent human being in order to save the life of another is wrong. That principle is not violated in at least some DCD cases.

Another strategy to justify overriding the dead donor rule on rare occasions would appeal to the view that organ donation is permissible if a prospective organ donor's neurological injuries are so severe that he lacks a future that would contain experiences he would value, provided the appropriate consent is in place. One might argue that, in such cases, an individual is not harmed by the removal of his vital organs, and ending his life therefore does not wrong him.[20] Here is another strategy. According to orthodox Catholic doctrine, it is always wrong intentionally to end the life of an innocent human being. Some leading scholars have tried to defend this Catholic doctrine by appealing to the principle that it is wrong to kill anyone with the basic natural capacity for rational agency.[21] Because fetuses have the basic natural capacity for rational agency, this principle does support the view that abortion is wrong. However, it is hard to see how it could support the wrongness of killing a typical DCD donor. The devastating neurological injuries that typically qualify one for candidacy for a DCD protocol have destroyed the basic natural capacity for rational agency. Therefore, the principle on which, according to some authors, Catholic doctrine is based is compatible with DCD donation even if DCD donors are not dead and killing them is incompatible with Catholic doctrine itself.

Are any of these proposals acceptable? I have offered no more than a sketch of any of them. To show any is acceptable would involve a far more careful description of that particular proposal than I have offered. Any such proposal requires a defense, which I have also not offered. Furthermore, an argument is available that none of these proposals is acceptable. One might argue that to remove the vital organs of a living human being to benefit another is to treat that human being as a means only, and not as an end. This, one might argue, is always wrong. It is a violation of human dignity, which, as Kant said, is a dignity that is beyond all price. Whether this argument carries the day requires much more analysis.

This essay has shown two things. It has shown that DCD donors are not known to be dead. It has also shown that we should engage in the difficult but very interesting discussion forced on us by that conclusion. The alternative is to pretend that DCD donors are dead when they are not known to be dead at all.

ACKNOWLEDGMENTS

This essay was begun while I was a Laurance S. Rockefeller Visiting Professor for Distinguished Teaching at the Center for Human Values at Princeton University. I am grateful to Princeton for the opportunity for research afforded by this appointment. I am also indebted to Rachel Sachs, Amanda Bowers, Jim Bernat, Jerry Menikoff, and Ron Stephens for helping me, in various ways, with this essay. I am also indebted to an anonymous referee for very helpful comments on an earlier draft.

NOTES

1. G.D. Curfman, S. Morissey, and J.M. Drazen, "Cardiac Transplantation in Infants," *New England Journal of Medicine* 359 (2008): 749–50.

2. M.M. Boucek et al., "Pediatric Heart Transplantation after Declaration of Cardiocirculatory Death," *New England Journal of Medicine* 359 (2008): 709–14.

3. J. Bernat et al., "Report of a National Conference on Donation after Cardiac Death," *American Journal of Transplantation* 6 (2006): 281–91.

4. Jim Bernat pointed this out to me in conversation. See his "The Boundaries of Organ Donation after Circulatory Death," in *New England Journal of Medicine* 359 (2008): 669–71, and the discussion in Curfman, Morissey, and Drazen, "Cardiac Transplantation in Infants."

5. There are reasons for skepticism concerning both the dead donor rule and this definition of death. However, I shall take both for granted in the main analysis of this essay.

6. R.M. Veatch, "Donating Hearts after Cardiac Death—Reversing the Irreversible," *New England Journal of Medicine* 359 (2008): 672–73.

7. J. Robertson, "The Dead Donor Rule," *Hastings Center Report* 29, no. 6 (1999): 12.

8. J. Bernat, C.M. Culver, and B. Gert, "On the Definition and Criterion of Death," *Annals of Internal Medicine* 94 (1981): 389–94, and J. Bernat, "A Defense of the Whole-Brain Concept of Death," *Hastings Center Report* 28, no. 2 (1998): 18. Bernat no longer holds this view. See his "Are Organ Donors after Cardiac Death Really Dead?" *Journal of Clinical Ethics* 17 (2006): 122–32.

9. Others have indicated that in DCD cases, permanence is what counts in declaring death. See M.A. DeVita, "The Death Watch: Certifying Death Using Cardiac Criteria," *Progress in Transplantation* 11 (2001): 59, and Bernat et al., "Report of a National Conference on Donation after Cardiac Death."

10. S.J. Youngner, R.M. Arnold, and M.A. DeVita, "When Is 'Dead'?" *Hastings Center Report* 29, no. 6 (1999): 16, quoting with approval T. Tomlinson, "The Irreversibility of Death: Reply to Cole," *Kennedy Institute of Ethics Journals* 3 (1993): 157.

11. Robertson, "The Dead Donor Rule." The bracketed explanation is mine.

12. Obviously, what counts as "circumstances that could obtain" needs analysis. That difficult analysis would take us too far afield because the subject of this essay is not the nature of dispositional properties.

13. R.M. Veatch, "The Death of Whole-Brain Death: The Plague of the Disaggregators, Somaticists, and Mentalists," *Journal of Medicine and Philosophy* 30 (2005): 353–78 and elsewhere.

14. Tomlinson, "The Irreversibility of Death," 161. My bracketed comment.

15. This is too simple, but the complications are unnecessary here. I believe that a case can be made for the view that we have obligations to those who do not exist now but will exist at a later time, and for the view that we have obligations to those who do not exist now but have existed in the past. These obligations are transtemporal obligations. These special cases concern obligations of existing beings (at one time) to existing beings (at another time). Therefore, they are not counterexamples to the above claim.

16. J.T. Potts, Jr., et al., "Commentary: Clear Thinking and Open Discussion Guide IOM's Report on Organ Donation," *Journal of Law, Medicine and Ethics* 26 (1998): 167, responding to Jerry Menikoff's objections to the DCD protocol in "Doubts about Death: The Silence of the Institute of Medicine," *Journal of Law, Medicine and Ethics* 26 (1998): 157–65.

17. F. Miller and R. Truog, "Rethinking the Ethics of Vital Organ Donations," *Hastings Center Report* 38, no. 6 (2008): 38–46.

18. Bernat, "Are Organ Donors after Cardiac Death Really Dead?"

19. Menikoff, "Doubts about Death."

20. D. Marquis, "Why Abortion Is Immoral," *Journal of Philosophy* 86 (1989): 183–202.

21. P. Lee and R.P. George, *Body-Self Dualism in Contemporary Ethics and Politics* (Cambridge, U.K.: Cambridge University Press, 2008), at 82, and F.J. Beckwith, *Defending Life* (Cambridge, U.K.: Cambridge University Press, 2007), at 161–62.

CHAPTER TWELVE

The Irreversibility of Death

Metaphysical, Physiological, Medical or Ethical?

TOM TOMLINSON

Current law in the United States, under the Uniform Anatomical Gift Act, prohibits the removal of vital organs for donation before the donor has been declared dead. This requirement raises a question about so-called "Donation after Cardiac Death" (DCD) organ procurement protocols. In such protocols, ethically warranted decisions are first made to withdraw a life-sustaining ventilator from patients who are severely brain-damaged but not brain dead, followed by agreement to organ donation. The withdrawal of the ventilator quickly leads to death in most cases, after which the organs may be removed.

The question concerns the standard condition in ethical and legal criteria of death that the loss of the vital functions, whether brain- or heart-oriented, be "irreversible." But when does death become irreversible in the DCD context? For example, the University of Pittsburgh Medical Center's protocol states that removal "cannot begin until the patient meets the cardiopulmonary criteria for death, that is, the irreversible cessation of cardiopulmonary function" (UPMC Policy 1993, A6). The procedures then go on to specify when "irreversible" cessation has occurred. When the patient's heart is unlikely to resume beating on its own—when "autoresuscitation" is unlikely to occur—the patient is dead. In the UPMC protocol, this is set at just two minutes after the heart has stopped beating. Thus, under the protocol, a patient whose cardiopulmonary arrest might well be reversible by means of standard CPR or by other medical means could nevertheless be declared dead for the purpose of organ removal.

This rapid determination of death serves the ultimate transplantation purposes of the protocol because it minimizes organ damage from warm ischemia. But does it do so by an ad hoc and objectionable redefinition of the proper meaning of "irreversible" in the standard definitions of death?

The answer to this question may seem to turn simply on what we mean by "irreversibility." But I will argue that there neither is nor should be a single fixed meaning of "irreversible" in determining when someone has died. The criteria for determining irreversibility will vary with the contexts in which determinations of death are made. A person who would properly be declared dead in one context might not be properly declared dead in another.

In what follows, I examine four types of criteria for determining the irreversibility of death: metaphysical, physiological, medical, and ethical. How does each fare in the variety of contexts in which death must be declared?

Metaphysical Irreversibility

David Cole thinks that the irreversibility condition in the standard definitions of death could only refer to a kind of metaphysical irreversibility—irreversible in all possible worlds one might say. Cole points out that since we cannot predict what future scientific and medical advances might be able to do with a "dead" body, we can't ever say with certainty that a person's loss of vital functions would never be reversible. If irreversibility were a necessary condition for death, it would then be impossible to ever determine that someone had died. Cole concludes that irreversibility cannot properly be part of the concept of death. The irreversibility condition should be jettisoned in favor of a more "ordinary" concept of death that permits declarations of death such as those permitted in DCD protocols:

> On my view, the ordinary concept of death involves loss of capacity for auto-resuscitation, but the concept is compatible with reversal by extraordinary therapeutic procedures. . . . Thus . . . the operational definition embodied in the criteria set forth in the UPMC protocol is closer, I think, to the ordinary concept of death than the explicit definition of death it purports to satisfy. (Cole 1993, 150–51)

Cole's reasoning is set out in more detail in an earlier article published in the *Journal of Medical Ethics*. Irreversibility cannot not be part of the ordinary concept of death, Cole argues, because otherwise it would be a plain contradiction to say, "*X* was dead but later was brought back to life" (Cole 1992, 27).

In addition, Cole argues that both strong and weak construals of an irreversibility requirement have unacceptable implications for our treatment of the "dead." If "irreversible" is taken in a strong sense to mean "can never be reversed," then "no one, on this strong construal of the irreversibility condition, is clearly dead . . . [because] . . . at some time in the future it may be possible to restore a body in very bad condition to life. . . . These future possibilities can certainly not be ruled out altogether" (Cole 1992, 27).

This kind of uncertainty is unacceptable since it "causes . . . moral problems: it hardly seems permissible, for example, to remove organs from persons who may or may not be dead" (Cole 1992, 27). Organ removal under this strong construal of "irreversible" would not be permissible because "if death is reversible, as in the ordinary concept, then what is done to a body after death may well affect the possibility of reversal . . . in particular, mutilation, as by the removal of vital organs, will undoubtedly make reversal more difficult" (Cole 1992, 29).

A weak construal, in which "irreversible" merely means "not reversible now" also runs into problems, according to Cole, due to its relativity to the present moment. A weak construal would imply that a person could be dead one minute (because at that moment his condition was not reversible), but not dead the next moment (because right then a radical medical breakthrough is pushed through the door); and that in the intervening minute it would be all right to harvest his organs, even though that would mean that the medical breakthrough would not work to bring him back from the dead (Cole 1992, 28).

So Cole concludes that there is no proper sense of "irreversible" acceptable for making determinations of death. Our definitions of death, then, should drop references to irreversibility and revert to a non-technical, ordinary concept. "Life is a natural process and is something that a normal organism is capable of sustaining, on its own, in the natural order of things. . . . When the life processes cease and the organism loses the capability of resuming them, it is dead" (Cole 1992, 29). Hence, Cole's conclusion that the Pittsburgh non-heart-beating donor is dead: without the possibility of auto-resuscitation, his life-processes have ceased, and so he is dead. Not because they have irreversibly ceased, mind you, since irreversibility can't be part of the concept of death. He is dead only because he is no longer capable of recovering his vital processes on his own.

Cole's argument raises two questions. First, let's ask whether Cole has shown that the concept of death need not include its "irreversibility." Then we'll ask whether the metaphysical sense of "irreversible" that Cole favors provides a plausible account of the ways we use the concept of death.

Must Death Be Irreversible?

Cole's first argument that the concept of death does not include irreversibility is unconvincing. Granted, "X was dead but later was brought back to life" is not a plain contradiction. But is that because the very concept of death essentially admits of reversibility, as Cole concludes? Or could it instead be because we are willing to read such a sentence with "dead" in raised eyebrow quotes, translating it variously as "presumed dead," "appeared dead," "determined to be dead by the best medical minds of the century," and so on?

A fact supporting this latter explanation, rather than Cole's, is his admission that many of the ordinary practices following death presume irreversibility: "It is natural to wish to view death itself as irreversible—otherwise, what could justify taking such irreversible actions involving the decedent's body and property" (Cole 1992, 27). Cole's claim that the concept of death must allow for reversibility would make the ordinary practices surrounding death at odds with the ways the concept is used.

Furthermore, as Ed Bartlett points out, "death is irreversible" appears to function like a logical truth: "if someone has been pronounced dead, and if, *mirabile dictu*, that person then rises up and asks to see the morning paper, it follows, as a matter of logic, that the pronouncement of death was in error" (Bartlett 1995, 273).

So irreversibility is implied by the concept of death, contrary to Cole. But this claim tells us nothing about what the concepts of death or of its irreversibility should be. "A bachelor is an unmarried male" is a logical truth, but that tells us nothing about what "unmarried" or "male" mean. The meanings of those terms are presumed in our understanding of the claim; they are not implied by it.

And "death is irreversible" tells us nothing about how we should determine whether those concepts have been properly applied in a given context. So Bartlett is wrong when he also says that "if someone has been properly pronounced dead, then it is logically impossible for his condition to be reversed" (1995, 273). Bartlett can't mean to say that someone is dead only if it is logically impossible for him to come back to life. This is Cole's metaphysical irreversibility—which we reject in the next section and which Bartlett rejects as well. So he means instead to assert the truth of the conditional. But the conditional is not true. Were the person's condition to be reversed, it would not contradict the logical claim that "death is irreversible." It would only disprove the claim that the patient was dead. It would not even disprove the claim that the patient had been properly pronounced dead, since up until this point we may have had sound reasons for relying on the criteria we followed. It would only make a factual point: that whatever those criteria might be, our criteria for determining whether the conditions for death had been irreversibly met went wrong.

In short, the logical claim that death is irreversible tells us little about either death or irreversibility, at either the conceptual or practical level. This is because the concept of death has two distinct components. First, the concept embodies a claim about what the vital functions are. These might be heartbeat and respiration, or the integrating functions of the brain stem, or what-have-you. The loss of those functions is a necessary condition for being dead. Second, it embodies a claim about the criteria under which the loss of those functions is considered irreversible. These might be any of the criteria I discuss below. Meeting these criteria is also a necessary condition for being dead. The two necessary conditions are jointly sufficient for being dead, but neither by itself constitutes the meaning of "death." We can specify the meanings of the two conditions however we want, without contradicting the claim that death is irreversible. I rely on this point repeatedly in what follows.

Is the Irreversibility of Death Metaphysical?

Now we get to the second question. Granted that death is irreversible, should we take "irreversible" to mean "not reversible in any possible world"? Cole has already given us good reasons to answer "no" to this question. If we took this to be the proper sense of "irreversible" it would confound our ordinary uses of the concept "dead." Cole's arguments against this sense of "irreversible" do not undermine the claim that death is irreversible, as he assumes. As we've seen, that claim is silent on the meaning of "irreversible." But he has shown that it can't mean "not reversible in all possible worlds."

If so, two further principles are implied. The first is that the proper sense of "irreversible" will be judged in some measure by its implications for our accepted practices surrounding the declaration of death. It is just such implications, and their ethical significance, that refute the metaphysical interpretation. The second is that since "irreversible" cannot be understood relative to all possible worlds, it will have to be understood relative to an actual world; that is, to some context.

Understood relative to what plausible contexts? Shaped by what practical implications? These are questions I pursue in the remainder of this essay.

Physiological Irreversibility

One way to understand the irreversibility of death is relative to the potential of the organism to revive itself. Once the vital functions have been lost (loss of cardiopulmonary functions; loss of whole-brain functions), the question will be whether those could resume spontaneously, by "auto-resuscitation." If the answer is "no," then the vital functions have been lost "irreversibly," and the organism is dead.

This is the sense of irreversibly that Cole resorts to, and the one used by the UPMC and some other DCD protocols. It is also endorsed by the Institute of Medicine in its various reports discussing DCD (e.g., Institute of Medicine 1997, 58).

Of course, to apply this criterion we need some empirically well-grounded test for determining when auto-resuscitation is no longer possible. Joanne Lynn's 1993 critique of the Pittsburgh DCD protocol emphasized how weak the evidence was for setting two minutes asystole as the limit of that possibility (Lynn 1993). More recent evidence purports to strengthen the case for it (DeVita et al. 2000; Sheth et al. 2012).

But regardless where the limit of auto-resuscitation is set, why should we use this criterion of irreversibility at all? Cole suggests one answer. If death is a natural process, reversibility should be one as well. The relevant potential is the potential of the organism to recover its vital functions. Let's call the loss of this potential "physiological irreversibility."

This was perhaps the traditional understanding of irreversibility. Before the development of effective measures to restore heartbeat and respiration, once these had stopped, bystanders could do little but watch and pray. The critical question was whether those vital functions might silently continue, or resume on their own sometime later. Reports of premature burial were common into the nineteenth century. Fear of awakening in the "blackness of the absolute Night" (Poe 1992, 263) motivated elaborate precautions against this fate. Actual burial was preceded by wakes, ritual washings, and other long ceremonies involving observation of the corpse, or by the appearance of signs of putrefaction. Mortuaries were built so that a watchful eye could be kept on the presumed dead. These and other precautions hoped to ensure that the departed was well and truly gone, and would not spring back to life in the tomb, or on the anatomy table. Confidence that physicians had the expertise to make this determination quickly and reliably did not emerge until the end of the nineteenth century (Alexander 1980).

Physiological irreversibility was the only practical sense of the concept available, until we developed the means to restore vital functions the body would not have regained on its own. Once we had effective methods of artificial resuscitation, another kind of reversibility became possible and, with it, another practical sense of "irreversible"—*medically* irreversible.

Before examining this next sense of irreversibility, let's consider a question. Mr. Smith, who lived in the eighteenth century, was declared dead shortly after his loss of vital functions became physiologically irreversible. If some centuries later we decided that medical irreversibility was necessary for the determination of death, would that mean that Mr. Smith might not have been really dead when the declaration was made? Put this way, the question is easy to answer. Mr. Smith would have been dead regardless of the sort of irreversibility employed, since in the eighteenth century we did not have the medical means to resuscitate him. His death was medically irreversible as well.

The question becomes more difficult when we consider contemporaneous cases. Once we have the medical ability to reverse the loss of vital functions, should medical irreversibility become the single standard, displacing the use of physiological irreversibility altogether? Or can two standards live alongside one another, so that another Mr. Smith might properly be declared dead when the loss of vital functions has become physiologically irreversible, even if they might be restored by medical means? I'll shortly give reasons to answer "No" to the first question, and "Yes" to the second.

Medical Irreversibility

The first thing to note about the move from physiological to medical irreversibility is that irreversibility has become a relational property. With physiological irreversibility, both the loss of the vital functions and the irreversibility of that loss are states of the body. Irreversibility is solely a product of the body's own potential to recover its vital functions.

With medical irreversibility, however, this is not the case. When irreversibility is understood in a medical sense, the loss of vital functions (however they might be understood) remains a state solely of the body, but the irreversibility of that loss—and hence the person's death—is not. That will also depend on the state of medical knowledge and ability. Note as well that the bodily states in question will be different between these two senses of irreversibility, once artificial resuscitation becomes possible. The bodily state that corresponds to physiological irreversibility will be that state in which auto-resuscitation is no longer possible. The bodily state that corresponds to medical irreversibility will be that state in which artificial resuscitation will not succeed. That latter bodily state will change as our resuscitative abilities advance.

This raises problems for a general principle Don Marquis wants to use: "If an individual is dead in virtue of his body being in state S, then all other individuals whose bodies are in the same state are also dead" (Marquis 2010, 29). As just noted, the nature of that state is subject to change, and so the principle doesn't hold across time. Physiologically, the patient in cardiac arrest who would properly have been declared dead in an emergency room prior to the development of the ventilator could be in the same state as a patient today, for whom such a declaration would be premature. Agreeing to this statement betrays no conceptual confusion, about either "death" or "(medical) irreversibility." Death can still be understood as the loss of the vital functions of heartbeat and respiration, when that loss is medically irreversible. The concepts that comprise the meaning of death remain unchanged. What has changed are the criteria for applying the concept of "medical irreversibility." Those criteria refer to different bodily states before and after the introduction of the ventilator.

Surely, though, isn't some logical inconsistency at work if we treat two contemporaneous patients differently? Marquis thinks so, and uses his principle to argue against declaring a DCD donor dead. A patient who entered the ER two (or even more!) minutes asystole wouldn't be declared dead on the spot, he points out. Such a patient could be "in the same physiological state as patients declared dead on the basis of the DCD protocol." Since "death is a state of the body . . . this consequence of DCD death declarations is unacceptable" (Marquis 2010, 29).

Marquis apparently thinks that medical irreversibility is the only legitimate sense of "irreversible." Without this assumption, the fact that medical irreversibility is the appropriate sense for use in the emergency room would by itself tell us nothing about what's to be done in DCD donations. Seeing how critical the assumption is to his argument, it's surprising that he never explicitly defends it.

Perhaps, like Ed Bartlett, Marquis thinks that " 'irreversible' is a common term in ordinary language whose meaning is straightforward, unambiguous, and on the tip of everyone's tongue. It means, not reversible, that is, not capable of being reversed" (Bartlett 1995, 274). This appeal to the dictionary doesn't get us very far, however, unless we already know, or think we know, what kind of "capability" is relevant in determinations of death.

Contrary to Bartlett, our use of "irreversible" is not straightforward and unambiguous. The evidence from our practice is that we quite readily make use of different kinds of irreversibility. As Marquis notes, in the emergency room (ER) death is not declared unless the patient is beyond the reach of medical resuscitation. It would be improper to declare dead every patient admitted to the ER in cardiac arrest. But what about a patient admitted to hospice? The cardiopulmonary condition of a hospice patient who has an anticipated cardiac arrest at the end of a terminal illness may be very similar to the patient entering the emergency room. And yet the hospice patient may be properly declared dead much sooner than the ER patient should be.

Now Marquis might say that the hospice patient's bodily state is not the same. His cardiac arrest is a result of a terminal illness, and that means that the prospects for a resuscitation attempt are very poor, even futile. No doubt that would be true for many such patients. But at least the short-term prospects for resuscitation will in all likelihood vary depending upon the nature of the patient's co-morbidities and the mechanisms producing the arrest. If that's true, and if the proper determination of medical irreversibility must identify a single bodily state regardless of context, then on Marquis's account, at least some hospice patients are being declared dead prematurely.

Marquis's methodology creates this problem for him. He wants to claim that death is a single state of the body in all instances. But then the question is, what physiological state is that to be? To answer that question, one must look to the circumstances in which we are all agreed that death has been properly declared, and determine what physiological state is present. Select declarations in the ER as your benchmark, as Marquis does, and you'll identify one sort of physiological state as the instantiation of death. Select declarations in hospice as your benchmark, and you identify another. The problem is that neither of these contexts is the benchmark, because there are no grounds for privileging only one of them.

Unlike the ER, the standards used to determine death in a hospice setting don't involve any determination of the prospects for resuscitation. Those prospects would be best evaluated in individual cases by a trial of resuscitation, just as it is most often evaluated in the ER. It is fitting to do this in the ER, but it would be bizarre to do it in hospice. Why?

The answer has to do with the differing goals and values of emergency medicine and hospice. The goal in the emergency room is to preserve life first, and ask questions later. It would frustrate this goal if physicians determined too easily that we could not be resuscitated, and so we rightly expect maximum efforts to precede a declaration of death. The goal in hospice is to facilitate a peaceful death, in keeping with the patient's wishes. It would frustrate this goal if physicians insisted on determining whether we could be resuscitated before declaring death. In the emergency room, death is declared on grounds of medical irreversibility. In hospice, death is declared without regard to medical irreversibility, in effect employing physiological irreversibility as the standard.[1]

We can't make sense of this difference solely in conceptual or logical terms, as commentators like Marquis and Bartlett insist we do. We must appeal to ethical considerations to understand why a criterion of irreversible that's appropriate in one context might not be in another. That gets us to the last kind of "irreversibility."

Ethical Irreversibility

As I've illustrated, the ethical implications of various criteria of irreversibility shape how they are used. This should not be a surprise. As Cole and many others observe, by its nature the determination of death authorizes decisions and actions that presume the deceased has lost most of the interests that she had in life, and that our former obligations to protect or account for those interests have ended. Like all other interests and obligations, these can be affected by the context in which death occurs, and by other obligations that we may owe to the person who has died.

Donation following cardiac death is one more such context. An essential element in DCD protocols is that the donor has volunteered to donate organs only after either the patient or someone authorized to act for him has exercised the patient's right to refuse any further life-prolonging treatments, including treatments aimed at resuscitation from cardiopulmonary arrest. To refuse to withdraw the life-prolonging respirator therapy or to institute other life-prolonging treatments would be a violation of the donor's wishes and of his rights, and so not ethically acceptable.

Such medical means for reversing his cardiopulmonary arrest are no longer ethically significant possibilities, any more than they are for the hospice patient. To the contrary, pursuing them would be ethically objectionable. Therefore, to ignore those possibilities in making the determination of death takes all due account of our obligations to the donor's interests, and so does no violence to the requirement of irreversibility once that requirement is properly understood. A donor under the Pittsburgh protocol who arrests and has been reliably determined to have lost the capacity for auto-resuscitation is properly determined to be "irreversibly" dead, despite the remaining possibilities of medical resuscitation.

This reasoning concerns criteria for the irreversibility of death; it does not concern criteria for *the loss of vital functions*, to use a distinction made earlier. To illustrate the difference here, imagine a possible counterexample. A patient is admitted in respiratory arrest from a drug overdose and placed on a ventilator. He shows all the clinical signs of "brain death" (we will suppose), although we don't yet know whether this reflects the condition of his brain or is caused by the drug he took. There is still the possibility that brain function will resume in twenty-four hours, after the drug levels have dropped. Subsequently, it comes to light that he has left clear and competent instructions not to continue ventilator therapy under precisely these conditions. Assume it would be ethically objectionable to continue ventilator therapy, the only means available for recovering his brain function. If so, the objection goes, his loss of brain function is irreversible on my account, and he is therefore dead. And yet this conclusion seems plainly wrong.[2]

But the conclusion that he would now be dead is not so plainly wrong once we distinguish two different sorts of losses suffered in brain death: physiological vs. functional. If by "death" we mean to refer to the destruction of the whole brain, then the patient in the counterexample has not yet suffered the loss of his vital functions, since we are not yet in a position to determine whether his brain has indeed been destroyed. Therefore, my account of the irreversibility condition would not imply that he is dead, despite the fact that his condition is (ethically) irreversible. If, on the other hand, by "death" we mean to refer to the loss of the brain's functions (of consciousness, responsiveness, organic integration, and what have you), then it is not so plainly wrong to refer to him now as "dead," since he has indeed lost all of the functions thought essential to being alive, and these are now irreversibly lost due to his treatment refusal. The purported counterexample gets its power from trading on an equivocation between these two conceptions. From the functional perspective, the patient would properly be determined to be dead on my account; but from the physiological perspective, that is a premature judgment. Settle on one or the other of these perspectives, and the problem dissolves.

Speaking against the position both I and John Robertson have taken (Tomlinson 1993; Robertson 1999), Marquis succumbs to a related confusion:

> Consider the following case. An individual is in a severe automobile accident and arrives in the emergency room. You are the emergency room physician. You judge that the patient's blood loss is so great that the patient will soon die unless she receives a blood transfusion. Her surrogates decline the transfusion because the patient is a Jehovah's Witness. You respect the refusal and she dies. You would say, of course: "Her condition was reversible! I wish I could have transfused her!"
>
> If the appeal-to-a-norm defense of the DCD protocol is sound, however, you would be wrong to say that. Robertson seems to be committed to the view that since reversing the patient's condition was not legally or morally permissible, the patient should have been viewed as being in an irreversible condition [i.e., dead]. (Marquis 2010, 29; brackets mine)

Here Marquis confuses the claim that this patient is irreversibly dying with the claim that she is (irreversibly) dead. Her preventable death cannot be ethically prevented, and so I agree she is irreversibly dying. But she is not dead until she meets the criteria for death; that is, until she loses her vital functions, however those might be understood; and that loss is irreversible, however that might be understood. I am claiming that the criteria for the irreversibility of death are properly shaped by ethical considerations, not that someone is dead whenever their death is not preventable. Irreversibility is only a necessary condition for death. It's not a sufficient condition, because it's not the only component in our concept of death.

So it is not conceptually confused for DCD protocols to use a physiological rather than a medical criterion of "irreversible." Neither is it unwarranted on ethical grounds. In a response to a letter to the editor I wrote, Don Marquis suggests that it is unwarranted:

> I would think that if you believe that vital organ donation is morally justified only if the donor is dead—that is, if you accept the dead-donor rule—then you would want to be quite certain that the donor is dead. (Marquis 2011, 10)

Indeed, you would want to be as certain as you need to be in order to preserve the ethical purposes of the dead-donor rule. So what are those purposes? Primary among them is to prevent taking vital organs under circumstances or in ways that ignore or thwart the interests of the donor in remaining alive or being rescued from death. It is with regard to this goal that so-called "uncontrolled" DCD organ

procurement in the emergency room is ethically suspect. Making DCD organ procurement a goal in the emergency room threatens patients with the prospect that
ER personnel may be motivated, however unconsciously, to declare patients dead
too quickly. Serving the ethical purposes of the dead-donor rule in that context
requires us to rely on medical irreversibility of a particularly stringent kind.

Being given up on too quickly is not a danger in the controlled DCD donation,
where the patient or someone acting in her name has requested the withdrawal of
life-prolonging treatment, preferring death to survival. Reliance on physiological
reversibility is sufficient in that context to protect the donor from the threat of a
premature declaration of death and is therefore in keeping with the goals of the
dead-donor rule.

Summary

Irreversible is indeed part of the meaning of *dead,* but it's a necessary condition only.
The irreversibility concerns the loss of the vital functions, not the condition of
dying. A person whose death is not preventable is not thereby dead.

The tautology "death is irreversible" tells us nothing about how *irreversible* should
be understood. The various senses of *irreversibility* must be evaluated by reference to
their ethical implications for our practices surrounding death. This means that the
context in which death is declared will shape which sense of *irreversible* is appropriate. In the DCD context, obligations to respect the donor's refusal of resuscitation support the use of a physiological irreversibility rather than a medical one, even
though that would not be the proper standard in the emergency room.

NOTES

This article draws from my earlier work (Tomlinson 1993) but differs from it in significant
respects.

1. This is implicitly acknowledged by the medical consultants to the President's Commission for the Study of Ethical Problems in Medicine and Biomedical and Behavioral
Research when they say that "irreversibility is recognized by persistent cessation of function
during an appropriate period of observation and/or trial of therapy"; they also note various
ways in which what is "appropriate" will vary with context (Medical Consultants 1981, 2185).

2. Thanks to Stuart Youngner for suggesting this counterexample.

REFERENCES

Alexander, M. 1980. The rigid embrace of the narrow house: Premature burial and the signs
of death. *Hastings Center Report* 10(3):25–31.

Bartlett, E. T. (1995). Differences between death and dying. *Journal of Medical Ethics* 21(5):270–76.

Cole, D. 1993. Statutory definitions of death and the management of terminally ill patients who may become organ donors after death. *Kennedy Institute of Ethics Journal* 3:145–55.

———. 1992. The reversibility of death. *Journal of Medical Ethics* 18:26–30.

DeVita, M. A., Snyder, J. V., Arnold, R. M., and Siminoff, L. A. 2000. Observations of withdrawal of life-sustaining treatment from patients who became non-heart-beating organ donors. *Critical Care Medicine* 6:1709–12.

Institute of Medicine. 1997. *Non-Heart-Beating Organ Transplantation: Medical and Ethical Issues in Procurement.* National Academies Press.

Lynn, J. 1993. Are the patients who become organ donors under the Pittsburgh protocol for "non-heart-beating donors" really dead? *Kennedy Institute of Ethics Journal* 3:167–78.

Marquis, D. 2010. Are DCD donors dead? *Hastings Center Report* 40(3):24–31.

———. 2011. The not-so-tell-tale heart (Reply). *Hastings Center Report* 41(2):4–11.

Medical Consultants. 1981. Guidelines for the determination of death. Report of the medical consultants on the diagnosis of death to the President's Commission for the Study of Ethical Problems in Medicine and Biomedical and Behavioral Research. *Journal of the American Medical Association* 246(19):2184–86.

Poe, E. A. 1992. The premature burial. In *The Collected Tales and Poems of Edgar Allan Poe.* New York: Random House.

Robertson, J. 1999. The dead donor rule. *Hastings Center Report* 29(6):6–14.

Sheth, K. N., Nutter, T., Stein, D. M., Scalea, T. M., and Bernat, J. 2012. Autoresuscitation after asystole in patients being considered for organ donation. *Critical Care Medicine* 40(1):158–61.

Tomlinson, T. 1993. The irreversibility of death: Reply to Cole. *Kennedy Institute of Ethics Journal* 3(2):157–65.

UPMC Policy. 1993. UPMC policy for the management of terminally ill patients who may become organ donors after death. University of Pittsburgh Medical Center, May 18, 1992. Rpr. *Kennedy Institute of Ethics Journal* 3(2):A1–A15.

CHAPTER THIRTEEN

On the Ethical Relevance of Active versus Passive Potentiality

JOHN P. LIZZA

The distinction between "active" and "passive" potentiality is often invoked in discussions about the ethical treatment of human beings at the beginning and end of life. In this essay, I raise two questions about this distinction. The first concerns whether an individual can be said to have an "active" potentiality as opposed to a "passive" potentiality apart from any arbitrary claims about the nature of a human being. The second concerns whether the distinction itself carries any moral weight. My discussion focuses mainly on potentiality at the end of life.[1]

Grounding their view in an Aristotelian metaphysics, in which things that exist by nature have innate principles to develop in certain ways, some bioethicists hold that the human embryo has the potential to develop characteristics, such as intellect and will, by virtue of the kind of thing it is. According to this account, as long as an individual is a member of the kind *human being*, its potentiality to develop in certain ways is not affected by any internal or external impediments. Moreover, in this understanding of potentiality, whether the individual has any realistic or practical probability of developing these characteristics does not affect its potential. In *Human Cloning and Human Dignity,* the U.S. President's Council on Bioethics illustrates this view of potentiality at the beginning of life:

> An embryo is, by definition and by its nature, potentially a fully developed human person; its potential for maturation is a characteristic it *actually* has, and from the start. The fact that embryos have been created outside their natural environment—which is to say, outside the woman's body—and are therefore limited in their ability to realize their natural capacities, does not affect either the potential or the moral status of the beings themselves. A bird forced to live in a cage its entire life may never learn to fly. But this does not mean that it is less of a bird, or that it lacks the immanent potentiality to fly on feathered wings. It means

only that a caged bird—like an in vitro human embryo—has been deprived of its proper environment. (President's Council 2002, 175)

D. Alan Shewmon (1997) expresses a similar view about potentiality at the end of life when he claims that artificially sustained human organisms with total brain failure retain the potential for intellect and will. Shewmon argues that the potential for intellect and will resides not in any organ, for example, the brain, but in the organism as a whole. Since he believes that the human organism as a whole may persist through the loss of all brain function, it retains the potential for intellect and will. He sees the loss of brain function (indeed, the destruction of the brain) as simply an impediment in the actualization of the potential for intellect and will that remains in the organism. Its loss does not affect whether the organism has the potential. He gives an analogy in support of his view: Before cataract surgery, people with cataracts still had the potential for sight. Moreover, he claims that if someone suffered enucleation of both eyes and even removal or infarction of the entire visual cortex, the person would still retain the potential for sight:

> As with potency for sight, the potency for these functions [human intellection and will] ultimately resides not in the organ, but in the organism. Theoretically, if brains could be reconstituted (e.g., through implanted futuristically transformed neuroblasts), a "brain-dead" person could be made to regain consciousness and other human functions, although perhaps with a clean mnemonic slate and new personality traits . . . .
>
> Thus, if "brain death" does not cause loss of somatic integrative unity (as it now seems not to), then neither does it cause a loss of essential human properties, i.e., a loss of potency for specifically human functions—potency at the most profound ontological level, at which the occurrence or note of substantial change is determined. (Shewmon 1997, 74–75; bracketed remarks added)

Proponents of this understanding of potentiality appeal to a distinction between "active" and "passive" potentiality. For Aristotle (*De anima,* 2.1.412, a28–29), active potentiality refers to an organism's intrinsic "power of setting itself in movement and arresting itself." For example, features intrinsic to seeds make it possible for plants to develop in the "natural" or normal course of events; this developmental activity is goal-directed by certain intrinsic features. While some theorists, such as Lee and George (2008, 52–59), maintain that the active potentiality for conceptual thought requires an immaterial principle, the potentiality is thought to lie in the human organism's genetic and epigenetic factors. Passive potentiality, in contrast, requires that the individual be acted upon in ways outside of the normal or natural course of events. For example, Aristotle gives the example of a block of wood having the potential to become a statue of Hermes (*Metaphysics*, 1048b1–3). There is no intrinsic motive principle in the block of wood that, in the natural or normal course of events, would direct it to become a statue of Hermes. The wood thus has a "passive" potentiality to become a statue. This distinction between active and passive potentiality is then used to distinguish, for instance, human embryos, either in vivo or in vitro, from human gametes or other human cells. Human gametes and other human cells lack the internal genetic and epigenetic factors that are necessary to develop naturally or normally into individuals with intellect and will, whereas normal human embryos have such factors. Gametes and other cells have to be acted upon in ways that change the kind of the thing that they are. While embryos need an appropriate environment to realize their potential, the realization of the potential does not involve a change in kind.

Despite agreement on a distinction between active and passive potentiality and the significance of something undergoing a change in kind, proponents who invoke this distinction differ on the necessary material conditions for something to have the active potentiality for intellect and will. For example, they disagree over whether anencephalic fetuses and infants have the biological substrate necessary for the active potential for intellect and will and therefore whether they should be accorded the same rights and respect as normal human beings.[2] They also disagree over which individuals have the active potentiality for intellect and will at the end of life. For example, in his discussion of whether a person who has undergone cryopreservation or total brain failure may retain the active potentiality definitive of human life, Jason Eberl (2008) points out how his view differs from that of van Inwagen and Shewmon. Van Inwagen holds that a cryopreserved organism remains "a living corpse":

> Before the cat was frozen, its life consisted of mostly chemical reactions and various relatively large-scale physical processes (the breaking and establishing of chemical bonds, the movement of fluid under hydraulic pressure, the transport of ions); when the cat was frozen, its life was "squeezed into" various small-scale physical processes (the orbiting of electrons and exchange of photons by charged particles). Its life became the sum of those subchemical changes that underlie and constitute chemical and large-scale physical change. But the life was *there*, disposed to expand into its normal state at the moment sufficient energy should become available to it. I, who am fond of oxymorons, would describe the frozen cat as a living corpse. (van Inwagen 1990, 146–47)

Eberl disagrees. He takes "the 'subchemical changes' that persist in a cryopreserved organism to constitute its structural integrity, but such changes are not equivalent to the vital metabolic processes definitive of life" (Eberl 2008, 70). According to

Eberl, the cryopreserved organism lacks "its own motive principle" by which it is able to reanimate itself and thus has at most a passive potentiality for reanimation. Eberl further notes (70–71) that subchemical changes at the atomic and subatomic levels also persist in a corpse. Therefore, he is concerned that van Inwagen's view absurdly entails that a corpse or even a human skeleton would retain the active potentiality for distinctly human traits. Van Inwagen tries to distinguish the cryopreserved body from a corpse on grounds that the cryopreserved body "is disposed to expand to its normal state at the moment sufficient energy should become available to it" (van Inwagen 1990, 147), whereas the same cannot be said about a corpse. Eberl, however, argues that the whole matter turns on "how the requisite disposition should be defined" and maintains that in terms of Aristotelian potentiality, "a cryopreserved body is not sufficiently disposed to be a living (ensouled) organism" (Eberl 2008, 71), since it no longer has the capacity to coordinate its vital metabolic functions (2008, 75).[3]

While I am not sure how Shewmon would weigh in on the question of whether a cryopreserved human body retains the active potential for intellect and will, he thinks that an artificially sustained, whole-brain-dead human body retains this potential and therefore rejects total brain failure as a criterion for determining death. Again, Eberl disagrees. He appeals to the difference between a body's vital functions being taken over by external support and a person being in control of those functions. Since he holds that a functioning brain is essential for a person to have control over vital functions (heartbeat and respiration), individuals who have irreversibly lost all brain functions are dead. Eberl (2008, 75) distinguishes cases of total brain failure from cases in which a patient may temporarily depend on artificial life-support, for instance, someone undergoing cardiopulmonary bypass surgery. In Eberl's view, the capacity or active potentiality of the bypass patient to coordinate vital functions remains intact "due to the fact that the patient's ability to engage in cardiac and respiratory activity under her own control can be restored with available technology and technique" (2008, 76). Eberl goes on to distinguish this case from the cryopreserved body by appeal to "a significant difference with respect to the degree of internal change the two types of bodies must undergo in order to live independent of life-sustaining technology" (2008, 76). Whereas metabolic functions persist in the bypass patient and the patient retains "some control" of vital functions, a cryopreserved body has undergone total arrest of all vital metabolic functions and has no control over those functions.

Eberl is right that whether an individual has an "active potentiality" as opposed to a "passive potentiality" turns on "how the requisite disposition should be defined." However, it is entirely unclear whether such a disposition can be defined in a nonarbitrary way to resolve the borderline cases. For example, while the bypass patient is certainly functioning metabolically, it is unclear what type of "control" the patient has over those functions and therefore whether the patient has, in Aristotle's terms, "in itself the power of setting itself in movement and arresting itself" (Eberl 2008, 68). Isn't it precisely the lack of such a "motive principle" that necessitates the bypass operation? Moreover, suppose a patient permanently required a mechanical ventilator, pacemaker or artificial heart. In Eberl's view, "If a person cannot actually perform his vital metabolic functions, then he is dead" (2008, 75). Many patients, however, have been permanently dependent on artificial life-support, for example, those who were dependent on "iron lungs," but it would be absurd to consider them dead. Are they no longer ensouled, when they can still exercise intellect and will albeit through artificial support? Shewmon would also challenge Eberl's view, since he holds that brain function is not necessary for organic integration. In Shewmon's view, artificially sustained human organisms with total brain failure may be organically integrated and therefore would still be alive.

I agree with Eberl's criticism of van Inwagen. If van Inwagen recognizes the cryopreserved body to have an active potentiality, then he would have to allow an inanimate but structurally preserved corpse to have the same potentiality. But this would be absurd. Neither being is going anywhere on its own. Both lack the supposed "motive principle" to develop in certain ways. Eberl would say that the cryopreserved body has at best a passive or "weak" potential to develop intellect and will. I have charged Shewmon with a similar difficulty (Lizza 2005; 2006, 99–110). If an artificially sustained human organism with no brain function has the potential for intellect and will, then I see no nonarbitrary grounds for not attributing this same potential to an artificially sustained decapitated human organism, the cryopreserved body, or to even a corpse. Perhaps instead of just implanting future neuroblasts, we also implant other materials and energy that generate the restoration of life in the cryopreserved body or corpse. Presumably, the kind of consciousness and other functions that would be restored would be human. Would we take this to mean that all along these individuals had the active potential for intellect and will? To do so, I think, would blur the distinction between active and passive potentiality and make the distinction useless for deciding the borderline cases.

Shewmon suggests that an active potentiality for X should be understood as a "capacity to develop the capacity for X" and that "to develop" should not be understood in the overly restrictive sense of being entirely spontaneous but should accommodate instances "where external elimination of some impediment is required for the development to proceed" (Shewmon 2010, 272). Thus, he argues,

So long as the assistance is truly the removal of an impediment and not a frank replacement, such a "capacity to develop a capacity" should be ontologically relevant. One can distinguish potential for *X* without assistance, potential for *X* with assistance, and performance of *X* by an external agent. The first is too restrictive a concept, and the third is not a potential of the organism at all. The second sense is the appropriate one for the question at issue.

For example, we should not adopt an interpretation of radical capacity so strict that the facts that the healing of large wounds requires sutures, the healing of fractures requires plates, and recovery from serious infections requires antibiotics would negate the body's radical capacity for self-healing. Similarly, the radical potential for sight should be understood as present in someone with dense cataracts, even though ophthalmologic surgery is necessary to actualize that potential. The hidden regenerative potentials of mammals, including humans, which are actualizable through epigenetic desuppression, are now beginning to come to light. If a certain kind of self-repair requires assistance to become actualized, that should not negate the existence of a radical capacity for self-repair, any more than requiring external assistance to survive negates being alive. (Shewmon 2010, 272)

Even if the distinction between "the potential for *X* with assistance" and "performance *X* by an external agent" is recognized, it is unclear how to apply this distinction, especially in the controversial cases. Using sutures and antibiotics seems clearly to assist in the self-healing process. The healing is not "performed by" the externally imposed factors, although the healing may be dependent on them. In addition, the sutures and antibiotics are not part of the normal or "natural" course of events which is all that is usually assumed in ascriptions of potentiality. However, there is a spontaneous internal impetus for self-healing that is triggered by the wound and is independent of the external factors.

The ophthalmic surgery and desuppression of epigenetic factors are more controversial, especially if the surgery or epigenetic intervention is unknown or unavailable. The problem is that if we construe these measures as "assistance" in helping an individual realize certain active potentialities, it may lead to ascribing the same active potentialities to other individuals that we are inclined to say do not have them and may therefore make the concept of active potentiality so "promiscuous" as to be useless. For example, if we allow for genetic and epigenetic intervention within the realm of "the potential for *X* with assistance," it is unclear why we should not attribute the potential for intellect and will to human gametes or every human cell. Why not construe cloning as assisting a human cell to realize its active potential for intellect and will, as opposed to "the performance of *X* by an external agent"? We cannot assist (at least given the current state of knowledge) the cells of an acorn to develop intellect and will because they lack the requisite internal genetic and epigenetic material. However, since this is much more realistically possible with human cells, isn't that an indication that they have different active potentialities from the acorn cells and therefore that they have the "potential for intellect and will with assistance"?

R. A. Charo (2001) has argued that with the advent of nuclear transfer cloning to actualize the potential of every somatic cell, there is no significant difference between the "assistance" that skin cells need to generate a baby and that of in vitro embryos:

> Both need a culture medium. For skin cells, that medium is found in the cyto-
> plasm of an enucleated cell, but a medium it is nonetheless. The skin cell needs an
> electric shock. Again, however, it is unclear why electricity, as opposed to the
> warmth of the incubator used in ordinary management of an in vitro embryo, is
> of ontological significance. (Charo 2001, 86fn2)

Charo's claim is that if there is no significant difference between the potential of skin cells and in vitro embryos, then, if we think that in vitro embryos have rights and should be protected because of their potentiality, every somatic cell would be deserving of the same rights and protections, which she thinks is absurd. Russell DiSilvestro (2006) challenges Charo's argument on the grounds that the effect of the assistance is different. In the case of assisting skin cells, the skin cells are transformed into a different kind of thing, a human organism. A new kind of being is "generated." In contrast, DiSilvestro argues, "when an in vitro embryo (x) develops into a baby (y), the embryo is numerically the same thing as the baby, and is the same kind of thing as the baby—namely an individual human organism" (2006, 149).

DiSilvestro, however, never explains why the distinction between something's having a potential for intellect and will and undergoing a change in kind to realize that potential is less morally significant than something's having the potential for these characteristics but not having to undergo a change in kind for their realization. I have more to say below about challenging the ethical relevance of an individual's having an active potentiality as opposed to a passive potentiality. However, even if appeal to the difference in change of kind can be used to distinguish skin cells from embryos, it is unhelpful in the debate about potentiality at the end of life. Since at issue is precisely whether the loss of all brain functions or cryopreservation entails the death of the human organism and therefore a change in kind, any appeal to the distinction between the human organism undergoing a change in kind versus a change in quality to resolve the issue of whether the individual has an active potentiality for intellect and will would be question begging. In short, there is no way to distinguish whether intervening in a whole-brain dead human organism to restore intellect and will would be intervening in an individual with the potential for intellect and will "with assistance" or intervening in an individual who lacks such potential "with assistance."

In conclusion, Shewmon tries to justify his view by appealing to the degree of organic integration that may be maintained, albeit artificially, in a whole-brain-dead body and claiming that because of that degree of metabolic functioning and organic integration, the individual retains the potential for intellect and will. Eberl, in contrast, tries to justify his view by claiming that the degree of organic integration that may remain in an artificially sustained, whole-brain-dead body is insufficient for that body to retain the active potential for intellect and will. He maintains that "since these patients no longer exhibit control over the primary metabolic functions of heartbeat and respiration, they are no longer rationally ensouled" (Eberl 2008, n.55, 77). There is, however, no way to determine when an individual retains or loses this active potentiality in these borderline cases. For Eberl, the fact that the artificially sustained whole-brain-dead body requires external support and control for circulation and respiration indicates that it no longer has the active potential definitive of human beings. However, this view leads to the absurd conclusion that patients permanently dependent on artificial support for these functions are dead.[4] For Shewmon, the external support is irrelevant, as he thinks that there is enough internal organic activity and integration to indicate that the individual retains the active potential definitive of human beings. However, this view leads to the absurd conclusion that artificially sustained, decapitated human bodies would be living human beings with the potential for intellect and will. Both positions are untenable. Thus, I do not see how this type of disagreement between Shewmon and Eberl can be resolved by appealing to the standard ways of distinguishing between active and passive potentiality. It is unclear in these borderline cases when we should say that the individual retains an active potentiality as opposed to its having merely a passive potentiality.

Part of the difficulty in answering this question stems from the Aristotelian-inspired notion of potentiality that these authors rely on and that involves ensoulment. At work is a spiritual principle that informs physical bodies and gives them the potentials they have. However, since souls or spiritual principles are not directly observable, any determinations of ensoulment and, therefore, active potentialities will be dependent on inferences from what is physically observable. While the tradition and these authors are clearly committed to the idea that not every bit of matter can be rationally ensouled and that the matter must be sufficiently organized to be rationally ensouled, the spiritual nature of the soul makes it impossible to give a determinate answer to the borderline cases. There is no more reason to think that an artificially sustained whole-brain-dead body retains the potential for intellect and will due to ensoulment than to think that it lacks such potential due to the separation of the soul from the body. Thus, even if one accepted that the actuality and potentiality for intellect and will could not be explained without appealing to a spiritual principle, as Lee and George maintain, the theory is no help in resolving borderline cases.

Another difficulty in determining when there is an active potentiality as opposed to a passive potentiality and, in fact, whether the distinction between these types of potentiality makes sense and has any ethical import stems from the nature of potentiality itself. Edward Covey (1991; reprinted in this volume) has suggested that part of what we mean when we say that X has the potential to become Y is that it must be *possible* for X to become Y. If this condition correctly captures part of the ordinary meaning of potentiality (and I believe that it does), it is then critical to understand the notion of possibility invoked in this condition. Feinberg (1974; reprinted in this volume) has pointed out that it cannot mean logical possibility, since that would make the concept of potentiality so "promiscuous" as to be useless. As Feinberg notes, any bit of matter is potentially anything. All we have to do is adjust the conditions.

I have followed Covey in suggesting that the kind of possibility assumed in ascriptions of potentiality must be "realistic" or "actual" possibility (Lizza 2007). Any sensible theory of potentiality must recognize that potentiality is at least dependent on certain internal factors, since those internal factors may affect whether a possibility is actual or not. Thus, Stone (1987), for example, correctly holds that the potentiality of a genetically defective human embryo *is* different from the potentiality of a normal, healthy one. The genetic defect, especially one that we have no idea how to correct, may make it realistically impossible for that embryo to develop intellect and will. In addition, while the possibility of correcting the genetic defect may be within the realm of physical possibility, its remoteness makes it and therefore any potentiality dependent on it ethically irrelevant. Similarly, brain damage may be so significant and the possibility of correcting that damage may be so remote that it makes no sense to ascribe the potentiality for intellect and will to such individuals.[5]

Ascriptions of potentiality are made against a background of assumptions about the external world. Thus, the potential for intellect and will is ascribed to human embryos, because in the natural or normal course of events, and if not interfered with, those embryos will actualize those potentials. If the world were radically different, such that in the normal or natural course of events, human embryos did not actualize those potentials, there would be no reason to ascribe such potentials to them. However, at this point, there is disagreement over whether ascriptions of potentiality are affected by the kind of external conditions that naturally or normally obtain for different kinds of things or by the actual external conditions that may obtain for the particular thing.[6] Singer and Dawson (1990) and Sagan and Singer

(2007; reprinted in this volume), for example, argue that because frozen embryos exist outside the "natural" course of development and therefore have no realistic or practical possibility for further development unless acted upon, they lack whatever natural potential in vivo embryos may have.

In contrast, others use the concept of potentiality in its Aristotelian sense, where it applies most clearly to biological species. For example, normal, healthy bees have the potential to build hives, because in a "normal" or "suitable" environment that is what they do. Bees differ from birds in that they have internal characteristics that, in a normal environment, cause them to build hives. Because the potentiality is thought to be intrinsic to the bees, the realistic possibility invoked is not affected by factors external to the bees that would prevent them from building hives. That some bees will be wiped out by a natural disaster before they ever get to build a hive does not affect their having the potentiality to do so. Similarly, although in vitro embryos may not realize their potential unless acted upon, they have the inherent motive principle to develop in a certain way, given the kind of thing they are. Nonetheless, the attribution of this potentiality to the bees makes certain assumptions about the natural or normal course of events. Indeed, if there were no assumptions about the natural or normal environment, it is unclear whether any ascriptions of potentiality would make sense.

As Michael Kottow has pointed out, an ascription of potentiality is

> a statement about an entity concerning those features that allow a prediction about future states of the entity. This statement disregards external influences on the entity and thus restricts the prediction. This is admittedly a narrow view of potentiality, since it disregards that outer influences and interactions do play strong roles in modulating potentiality. But they cannot create it and therefore it is important to restrict potentiality statements to those prospective states or actions that can be directly derived from analyzing the being under scrutiny. One advantage of this approach consists in making potentiality statements more empirical and therefore, less prone to the naturalistic fallacy of attaching ethical considerations to empirical data. (Kottow 1984, 295)

Kottow is trying to capture the idea that an entity's potentiality is not affected by things external to it, particularly by how external things may affect the possibility or probability of the realization of the potential and, especially, if ethical decisions affect such possibilities or probabilities. Ideally, for Kottow, ascriptions of potentiality should focus on the inherent characteristics of the entity in question, independent of what is external to the entity.

While this latter view coheres with the assumption that potentialities are a kind of power or disposition intrinsic to entities, it cannot be correct. Predictions entail beliefs about possibility. However, as Kottow himself observes, possibility statements "refer to entities as systems seen in the context of their relationships and interactions" (Kottow 1984, 297). Hence, insofar as ascriptions of potentiality necessarily refer to possible future states of the entity, potentiality cannot be understood completely in terms of the internal features of the entity. Instead, ascriptions of potentiality to an entity must always be understood against a background of assumptions about the entity's relation to the world and the possibility that it may be actualized.

As noted above, Covey (1991, 237) has suggested that the sense of possibility assumed in ascriptions of potentiality must be physical possibility, not logical possibility. This is because considerations of logical possibility rather than physical possibility would make the concept, in Feinberg's terms, so "promiscuous" that it would be useless, for any practical matter. Covey contrasts physical possibility with logical possibility and analyzes the former in terms of nomic regularities, that is, "an event or state of affairs is nomically possible just in cases its coming about is in accordance with the laws of nature, given the initial state of affairs which actually obtains in the world" (237).[7] To illustrate the distinction, Covey cites the example from Nicholas Rescher that it is logically possible or conceivable that an acorn could develop into a tree that produces pears, but it is not nomically possible that it can.

Covey, however, goes on to draw another distinction within the category of nomic possibility, which qualifies his treatment of the example cited from Rescher. He observes that sometimes we make conjectures about what might be nomically possible but which fall short of the lawlessness of logical possibility. For example, although it is absolutely nomically impossible for two masses to be near one another without being affected by gravity, as this would be inconsistent with the most basic physical laws in the actual world, it is not absolutely nomically impossible for an acorn to grow into a tree that produces pears. While respecting the laws of nature, it is possible that people could exploit them by developing techniques of genetic alteration, which reprogram acorns with pear genes (240). However, Covey observes that given our existing state of knowledge about genetics, it is actually nomically impossible for a particular acorn starting to germinate at this time to produce pears. In these cases, certain absolute physical possibilities, for example, that we could manipulate the genes of the acorn to get pears, fail to generate actual possibilities about, let us say, currently existing acorns. In other words, the possibility of a possibility does not yield an actual possibility. Thus, certain potentialities are ruled out because of consideration of actual possibility.

Although Covey's example involves what some would say is a "passive" potentiality of the acorn to grow into a tree that produces pears, his point also applies to purported "active" potentialities. For example, normal, healthy bees have the potential to build hives and produce honey, because in a "normal" or "suitable" environment it is physically possible that that is what they will do. In contrast to birds, there is a realistic physical possibility that bees will build hives. However, if a swarm of bees were destined to be wiped out by a natural disaster before they could possibly build a hive and produce honey, that is, if it is only logically or absolutely possible that they could build a hive and produce honey, then those particular bees would have no more actual possibility and hence no more potentiality of building a hive and producing honey than a flock of birds. Assuming that we value bees that have the potential to produce honey but that it is actually physically impossible for those bees to produce honey, there would be no more reason to value those bees as a source of honey than a flock of birds. The same can be said of some human embryos, whole-brain-dead individuals, and individuals in a permanent vegetative state who have no actual possibility to develop intellect and will, due to external conditions beyond our control. Based on considerations of potentiality, there is no more reason to value them as potential or actual beings with intellect and will than a flock of birds.

Even if one rejected Covey's claim that the ascription of any kind of potentiality requires actual possibility and held that these individuals had an active potentiality for intellect and will, it would not follow that they would have more value than individuals who had merely a passive potentiality for intellect and will. For example, suppose that we allow for Shewmon's distinction (2010, 273) between an embryo's having "the potential with assistance" (active potentiality) and a potential due to "the performance of *X* by an external agent" (passive potentiality). Suppose further that we categorize an anencephalic embryo as a human embryo with the active potential for intellect and will *with assistance* and a human skin cell as having only a passive potential for intellect and will because it would need to undergo a transformation in kind caused by an external agent, for instance, cloning. Suppose that the assistance provided to the anencephalic involved correcting some genetic defect and that the correction, because it is only "assistance," would preserve the identity of the embryo over time. In contrast, suppose that the cloning of the skin cell would not preserve its identity but would create a new kind of being. Although a human being with the potential for intellect and will might result from the cloning procedure, that individual would not be identical to the skin cell. Does active potentiality and identity preservation make a moral difference in how the anencephalic embryo and skin cell should be treated? The answer would seem to depend on other relevant facts, rather than whether the potentiality is active and the procedure is identity preserving.

For example, suppose that we have the knowledge and technology to clone the skin cell but lack the knowledge and technology to correct the genetic defect in the anencephalic embryo. Suppose further that we had some dire need to increase the human population and that the cloning technology was in very limited supply. Even though the anencephalic embryo might be said in Shewmon's view to have the active potential for intellect and will with assistance, we would not value it as much as the skin cell and cloning technology that could "produce" a human being. If one had to perform triage and devote resources to either the anencephalic embryo or the skin cell, it would be ethically justified to devote those resources to the skin cell rather than to the embryo. Thus, what is ethically significant about potentiality is not whether it is active or passive but whether there is an actual possibility for the potentiality to be realized.

In addition, suppose again, contra Covey, that actual possibility is not required for active potentiality. Suppose the embryo was not anencephalic but normal and therefore had the requisite genes for further development. It might be said to have an unqualified "active potentiality" in the sense that it does not require the type of "assistance" that Shewmon would say an anencephalic embryo might require. However, suppose the embryo is in an environment that will in fact prevent the embryo from actually realizing its potential and there is nothing that can be done to change the requisite environmental conditions, for example, the embryo may be situated in a uterus that is so scarred that implantation is physically impossible and there is nothing physically possible that could be done to save the embryo.[8]

If it is only absolutely possible but not actually possible to change the requisite external conditions, the embryo would lack the actual possibility for the potential to be realized but would nonetheless be said to have the active potentiality for intellect and will. What would be the ethical significance of such an active potentiality? The absolute but not actual possibility of the embryo's realizing such a potentiality would make it so remote that it would lose whatever ethical significance it might have, if the potentiality were more proximate. Again, if there were some urgent need to increase the human population, we would value a human skin cell that, through available cloning technology, would have a more proximate potentiality to become a being with intellect and will than a human embryo that had a more remote active potentiality to develop intellect and will. Thus, when the remoteness of a potentiality is out of our hands and fixed by external physical conditions, whether a potentiality is "active" or "passive" becomes ethically irrelevant.

The situation is more complicated when it comes to individuals who may have an actual physical possibility of realizing some active or passive potentiality but there are external impediments to the realization of the potential due to social or individual decisions. For example, suppose, as advocates of the potentiality argument in the abortion debate maintain, that many in vivo and in vitro human embryos, in contrast to whole-brain-dead individuals and individuals in permanent vegetative state, have the active potential for intellect and will but may not realize their potential due to decisions such as abortion, a refusal to allow a frozen embryo to be implanted, or a refusal to adjust the external conditions in ways that will enable them to realize their potential. In such cases, these embryos have an actual physical possibility of realizing their potential for intellect and will, and it is "up to us" whether we provide the requisite external conditions for their realization. Does the potentiality of all such embryos give these embryos the same ethical significance? Indeed, does their having such a potentiality give them such ethical significance that it would be wrong not to provide the conditions for their development?

Consider a normal embryo situated in a womb that is so scarred that physical implantation in that womb is not actually possible. However, suppose further that it is actually possible to flush the uterus, harvest the embryo, and implant it in a surrogate mother. Suppose that the technology to do this transfer is readily available and that there is a willing surrogate. Would such an active potentiality be so ethically significant that it would warrant the transfer and implantation, even if the woman in which the embryo was gestating refused to allow the transfer? Would her refusal to allow the transfer be tantamount to child neglect and murder? Indeed, if the active potentiality of an embryo for intellect and will were sufficient to make it a person with basic rights, then it seems that we ought to be taking measures to detect and rescue such embryos. Shouldn't we be doing much more to rescue embryos that are destined to be destroyed due to external factors that will prevent their development? Just as we might initiate a search mission to save someone we believe may be lost at sea, shouldn't we search for embryos that might be miscarried due to external conditions that are in our power to rectify? If an embryo's having the active potentiality for intellect and will were sufficient for the embryo to have the same moral standing as any other person, then it is hard to see why such conclusions would not follow. However, since we do not and should not engage in search missions to rescue endangered embryos or compel women to allow endangered embryos to be harvested, the presence of an active potentiality without consideration of the ethical implications of what it takes to realize the potentiality does not have the ethical significance that some proponents of the potentiality argument assume it to have.

Assuming for the sake of argument a distinction between active and passive potentiality, an embryo with an active potentiality as opposed to something with a passive potentiality (for example, a skin cell), will normally require less external intervention to realize its potential. Many of the causal factors that lead to the realization of the potential are inherent in the embryo. Therefore, *ceteris paribus*, it has a greater probability of realizing the potential than the skin cell. This makes its potentiality more proximate than something with merely a passive potentiality. Moreover, it is the proximity of realization that may make it more ethically significant. If there are factors that make its realization more remote and, at the extreme, not actually possible, its ethical significance would be diminished.

As noted above, a human embryo in a womb that is so damaged that it will prevent implantation may have an active potentiality for intellect and will. However, if there is nothing that can be done to correct the situation, its possibility of realizing this potential would be so remote that it would have little ethical significance. If there is an actual possibility of the embryo's realizing its potentiality, but it would require intervention that would involve violation of some law or moral principle that we ought to respect, those legal and moral obstacles create conditions that make the potentiality more remote and consequently less ethically significant. Thus, if the actual possibility of an embryo located in an inhospitable womb to realize its potential were dependent on compelling a woman against her will to undergo the harvesting of the embryo, the potentiality of that embryo would be more remote than that of an embryo in a similar predicament with a woman who was willing to undergo the procedure. Since respect for the autonomy and bodily integrity of women prevents us from intervening without their consent, the lack of consent makes the potentiality of that embryo more remote and therefore less ethically significant. Because potentiality is dependent on assumptions about conditions of its realization, it does not have ethical significance in and of itself. Its ethical significance is bound up with the possibility of its realization.

To reinforce this claim, consider how what is usually considered a "passive" potentiality can have ethical significance. Someone might say, "That hunk of marble has the potential to become a great sculpture, as Michelangelo intends to start working on it tomorrow." Appeal to such potentiality may be used to justify certain moral claims, for example, "I don't care about the granite but *be very careful* when moving that hunk of marble." In this context, potentiality refers to the internal properties of the marble that are part of the causal story involved in the actual possibility that some end may be realized. The marble is not in itself valuable, but its value is inextricably bound up with the actual possibility of its being transformed into a sculpture by Michelangelo. So too, an active potentiality is not in itself valuable or ethically relevant independent of the actual possibility of its being realized. Just as the hunk of marble would become less valuable if it were unlikely that Michelangelo would work on it, an active potentiality may have less value or moral significance if it is unlikely or, at the extreme, not actually possible that it will be realized. The point is that any appeal to potentiality, active or passive, as having some ethical relevance involves assumptions about the actual possibility of the potential being realized. If there are physical conditions or respect for ethical rules that impede the realization of the potential, whatever ethical significance the potentiality has cannot be evaluated independently of consideration of whether those impediments can or should be removed.

These considerations bear on our ethical evaluation about potentiality at the end of life. For example, critics of non-heart-beating organ donation, such as Joanne Lynn (1993), Robert Veatch (2008), and Don Marquis (2010; reprinted in this volume), have questioned whether such donors are really dead after, say, two or even five minutes of their heart stopping. Their concern can be rephrased as one about potentiality: How can these donors be "irreversibly" dead, if there is the potential for their circulatory and respiratory functions to resume? These critics are correct that there is some uncertainty that two or even five minutes of asystole renders the cessation of circulatory and respiratory functions irreversible. Also, if we consider the possibility of performing cardiorespiratory resuscitation on these patients, then the physical condition alone is insufficient to conclude that the cessation of functions is irreversible. Many of these donors would have an actual possibility and therefore potential to be revived. However, these critics ignore ethically justified decisional factors that put real restrictions on the possibility of the resumption of functions, for example, a patient's advance directive not to be resuscitated. Respect for the advance directive diminishes the ethical relevance of any potential that the individual may have for the resumption of circulatory and respiratory functions. The ethical relevance of the potential for functions to resume in a patient in the same physiological state but with an advance directive to be resuscitated would be different, since the individual and social decisions make the possibility of the realization of the potentiality more or less remote.

That modern resuscitative techniques allow us to reverse conditions that were earlier irreversible complicates the determination of death, because the background conditions for the ascription of the disposition of the irreversible loss of circulatory and respiratory functions have changed. Whereas the earlier account of irreversibility of such functions was based on the natural history of the biological organism on its own—whether it had the internal power to reverse its loss of circulation and respiration, the modern account must take into consideration the possibility of external intervention. In the context of declaring death, the irreversibility of the loss of such functions is thus no longer determined exclusively by the intrinsic, physical condition of the organism. It is partly determined by whether we decide to intervene with resuscitative techniques. Moreover, these decisions affect the remoteness or proximity of the potential for the resumption of functions, since they restrict the conditions for human intervention to reverse the cessation of functions. Because of the decisional factors, whatever remote potential a DCD donor might have for the cessation of her circulation and respiration to be reversed is therefore ethically irrelevant to the determination of death in these cases.

In short, because extrinsic factors now affect whether a condition is irreversible, death, understood as an irreversible loss of functions, is no longer a strictly biological condition intrinsic to the organism. In addition, the potentiality for the resumption of functions can no longer be understood in terms of a "natural or normal course of events." Indeed, advancement in resuscitative technology has altered the "natural or normal course of events," such that the background conditions for the ascription of the potential for the resumption of functions now include the possibility of extrinsic intervention. Since the application of the technology is also subject to human decisions, those decisions also become part of the set of background conditions for what "irreversibility" means and whether whatever reversibility may exist is ethically relevant to the determination of death.

Clearly, an individual is dead when the loss of circulation and respiration is beyond the point of any known or perhaps conceivable method of reversibility. Hours or days after rigor mortis sets in, the condition is physiologically irreversible. Nothing intrinsic or extrinsic can possibly restore circulatory and respiratory functions. In such cases, the organism undergoes changes incompatible with the possibility of the resumption of functions. However, such clear cases of irreversibility are not what are at issue. In common medical practice, we don't wait for rigor mortis to set in to declare individuals dead. Death is often declared even though we have not ruled out all possibility of reversing the loss of circulatory and respiratory functions. What we mean by "irreversibility" in the definition of death is thus defined by the context in which the declaration of death is made.

In conclusion, even if there is a distinction between something's having an active as opposed to passive potentiality, the distinction is irrelevant to whatever ethical significance potentiality has. In cases in which there is no actual possibility for an active potentiality to be realized due to either internal privation or external barriers that cannot be rectified, the potentiality has little or no ethical significance. Since we cannot do anything to help the thing realize its potential, it has little bearing on how we ought to act. In cases in which we could do something to rectify the internal privation or remove the external barriers, the ethical significance of the potentiality cannot be determined independently of an ethical evaluation of whether our intervention to correct the privation or remove the external barriers is justified. If there are strong ethical reasons for thinking that intervention should not take place or that the barriers should not be removed, the potentiality will and ought to have little ethical significance in our deliberations.

NOTES

1. I would like to thank Jason Eberl for comments on an earlier draft of this essay and Allan Bäck for helpful discussion of some of the issues. I also thank the editors of the *American Philosophical Association Newsletter for Philosophy and Medicine* for permission to republish most of this content, which initially appeared under the same title in the Fall 2011 issue of *APA Newsletter for Philosophy and Medicine* 11(1): 22–28.

2. Contrast, for example, the Catholic positions articulated in Smith (1989), 275–76, and in Ashley and O'Rourke (1986), chap. 11, sec. 2 and (1989), 311–12.

3. If the frozen cat were reanimated, van Inwagen would consider it to be the same organism. In contrast, Eberl holds that it would be a new organism, since the cat underwent a substantial change when it was frozen.

4. Eberl has responded that "patients who are permanently dependent on artificial support for circulation and respiration are not dead, but that the parts that compose them may be less in number. Thus, before his death, the quadriplegic Christopher Reeve was composed of only his head. The rest of his body was merely structurally but not functionally conjoined to him. Just as if his head were completely decapitated and hooked up to a machine that kept him alive, the machine would not be a part of him in such a case but a source of external support" (pers. comm.; see further Eberl [2005]). In this case, it is unclear to me whether such a radical change in the parts that compose the person following Reeve's accident would involve a substantial change. If the change is substantial, then, for Eberl, after becoming quadriplegic Christopher Reeve would be a different kind of being than he was before the accident. If the change is not substantial, then, assuming an artificially sustained head is not a human organism, it is unclear whether Reeve was ever essentially a human organism. However, this implication would conflict with the assumption that on the Aristotelian-inspired view that Eberl defends, Reeve is essentially a human organism.

5. Individuals with total brain failure and individuals in *permanent* vegetative states should be distinguished from some individuals in a vegetative state, where there may be a realistic possibility of their transitioning to a minimally conscious state and undergoing further improvement.

6. There are two other complications concerning "external" conditions of potentiality. First, proponents of the potentiality argument believe that the active potentiality of the human embryo resides in the genetic and epigenetic material of the embryo. While the genetic material (DNA) may be construed as internal or intrinsic to the embryo, this is not true of the epigenetic factors. Due to environmental influences, epigenetic factors are not static and change as the organism develops. If the epigenome is determined as much by factors external as internal to the embryo, it cannot be understood as an intrinsic power or motive principle of the embryo, i.e., an active potentiality, in the way that the DNA can be so understood. Moreover, if the epigenome is essential to the developmental trajectory of the embryo, the distinction between whether an embryo has an "active" or "passive" potentiality to develop in certain ways becomes blurred. There is no more reason to think of the epigenome as the material conditions for an active potentiality than for a passive potentiality. Thus, if the distinction between active and passive potentiality turns on whether the power or motive principle is intrinsic or extrinsic, the distinction may be nonsensical when it comes to the epigenome. In short, it would not make sense to talk about the potentiality of the

embryo to develop in certain ways independent of the environmental conditions that bear on the determination of the epigenome.

Second, since persons are not simply biological beings but social and cultural beings as well, it is unclear how any account of what a "normal" or "suitable" environment is can be given independently of social and cultural considerations. To do so would involve a distortion of the nature of persons. In contrast to other biological beings, we can shape our environment based on rational consideration of the good and how to best realize it. Thus, it is hard to see how the attribution of potentialities to persons can be given without considering at the same time the nature of a good or suitable environment, which seems to take us beyond strictly biological considerations.

This same complication is raised in another way by Roy Perrett (2000). According to Perrett, a major problem for the standard potentiality argument is that it appeals to the "naturalness" of the kind of potentiality of an embryo to develop in certain ways but does not provide a justification for why we should conform to nature. Perrett argues as follows:

> Descriptive facts about biological functions do not by themselves entail any prescriptive claims. What has to be added is something like the Thomistic distinction between *laws of nature* and *natural laws*, where the former are descriptive statements derived from scientific observation of regularities in nature and the latter are prescriptive statements derived from metaphysical knowledge of the essential properties of human nature. Knowledge of our essences is then supposed to tell us how we *ought* to behave because of our nature as human beings. (2000, 193)

He expresses skepticism that natural-law theorists have been able to make sense of the obscure distinction between laws of nature and natural laws and justify why we should not interfere with anything that is "natural." In particular, he takes issue with Stone's argument that the potential of the embryo grounds an interest in continued life, because the embryo has a nature that, when actualized, involves conscious goods. Perrett claims that Stone's argument (Stone 1987, 821) assumes the undefended and unobvious claim that "we have a prima facie duty to all creatures not to deprive them of the conscious good which it is their nature to realize."

7. This paragraph and the following are drawn from Lizza (2005).

8. Suppose the embryo will die if not implanted in a surrogate and that there is no available technology or surrogate to accomplish the transfer.

REFERENCES

Aristotle. 1984. *De anima* and *Metaphysics*. In J. Barnes (ed.), *The Complete Works of Aristotle*. Princeton: Princeton University Press.

Ashley, B. M., and O'Rourke, K. D. 1986. *Ethics of Health Care*. St. Louis: Catholic Health Association of the United States.

———. 1989. *Health Care Ethics*. 3rd ed. St. Louis: Catholic Health Association of the United States.

Charo, R. 2001. Every cell is sacred: Logical consequences of the argument from potential in the age of cloning. In P. Lauritzen (ed.), *Cloning and the Future of Human Embryo Research*, 82–92. New York: Oxford University Press.

Covey, E. 1991. Physical possibility and potentiality in ethics. *American Philosophical Quarterly* 28(3):237–44.

Di Silvestro, R. 2006. Not every cell is sacred: A reply to Charo. *Bioethics* 20(3):146–57.

Eberl, J. 2005. Aquinas's account of human embryogenesis and recent interpretations. *Journal of Medicine and Philosophy* 30(4):379–94.

———. 2008. Potentiality, possibility, and the irreversibility of death. *Review of Metaphysics* 62(1):61–77.

Feinberg, J. 1974. The rights of animals and unborn generations. In W. T. Blackstone (ed.), *Philosophy and Environmental Crisis*. Athens, GA: University of Georgia Press.

Kottow, M. 1984. Ethical problems in arguments from potentiality. *Theoretical Medicine and Bioethics* 5(3):293–305.

Lee, P., and George, R. P. 2008. *Body-Self Dualism in Contemporary Ethics and Politics*. Cambridge: Cambridge University Press.

Lizza, J. 2005. Potentiality, irreversibility, and death. *Journal of Medicine and Philosophy* 30:45–64.

———. 2006. *Persons, Humanity, and the Definition of Death*. Baltimore: Johns Hopkins University Press.

———. 2007. Potentiality and human embryos. *Bioethics* 21(7):379–85.

Lynn, J. 1993. Are the patients who become donors under the Pittsburgh protocol for "non-heart-beating-donors" really dead? *Kennedy Institute of Ethics Journal* 3:167–78.

Marquis, D. 2010. Are DCD donors dead? *Hastings Center Report* 40(3):24–31.

Perret, R. W. 2000. Taking life and the argument from potentiality. *Midwest Studies in Philosophy* 24:186–97.

President's Council on Bioethics. 2002. *Human Cloning and Human Dignity: An Ethical Inquiry*. Washington, DC: U.S. Government Printing Office.

Sagan, A., and Singer, P. 2007. The Moral Status of Stem Cells. *Metaphilosophy* 38(2–3):264–84.

Shewmon, D. A. 1997. Recovery from "brain death": A neurologist's apologia. *Linacre Quarterly* 64(1):31–96.

———. 2004. The "critical organism" for the "organism as a whole": Lessons from the lowly spinal cord. In C. Machado and D. A. Shewmon (eds.), *Brain Death and Disorders of Consciousness*, 23–41. New York: Kluwer.

———. 2010. Constructing the death elephant: A synthetic paradigm shift for the definition, criteria, and tests for death. *Journal of Medicine and Philosophy* 35:256–98.

Singer, P., and Dawson, K. 1990. IVF technology and the argument from potential. In P. Singer et al. (eds.), *Embryo Experimentation*. Cambridge: Cambridge University Press.

Smith, R. E. (ed.) 1989. *Critical Issues in Contemporary Health Care: Proceedings of the Eighth Bishops' Workshop, Dallas, Texas*. Braintree, MA: Pope John Center.

Stone, J. 1987. Why potentiality matters. *Canadian Journal of Philosophy* 17:815–30.

van Inwagen, P. 1990. *Material Beings*. Ithaca, NY: Cornell University Press.

Veatch, R. 2008. Donating hearts after cardiac death—reversing the irreversible. *New England Journal of Medicine* 359:672–73.

EDWARD COVEY, independent researcher, Iowa City, Iowa

JASON T. EBERL, Semler Endowed Chair in Medical Ethics, College of Osteopathic Medicine and Marian University, Indianapolis, Indiana

JOEL FEINBERG, former Regents Professor Emeritus of Philosophy and Law, University of Arizona, Tucson, Arizona

EDWARD LANGERAK, Professor Emeritus of Philosophy, St. Olaf College, Northfield, Minnesota

MARGARET OLIVIA LITTLE, Associate Professor of Philosophy and Director of the Kennedy Institute of Ethics, Georgetown University, Washington, D.C.

JOHN P. LIZZA, Professor of Philosophy, Kutztown University of Pennsylvania, Kutztown, Pennsylvania

BERTHA ALVAREZ MANNINEN, Associate Professor, School of Humanities, Arts, and Cultural Studies, Arizona State University West, Glendale, Arizona

DON MARQUIS, Professor of Philosophy, University of Kansas, Lawrence, Kansas

MOHAN MATTHEN, Professor of Philosophy and Senior Canada Research Chair, University of Toronto, Ontario, Canada

JENNIFER MCKITRICK, Professor of Philosophy, University of Nebraska–Lincoln, Lincoln, Nebraska

JEFF MCMAHAN, Professor of Philosophy, Rutgers University, New Brunswick, New Jersey

AGATA SAGAN, independent researcher, Warsaw, Poland

PETER SINGER, Ira W. DeCamp Professor of Bioethics at the University Center for Human Values, Princeton University, Princeton, New Jersey and Laureate Professor, School of Historical and Philosophical Studies, University of Melbourne, Melbourne, Australia

TOM TOMLINSON, Professor of Philosophy and Director of the Center for Ethics and Humanities in the Life Sciences, Michigan State University, East Lansing, Michigan